Stroke Rehabilitation

Guidelines for Exercise and Training to Optimize Motor Skill

Janet H Carr EdD FACP

Honorary Associate Professor,
School of Physiotherapy,
Faculty of Health Sciences,
The University of Sydney, Australia

Roberta B Shepherd EdD FACP

Foundation Professor of Physiotherapy,
Honorary Professor,
School of Physiotherapy,
Faculty of Health Sciences,
The University of Sydney, Australia

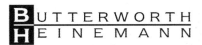
BUTTERWORTH
HEINEMANN

BUTTERWORTH-HEINEMANN
An imprint of Elsevier Science Limited

First edition 2003
  Reprinted 2003

ISBN 0 7506 4712 4

British Library Cataloguing in Publication Data
A catalogue record for this book is available from the British Library.

Library of Congress Cataloging in Publication Data
A catalog record for this book is available from the Library of Congress.

Note
Medical knowledge is constantly changing. As new information becomes
available, changes in treatment, procedures, equipment and the use of
drugs become necessary. The authors and the publishers have taken care
to ensure that the information given in this text is accurate and up to
date. However, readers are strongly advised to confirm that the
information, especially with regard to drug usage, complies with the
latest legislation and standards of practice.

your source for books,
journals and multimedia
in the health sciences

www.elsevierhealth.com

The
publisher's
policy is to use
**paper manufactured
from sustainable forests**

Printed in China
N/02

Stroke Rehabilitation

For Butterworth Heinemann:

Senior Commissioning Editor: Heidi Allen
Project Development Editor: Robert Edwards
Project Manager: Jane Dingwall/Pat Miller
Design Direction: George Ajayi

Contents

Preface vii

Acknowledgements ix

Section 1 Introduction **1**
 1 Brain reorganization, the rehabilitation environment,
  measuring outcomes 3

Section 2 Training guidelines **33**
 2 Balance 35
 3 Walking 76
 4 Standing up and sitting down 129
 5 Reaching and manipulation 159

Section 3 Appendices **207**
 6 Impairments and adaptations 209
 7 Strength training and physical conditioning 233
 8 Overview 259

References 267

Index 293

Preface

In this book we have set down guidelines for training critical motor actions after stroke: walking, reaching and manipulation, balancing in sitting and standing, and standing up and sitting down. The guidelines are designed to optimize motor performance, in other words, skill. They are science-based in that we have preceded each set of guidelines with a brief résumé of scientific findings relevant to the action, including a description of major biomechanical characteristics, and of muscle activity, and the changes that occur in performance due to impairments and adaptations. Since stroke is the model used, details of age-related changes in performance are also provided. The guidelines themselves include methods of task-oriented training of motor control to maximize skill, environmental manipulations to foster cognitive engagement and enhance skill learning, and methods of increasing muscle strength, soft tissue flexibility, endurance and fitness. A short list of appropriate methods of measurement is included. The guidelines are based on the limited evidence so far available from clinical outcome studies, and each training chapter includes a table of recent clinical trials we consider are of particular clinical interest, trials in which the interventions are clearly outlined. The mechanisms of impairments and adaptations and their impact on performance, the task-dependence of strength training and conditioning, and a brief overview of the role of physiotherapy in the early care of individuals who have had a stroke, are included in appendices.

Bridging the gap between science and practice is an overwhelming task for the clinician, who must endeavour to keep up to date in scientific findings in a wide range of subjects, as well as work out how to use the information to intervene with clinical problems. Illustrating ways of bridging the gap has therefore been a critical aim for us in writing textbooks over the last two decades. It is 20 years since we published the first edition of *A Motor Relearning Programme for Stroke*, with an updated version in 1987. This book was an early attempt to demonstrate rational guidelines for task-oriented motor training in a format enabling clinical testing. We were aiming to present not another approach to intervention to compete with the eponymous approaches of the mid twentieth century but an illustration of what would undoubtedly be a new direction for neurophysiotherapy. This direction would involve ongoing changes to practice based on developments in scientific understanding and the results of clinical outcome trials. The current book represents a considerable development, since the amount of material relevant to motor training is increasing exponentially, and evidence of what interventions are effective and what are not is beginning to emerge. It has become necessary for us to reconsider methods of practice for which there is no positive evidence of effectiveness and for which there is little scientific basis. As a result practice is making considerable change and the neurophysiotherapy in many rehabilitation units today would be unrecognizable to the forerunners of our profession.

There is currently, therefore, considerable focus in physiotherapy on the need for evidence-based practice, defined by Sackett and colleagues (2000) as 'the conscientious, explicit and judicious use of current best evidence in making decisions about the care of individual patients'. As they point out, a concerted effort is being made to find answers to questions that continually arise in clinical practice. The best evidence is provided by randomized controlled trials and systematic reviews. However, clinical trials and systematic reviews are only as good as the scientific rationale underlying the intervention and the design of the trials themselves. It is unlikely, for example, that we can develop evidence-based physiotherapy practice if we have not first developed scientifically rational practice. Development of the hypothesis and its embedding within a coherent and rational body of knowledge is a critical element in research. In addition, for research findings to be meaningful, the detailed nature of the interventions tested must be clear (methods, intensity, dosage). Where standardized guidelines and protocols are tested, the reader knows what it is that is effective and what is not.

As Herbert and colleagues point out (2001), basing clinical practice on evidence differs from traditional models of practice in which there may be priority given to clinical experience as a form of evidence. With measurement of progress becoming mandatory in the clinic, it is becoming more acceptable for clinicians to follow a clearly identified set of guidelines as an aid to identifying the interventions that were carried out.

Physiotherapy, together with the other health professions, is undergoing a large degree of change with rapid growth in technology and changes in methods of delivery. We hope this text will be an aid to clinicians and give them food for thought.

2003   Janet Carr
                                                                                Roberta Shepherd

Acknowledgements

We particularly wish to thank the neurological physiotherapy teaching team at The University of Sydney for many stimulating discussions over the years and for their ongoing comments on our work: Dr Louise Ada, Dr Colleen Canning, Dr Cath Dean, Virginia Fowler and Dr Sharon Kilbreath. We particularly thank Dr Kilbreath for discussions on early drafts of several chapters.

We also thank the people who so kindly agreed to be photographed for this book, and their physiotherapists from Sydney hospitals who gave us generous support, in particular Karl Schurr, Simone Dorsch and colleagues at Bankstown-Lidcombe Hospital; Sarah Crompton and colleagues at Prince Henry Hospital; Lynne Olivetti and colleagues at War Memorial Hospital; also Ruth Barker, University of Queensland, Claire Lynch, Physiotherapy Department, Ipswich Hospital, Queensland, and Fiona Mackey, Physiotherapy Department, Illawarra Area Health Service.

David Robinson provided valuable assistance and advice with photography. Dr Jack Crosbie, Head of School of Physiotherapy, The University of Sydney, provided technical assistance in the collecting of some biomechanical data.

The authors and publishers express their appreciation for being granted permission to reproduce figures as indicated throughout the book. We also thank PRO-ED Inc., Austin, Tx for granting permission to reproduce Figures 1.1, 2.11b, 3.17b, 3.26, 5.9b, 5.12 and 5.19c.

Introduction

**SECTION
CONTENTS**

1 **Brain reorganization, the rehabilitation environment,
   measuring outcomes**   **3**

Brain reorganization, the rehabilitation environment, measuring outcomes

CHAPTER CONTENTS

- **Introduction**
- **Brain reorganization and functional recovery**
- **The rehabilitation environment**
  Structuring a practice environment
  Optimizing skill

- **Measurement**
  Measures of motor performance
  Functional outcomes
- **Circuit training: example of organization**

INTRODUCTION

Optimal functional recovery is the ultimate aim of neurorehabilitation after acute brain lesion. The focus of this book is on the contribution of physiotherapy to this process using stroke as a model. The unique contribution of physiotherapy to the rehabilitation of individuals following stroke is the training of motor control based on a contemporary understanding of impairments and secondary adaptations, biomechanics, motor learning, exercise science and factors that influence brain reorganization after injury.

The major objective of physiotherapy is the optimization of motor performance in functional actions. Guidelines for task- and context-specific exercise and training of critical everyday actions based on a scientific rationale and on clinical research are outlined in Chapters 2–5. In these chapters, the explication of normal and impaired motor performance is largely based on biomechanical and muscle data. The guidelines emphasize the training of effective functional motor performance using methods that provide both a stimulus to the acquisition of skill, and increase strength, endurance and fitness.

Biomechanics provides the major foundation for understanding motor performance. Without a knowledge of biomechanics, the clinician has only observation upon which to base the analysis and training of motor performance. It is widely recognized that analysing complex actions without a knowledge of biomechanical characteristics is difficult and may be inaccurate. Biomechanics also provides methods of measuring motor performance in clinical research, enabling the formulation and testing of interventions.

Musculoskeletal anatomy has, from the origins of physiotherapy, been a critical area of knowledge for clinicians. Combining a knowledge of anatomy and of the dynamics of multisegment movements is now a major requirement for physiotherapists who wish to play a significant motor training role in neurorehabilitation.

At this stage of the development of neurorehabilitation, the focus is on the need for evidence-based clinical practice. Currently there is a wide variation in practice and continued controversy about methods used. To some extent this may be due to a lack of standardized treatment guidelines and protocols, together with a paucity of outcome measurement in rehabilitation centres, which results in little ongoing feedback about the effectiveness (or otherwise) of interventions. This can result in a lack of awareness of the need to change or fine tune practice to keep up with new information.

One aim in writing a text of guidelines is to illustrate an important step in the process of improving patient outcomes: the translation of scientific knowledge and clinical evidence into clinical practice. There is now increasing evidence about which interventions are effective and which are not that allows clinicians to make considerable change to methods of delivery. As Rothstein (1997) has urged, once there is some evidence it is critical that this evidence is used in clinical practice.

One of the difficulties in doing clinical research and collecting data for clinical audits is the categorization and standardization of interventions, their frequency, duration and intensity – what could be called the dosage. In this book we have categorized interventions, basing the guidelines on the available empirical data that are known to us. Where available these data are used to support the guidelines; where they are not, reliance is placed on biological rationale.

This chapter starts with a brief examination of the interaction between postlesion brain reorganization and the process of rehabilitation. Since there are no widely available medical or surgical interventions that consistently reduce the extent of neuronal damage following stroke, rehabilitation remains the mainstay of improving outcome in these patients. Despite its importance, until recently very little research had been undertaken on understanding how therapy input may influence the process of recovery from stroke at the neurological level. Functional brain imaging techniques now provide a way of studying in vivo both cerebral plasticity after stroke and the influence of interventions on the reorganization and on functional recovery.

Since there are signs that physical activity in an enriched environment facilitates brain reorganization, this chapter also examines the typical rehabilitation environment, suggesting ways of providing more effective and efficient methods of service delivery and of building an environment that promotes physical and mental activity and skill acquisition. In such an environment the individual can be an active learner with opportunity for intensive exercise and training.

Collection of objective data in the clinic using valid and reliable tests is critical for the development of effective interventions. Valid, reliable and functional tests of motor performance are included in Chapters 2–5. This present chapter includes a section on measuring quality of life and self-efficacy since it is now recognized that patients' views about their functional abilities and their own perceptions of their lifestyle are essential to planning future follow-up and rehabilitation.

BRAIN REORGANIZATION AND FUNCTIONAL RECOVERY

New brain imaging techniques are making it clear that the neural system is continuously remodelled throughout life and after injury by experience and learning in response to activity and behaviour (e.g. Jenkins et al. 1990, Johansson 2000, Nudo et al. 2001). The possibility that neural cortical connections can be remodelled by our experience was suggested by Hebb over half a century ago. Modern cortical mapping techniques in both non-human and human subjects indicate that the functional organization of the primary motor cortex is much more complex than was traditionally described. Nudo and colleagues summarize this complex organization, pointing out the extensive overlapping of muscle representation within the motor map, with individual muscle and joint representations re-represented within the motor map, individual corticospinal neurons diverging to multiple motoneuron pools, and horizontal fibres interconnecting distributed representations. It is their view that this complex organization may provide the foundation for functional plasticity in the motor cortex (Nudo et al. 2001).

Support for the hypothesis that changes in the nervous system may occur according to patterns of use comes from studies of human subjects performing actions in which they are skilled. For example, the sensorimotor cortical representation (map) of the reading finger is expanded in blind Braille readers (Pascual-Leone and Torres 1993) and fluctuates according to the extent of reading activity (Pascual-Leone et al. 1995). Right-handed string players show an increased cortical representation of flexor and extensor muscles for the fingers of the left but not the right hand, and, with regular performance, the representational area remains enlarged (Elbert et al. 1995). Such studies reflect the changes associated with skill development that are provoked by active, repetitive training and practice, and by the continued practice of the activity.

Conversely, restriction of activity, examined in association with immobilization (Liepert et al. 1995) or amputation (e.g. Cohen et al. 1991, Fuhr et al. 1992), also induces alterations in cortical representation. A significant decrease in the cortical motor representation of inactive leg muscles was found after 4–6 weeks of unilateral ankle immobilization and was more pronounced when the duration of immobilization was longer (Liepert et al. 1995). Early investigation following amputation of part of one upper limb found that the remaining muscles in that limb received more descending connections than the equivalent muscles of the intact limb (Hall et al. 1990). It seems, therefore, that the neural system is inherently flexible and adaptive, responding according to many factors, including patterns of use.

Throughout the past century, neuroscientists have attempted to understand the neurophysiological and neuroanatomical bases for functional recovery after brain injury. It was assumed that other parts of the motor system must 'take over' the function of the damaged cortex but neural models for recovery of function were based on poorly understood processes (Nudo and Friel 1999). Over the past 10–15 years, however, neuroimaging and non-invasive stimulation studies – positron emission tomography (PET), functional magnetic resonance imaging (fMRI) and transcranial magnetic stimulation (TMS) – have confirmed that the cerebral cortex is functionally and structurally dynamic, that neural reorganization occurs in the human cortex after stroke, and that altered neural activity patterns and molecular events influence this functional reorganization (Johansson 2000).

Broadly speaking, two types of process have been suggested to underlie functional recovery from hemiparetic stroke: reorganization of affected motor regions and changes in the unaffected hemisphere. Following a lesion, there are a number of physiological, pharmacological and anatomical events that occur in widespread regions of the cortex (Schiene et al. 1996), ranging from the intact peri-infarct zone to more remote cortical motor areas of the unaffected hemisphere (Furlan et al. 1996, Cramer et al. 1997). Potential mechanisms include changes in membrane excitability, growth of new connections or unmasking of pre-existing connections, removal of inhibition and activity-dependent synaptic changes. Plastic changes have also been demonstrated in subcortical regions.

Knowledge of the potential capability of the brain to adapt following a lesion and of the probability that patterns of use and disuse affect this reorganization provides a stimulus to the design of optimal stroke rehabilitation (Carr and Shepherd 1998, Shepherd 2001). Studies of animals and humans with brain lesions provide insight into the process of functional recovery and reflect a relationship between neural reorganization and the rehabilitation process. A series of studies of squirrel monkeys that modelled the effects of a focal ischaemic infarct within the hand motor area of the cortex, found that there was further loss of hand representation in the area adjacent to the lesion when monkeys had no post-infarct intervention (Nudo and Milliken 1996). This suggested that further tissue loss could have been due to non-use of the hand and this was confirmed by a follow-up study which showed that not only could tissue loss be prevented when the unimpaired hand was restrained and the monkey had daily repetitive training in skilled use of the impaired hand, but there was also a net gain of approximately 10% in the total hand area adjacent to the lesion (Nudo et al. 1996). In a further study, in which the unimpaired hand was restrained but no training was given, the size of the total hand and wrist/forearm representation decreased, indicating that restraint of the unimpaired hand alone was not sufficient to retain the spared hand area (Friel and Nudo 1998). The results of these studies point to the necessity for active use of the limb for the survival of undamaged neurons adjacent to those damaged by cortical injury, and suggest that retention of the spared hand area and recovery of function after cortical injury might depend upon repetitive training and skilled use of the hand (Nudo and Friel 1999).

Human studies also provide evidence for functional plasticity after stroke associated with meaningful use of a limb (for review see Cramer and Bastings 2000) involving task-oriented repetitive exercise (Nelles et al. 2001). The results of a recent study using TMS suggest a relationship between physiotherapy intervention and reorganization of the cerebral cortex in persons several years after stroke (Liepert et al. 2000). The authors examined the output area of the abductor pollicis brevis muscle in the affected hemisphere after constraint-induced (CI) therapy which involved restraint of the unimpaired hand and training of the impaired limb. They reported a significant enlargement in the size of this area which was associated with improved motor performance of the impaired hand. These changes were maintained 6 months later, with the area of the cortical representation in the affected hemisphere almost identical to the unaffected side. The results of several other studies also support the idea that there is considerable scope for use-dependent functional reorganization in the adult cerebral cortex after stroke (e.g. Weiller et al. 1992, Cramer et al. 1997, Kopp et al. 1999).

It has been noted that soon after stroke the excitability of the motor cortex is decreased and cortical representations are reduced. This probably occurs as a result of diaschisis-like effects (Nudo et al. 2001). The recovery of function occurring early following stroke reflects reparative processes in the peri-infarct zone adjacent to the injury. These include the resolution of local factors such as oedema, absorption of necrotic tissue debris and the opening of collateral channels for circulation to the lesioned area. It is thought that this takes place over a relatively short period, perhaps 3–4 weeks (Lee and van Donkelaar 1995). However, the principal process responsible for functional recovery beyond the immediate reparative stage is likely to be use-dependent reorganization of neural mechanisms. What is certain is that adaptive plasticity is inevitable after an acute brain lesion, and it is very likely that rehabilitation may influence it, with the possibility of positive or negative consequences.

It is reasonable to hypothesize that repetitive exercise and training in real-life tasks following a stroke may be a critical stimulus to the making of new or more effective functional connections within remaining brain tissue. Training and practice using methods that facilitate motor learning or relearning would be essential to the formation of new functional connections. Increase of synaptic efficacy in existing neural circuits in the form of long-term potentiation and formation of new synapses may be involved in earlier stages of motor learning (Asanuma and Keller 1991). It seems certain from current research that if rehabilitation is to be effective in optimizing functional recovery, increased emphasis needs to be placed on methods of forcing use of the affected limbs through functionally relevant exercise and training, including specific interventions such as treadmill walking and constraint-induced training of the affected upper limb.

There are many complex issues arising from the studies cited here and from others. However, the evidence to date is very compelling in terms of the importance of intensive training in behaviourally relevant tasks in a stimulating and enriched environment after cortical injury. What is certain is that the brain reorganizes after injury. The changes, however, may be either adaptive or maladaptive in terms of function. Given the evidence from differential and context-dependent effects of reorganization, it is possible to hypothesize that the nature of organization depends on the inputs received and outputs demanded. To what extent functional imaging data correspond to outcome data needs further evaluation (Nelles et al. 1999). If we can understand the underlying processes and the interactions between brain reorganization, training and motor learning, interventions can be designed on neurobiological principles that may direct intact tissue to 'take over' the damaged function.

Although there is mounting evidence indicating that patterns of use affect reorganization, and increasing acceptance of a link between brain reorganization and recovery of function, it is still not generally accepted in medical or therapy practice that there might be a link between specific rehabilitation methods and functional recovery. Many clinicians would argue that rehabilitation is critical after stroke but only a few would take the next step and argue that it is the nature and the process of rehabilitation and the methods used that affect recovery, that some methods in use may be a waste of time or may actually inhibit recovery.

In summary, there is evidence of substantial potential for functional brain reorganization after stroke. Although the exact mechanisms are still unclear, results from animal and human studies suggest that a substantial substrate exists for influencing the recovery of an injured brain. Although the size of tissue loss has been equated with outcome, Johansson (2000) comments that 'it is not only the number of neurons left, but how they function and what connections they can make that will decide functional outcome'.

THE REHABILITATION ENVIRONMENT

If brain reorganization and functional recovery from brain lesions are dependent on use and activity, then the environment in which rehabilitation is carried out is likely to play an important role in patient outcomes. The rehabilitation environment is made up of:

1. the physical or built environment (the physical setting)
2. the methods used to deliver rehabilitation
3. the staff, their knowledge, skill and attitudes.

We argue in this section that the physical environment must offer possibilities for intensive and meaningful exercise and training; that the delivery methods should vary and include supervised one-to-one practice with the therapist, group practice and independent practice; and that therapists can be major facilitators of motor learning.

Evidence from animal experiments suggests that the nature of the environment and its physical structure, together with the opportunities it offers for social interaction and physical activity, can influence outcome after a lesion. Environmental enrichment after a brain lesion in rats can increase cortical thickness, protein content, dendritic branching, number of dendritic spines and size of synaptic contact areas (Kolb and Gibb 1991, Pritzel and Huston 1991, Will and Kelche 1992). Conversely, the mechanisms of brain plasticity are also affected by an impoverished environment. It has been suggested that environmental enrichment may affect a general factor or a host of specific factors that relate to the general adaptive capacity of the organism, i.e. its ability to cope with a variety of situations and problems of a general nature (Finger 1978).

Animal experiments have shown that exposure to a particular type of environment may either enhance or restrict opportunity for general experience. Rats housed in an enriched environment, with the opportunity for physical activities and interaction with other rats, performed significantly better on motor tasks than rats housed in a standard laboratory environment, alone and with no opportunities for interesting activities (Held et al. 1985, Ohlsson and Johansson 1995).

In animal research, the aspects of the enriched environment which appear to be critical as enhancers of behaviour are social stimulation, interaction with objects that enable physical activity (Bennett 1976) and an increased level of arousal (Walsh and Cummins 1975). It is of interest, therefore, to consider what effects a typical rehabilitation environment may have on the behaviour of humans, and observational studies of rehabilitation settings provide some insights. They suggest the environment may not be sufficiently geared to facilitating physical and mental activity or social interaction, and that the rehabilitation setting may not function as a learning environment (Ada et al. 1999).

Several studies investigating how stroke patients spend their time have shown that a large percentage of the day was spent in passive pursuits rather than in physical activity. Even less physical activity occurred on weekends compared with weekdays and there was little evidence of independent exercise. Patients were noted to remain solitary and inactive for long periods, watching others or looking out of the window. Although what physical activity occurred was in the therapy area, therapy was noted to occur for only a small percentage of the day (Keith 1980, Keith and Cowell 1987, Lincoln et al. 1989, Tinson 1989, Mackey et al. 1996, Esmonde et al. 1997). It is disappointing to see that over the nearly two decades spanned by these studies there was little change in the amount of time spent in physical activities.

Structuring a practice environment

The goals of physiotherapy are to provide opportunities for an individual to regain optimal skilled performance of functional actions and to increase levels of strength, endurance and physical fitness. For the able-bodied and the disabled, it is recognized that practice is the way to achieve these aims.

Skill in performing a motor task increases as a function of the *amount* and *type of practice* as does strength, endurance and fitness. Although the amount of practice is critical and more practice is better than less, recent research into motor learning and strength training suggests that the amount of practice may not be the only variable influencing any improvements in performance. There is some clinical evidence (e.g. Parry et al. 1999a) that merely increasing the time spent in therapy may not necessarily improve outcome. It is probably the *type of practice* rather than simply its occurrence that reshapes the cortex following a brain lesion (Small and Solodkin 1998).

The issue of how much time is spent in physical activity, including practice of motor tasks and how this time is organized, is a critical one for rehabilitation. The results of observational studies on how patients spend their day raise the question of whether the typical rehabilitation environment is sufficiently stimulating, providing opportunity for intensive and meaningful training and exercise. In other words, are the physical structures, organization and attitudes required to encourage active participation, exercise, independent practice and learning, in place? If they are not, a change in both staff attitude and work practices may need to be considered.

What the patient is actually doing in rehabilitation must itself be effective if increasing the amount of time spent practising is to improve outcome and there is increasing evidence of which methods can be effective. What the patient practises outside the time allotted to training and practice is also likely to impact significantly on outcome. As an example, self-propulsion in a one-arm drive wheelchair using unimpaired limbs is at odds with treatment goals to increase strength and control of impaired limbs (Esmonde et al. 1997). If the patient spends more time in this activity than in exercising the impaired limbs, it is not hard to guess the probable outcomes.

Delivery of physiotherapy

It is clear from studies of rehabilitation environments that only a small part of the day may be made available for practice and training. To some extent this reflects work practices. One way of increasing the amount of training and practice is for therapists to move away from reliance on hands-on, one-to-one therapy, to a model in which the patient practises, not only in individualized training sessions with the therapist, but also in a group with less direct therapist supervision (Fig. 1.1). One or two therapists with the assistance of an aide can oversee several individuals, with relatives and friends helping if they are willing. Such organization can improve efficiency of delivery by increasing the time the patient spends practising without substantially increasing the therapist's load. This ensures better use of the short time allowed for intensive inpatient rehabilitation (Fig. 1.2).

Group training can enable each individual to exercise independently or with another patient at specially designed work stations set up to enable practice of specific motor activities and with technological and other aids to promote strength and skill. Work stations can provide videotapes and/or photographs of the action to be practised, lists of some common problems and what to do about them.

Group training and exercise can be organized as a circuit class (see note at end of chapter). Circuit training in able-bodied individuals often involves two people working together, one observing and one physically practising. Alternating practice with a partner can be more effective than individual practice (Shea et al. 1999). Practising with another person in an interactive way may increase the learner's motivation by adding both competitive and cooperative components to the practice situation (McNevin et al. 2000), and there are benefits to be gained from observing another person learning a task (Herbert and Landin 1994).

FIGURE 1.1 *Group training: (a) Step-up exercise class. Safe independent practice is ensured by having a high table nearby for support when necessary. (b) Standing up and sitting down class. Seat height is customized to individual's lower limb strength.*

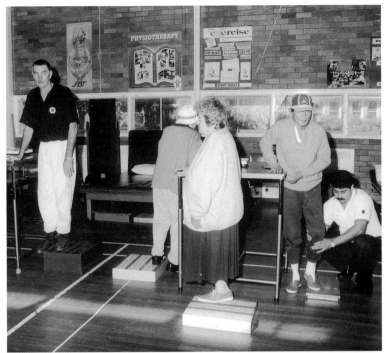

(a)

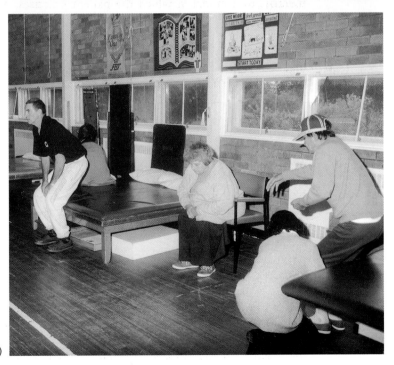

(b)

FIGURE 1.2   *Indirect supervision. (a) Simple reaching tasks in a harness can be progressed to reaching in a tandem foot position and to stepping out in order to reach further. (b) Repetitive practice of standing up and sitting down. (c) Repetitive leg exercises on a pedal machine. The paretic foot can be bandaged on to the pedal if necessary.*

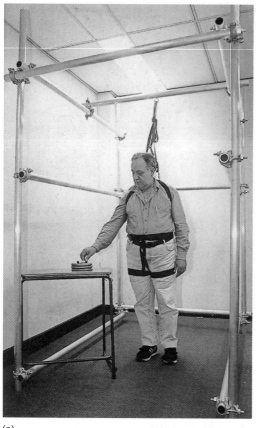

(a)

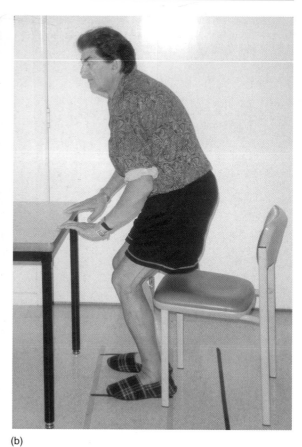

(b)

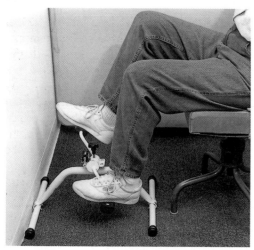

(c)

FIGURE 1.3	*Overview of an upper limb circuit class at a Queensland hospital. The work stations include reaching to attach stick-ons high on the wall, pegging playing cards on a line, modified (supported) reaching to push bean bag over the edge, playing a game with an opponent. (Courtesy of C Lynch, Physiotherapy Department, Ipswich Hospital.)*

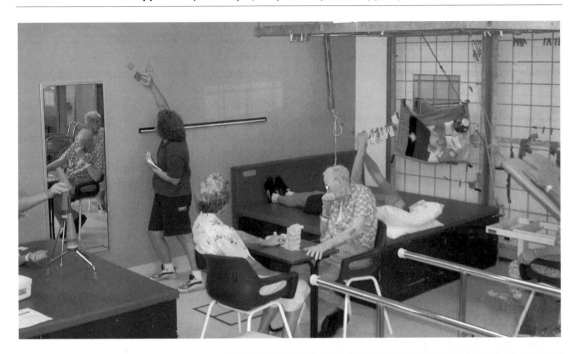

Working with another person provides rest intervals, especially when training is physically demanding, yet the individual has to remain focused in order to assist his/her partner. Moving on from one set of tasks to another in a circuit class is also a way to keep up alertness and enthusiasm.

These methods of delivery fit well within an exercise and training model of rehabilitation, and in the clinic such group training is being used by therapists (Fig. 1.3), with evidence that exercise classes and circuit training can be both efficacious and feasible (Taub et al. 1993, Dean et al. 2000, Teixeira-Salmela et al. 1999, 2001). Although the therapist's supervision is necessary, patients may benefit also from the experience of their peers (McNevin et al. 2000) and from helping each other. The presence and input from other patients with similar disabilities may motivate and encourage individuals to do better. In a recent study, it was found that the introduction of group exercise classes increased the level of social interaction throughout the day (De Weerdt et al. 2001). Such partially supervised practice can bridge the gap between individualized training and unsupervised practice in hospital and at home. Giving patients some control over practice conditions by empowering them to view the therapist as a resource person may encourage their problem-solving abilities (McNevin et al. 2000).

Actively involving patients and giving them a sense of responsibility in their exercise and training programme enables them to take some control over events that affect their lives. Although the patient's level of disability would influence the amount of independent practice that is possible, once the therapist and patient have decided how much practice can be expected, strategies to enable this to occur can be developed. Brief exercise lists with diagrams for independent practice, stored on computer, can be printed as appropriate for the individual. Monitoring needs to be put in place to determine whether or not the desired activity levels are being achieved, and individual work books with simple check lists can provide evidence of what each person has done and for how long in 1 day, or 1 week. There have been reports that, from the patients' point of view, perceived barriers to exercise programmes include lack of positive feedback and the perception that exercises are not adapted to their particular situation or daily routine. Patients who reported that their physiotherapists were very satisfied with progress were more likely to participate than patients who did not know whether or not the therapist valued their efforts (Sluijs et al. 1993).

Some therapists express concern about reducing hands-on therapy and increasing semi-supervised and unsupervised practice because patients may practise 'incorrectly'. However, it is well known that people do not learn to perform an action unless they have a chance to practise it themselves. It is only by attempting to carry out a movement to achieve a goal voluntarily that an individual knows whether the action attempted is successful. Motivation is known to be low when the learner cannot make mistakes during practice. In other words, learning requires an element of trial and error. Practice conditions can be organized to enable practice of the action even in patients with muscle weakness and poor limb control. For example, walking on a treadmill with partial body weight support has been shown to be more effective in improving gait than restricting walking practice in order to avoid the patient practising incorrectly, i.e. making errors (Hesse et al. 1995).

There is increasing understanding of the importance of strength training and exercise in stroke rehabilitation. However, the intensive and repetitive practice required to improve performance may not be demanded if patients are perceived to fatigue easily, particularly if they are elderly. Fatigue may be viewed as contraindicative and necessitating rest, instead of as a manifestation of the need to get stronger and develop more endurance. The past decade has seen an accumulation of data that provide reassurance of the safety of exercise and physical conditioning programmes following stroke (Ch. 7). The beneficial effects of such programmes include not only improved physiological responses but also improved functional motor performance. Simple ways to increase exercise tolerance and endurance, even in the early stages, may include setting goals such as increasing the speed of movement and the number of repetitions. The results can be graphed, providing the patient with feedback information and motivation.

Challenges to customary delivery of intervention can be difficult for clinicians because such practices have been built on long-standing traditions and beliefs and a culture which has not until recently demanded evidence of efficacy. The attitude that the critical method of therapy delivery is a one-to-one interaction, with emphasis on physical handling of the patient in order to facilitate more normal movement, does not fit well with modern views of the patient as active learner and the therapist as teacher or coach. Increasing numbers of clinical studies are supporting the use of more varied methods of delivery and more active methods of intervention.

Optimizing skill

Skill has been defined as 'any activity that has become better organized and more effective as a result of practice' (Annett 1971) and also as 'the ability to consistently attain a goal with some economy of effort' (Gentile 1987). Everyday activities, even such apparently simple ones as standing up from a seat, constitute motor skills. They are complex actions, made up of segmental movements linked together in the appropriate spatial and temporal sequence. The person with motor impairments following a neural lesion needs to learn again how to control segmental movement so that the spatial configuration and temporal sequencing of body movements brings about an effective action, thereby achieving the individual's goal with minimum energy expenditure. Task-oriented training is critical to gaining the necessary control. In attempting to regain movement control, however, the degree of muscle weakness may be such that initially the patient also has to practise exercises for activating and sustaining activity in specific muscle groups.

An important characteristic of acquiring skill is that learning seems to take place in overlapping stages. Two models that have been proposed give insights useful to the clinic. An early study described three stages of learning: an early or cognitive stage, an intermediate or associative stage and a final or autonomous stage (Fitts and Posner 1967). The learning stages have also been described as first getting the idea of the movement, then developing the ability to adapt the movement pattern to the demands of the environment (Gentile 1987). In both cases the initial stage is cognitive.

Early after stroke, patients with a lesioned system are struggling to learn again how to perform even simple movements as well as everyday actions. They need to practise repetitively in order to get the idea of the action they are (re)learning and to train the neural coordination necessary for effective performance. As they gain more strength and control, less attention can be directed toward performing the action and more attention to the goal and relevant environmental cues.

As motor control and skill develop, changes occur at different levels. For example, with more intersegmental control there is less tendency to 'freeze' the degrees of freedom. There is also a decrease in energy expenditure. The focus of attention shifts. In walking, the focus of visual attention shifts from the feet to the surrounding environment; 'star billing' for sit-to-stand changes from foot placement and speed of trunk rotation to steadying a glass of water while standing up. Being aware of the characteristics of each stage enables the therapist to provide the appropriate practice conditions to optimize performance.

For movement to become more automatic, intensive practice is required in order to increase endurance as well as the opportunity to practise adapting the action to varying environmental demands – for example, walking in different environments, coping with several simultaneous demands such as doing two things at once.

Focusing attention

Attentional abilities required for everyday functioning include the ability to focus attention on a task, to sustain concentration, to shift attention if additional task-relevant material comes along but to ignore distracting, irrelevant inputs. Training techniques to overcome these deficits involve highlighting the task to bring it to the patient's attention, reinforcing maintenance of attention to task and its relevant cues, and adding distractions to the environment then reinforcing the 'filtering out' of such inputs (Adams 1990).

Learning of motor skills involves two critical components, particularly in the early stages:

1. identifying what is to be learned
2. understanding the ways through which the goal can be accomplished.

A number of recent studies demonstrate that the person's attentional focus can have a decisive influence on motor performance and learning (Wulf et al. 1999a). It is important to decide what the patient should pay attention to during practice. Two methods of directing the focus of attention are demonstration (both live and recorded) and verbal instruction.

Demonstration.   Demonstration, or modelling of an action, gives the therapist the opportunity to point out the key components of the action. A demonstration assists the patient to get the idea of the spatial and temporal features of the action, the 'shape' or topology of the movement (Fig. 1.4).

Instructions.   In the early stages of learning, instructions should be brief, with no unnecessary words. They should cue the patient to concentrate on one or two critical features of the action (Fig. 1.5). In standing up practice, for example, the patient is drilled to place feet back, swing upper body forward at the hips and stand up, and can verbalize this sequence while practising. A stick figure drawing can reinforce these key elements. Asking the patient to list what cues they are to focus on aids mental rehearsal and enables the therapist to judge what the patient has gained from both instruction and demonstration. Gradually the patient internalizes these details and can start to think more of the goal of the action (e.g. to stand up and walk to another chair) while practising in a more complex environment.

At this later stage, instructing the patient to focus on the details of their performance may actually be detrimental. There is increasing evidence that directing learners to the effects of their movements, i.e. whether or not the goal is achieved, may be more effective than attending to the movement itself (Singer et al. 1993, Wulf et al. 1999a). Similarly, at this stage of learning, verbal instructions are used in directing attention to specific environmental features or events.

FIGURE 1.4   *Demonstrating the extent of trunk flexion at the hips in standing up: (a) beside the patient so that he can line his shoulders up with hers; (b) a sagittal plane view to show him how far forward the shoulders are moved.*

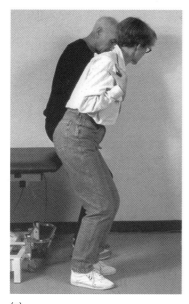

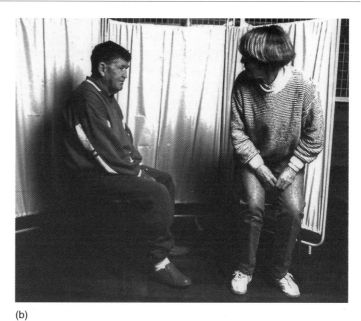

(a)   (b)

FIGURE 1.5   *The drawing illustrates in a simplified form the critical features of the action.*

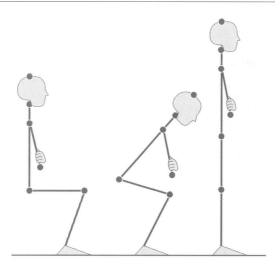

A typical approach to the question of what a person should attend to during practice has been to tell learners to be aware of what they are doing by paying attention to the 'feel' of the movement (Singer et al. 1993). This has also been a common approach in clinical practice. Singer and colleagues (1993) compared the influence on performing and learning a throwing task of consciously attending to the movement (awareness strategy) or focusing on one situational cue and ignoring the movement (non-awareness strategy). The findings indicated that, for able-bodied subjects, the non-awareness strategy led to higher achievement than the awareness strategy. Similar results have been found in several recent studies (see Wulf et al. 1999b for discussion). It may, therefore, be beneficial at times for the therapist to suggest a focus of only one cue, following this with a 'Now – just do it'.

Setting goals.   The goal to be achieved should be meaningful and worthwhile to the individual, reasonably challenging yet attainable. Some goals seem to facilitate action more readily than others. As an example, tasks that have goals directed toward controlling one's physical interaction with objects or persons in the immediate environment (concrete tasks) seem to have more meaning and be more motivating than goals directed at movements for their own sake (abstract tasks). Performance has been shown to improve significantly when an individual is presented with a concrete goal compared with an abstract goal. The facilitatory effect of a concrete goal has been demonstrated in several clinical studies, including one study of adults with restricted range of motion in the elbow or shoulder as a result of injury (Leont'ev and Zaporozhets 1960), and another of children with cerebral palsy (van der Weel et al. 1991). Furthermore, kinematic analysis has clearly demonstrated the different movement characteristics when a task is performed without the relevant object (Mathiowetz and Wade 1995, Wu et al. 2000). Wu et al. (2000) examined a group of individuals after stroke and an able-bodied group scooping coins off a table with and without the coins present. For both groups, reaching for the coins elicited faster movement compared with reaching without the coins. The data showed a greater percentage of reaches where peak velocity occurred, and smoother and straighter movement, all signs of a coordinated well-learned movement.

There may be several explanations for these results. Abstract and concrete tasks differ in the degree to which the action is directed toward controlling physical interaction with an object as opposed to merely moving a limb. The presence of an object provides clear visual information before starting the movement as well as providing feedback about performance and outcome. A functional task that is also familiar is more likely to produce more effective performance than an abstract task. A task that is relatively difficult to attain but achievable may provide more motivation, challenging the patient to succeed.

It has been rather a common practice in physiotherapy to have the patient practise abstract movements such as weight shift sideways in standing rather than the more concrete and meaningful task of reaching sideways for an object, or placing one foot on a step. In the former, the patient has to 'believe' the therapist's feedback about whether or not the goal was achieved. For the latter, there are observable outcomes. Examples of providing concrete goals to improve functional performance are given in Chapters 2–5.

Feedback

An essential aspect of skill acquisition is the feedback that learners receive about their performance of an action. There are two principal forms of feedback: intrinsic, which is the naturally available sensory feedback (visual, proprioceptive, tactile) occurring as part of the action, and augmented feedback, providing knowledge of the results of the action (KR) and knowledge of the performance itself (KP). Augmented feedback comes from external sources, such as the therapist or coach, and adds to or enhances intrinsic feedback. Augmented feedback can be positive or negative, qualitative or quantitative, and can provide motivation when presented in a way that influences the learner to persist in striving toward the goal.

The most commonly used form of augmented feedback is verbal feedback from the therapist or teacher. Feedback can involve instrumentation, and may include videotape replay or graphed representation of kinematics (path of body parts, joint angle displacement) or kinetics (amplitude and timing of vertical force) as a means of providing information about some aspect of performance. Electromyography (EMG) biofeedback is a commonly used method of providing information about physiological processes underlying the action.

Augmented feedback can have various effects on skill performance depending on the type of information given, how it is given and the skill being learned. In providing feedback about performance, the challenge for the therapist is to select the appropriate feature of performance on which to base that feedback. It is, therefore, important to prioritize biomechanical components so that feedback is confined to these key characteristics of the movement. The patient's attention is directed to the part of the action to be changed in order to improve the next attempt. As skill in performance increases, feedback changes from prescriptive in the early stages to descriptive, which may be more appropriate in the later stages.

The experience a person has in making and correcting errors is part of skill learning. Not every attempt needs to be 'perfect'. There is a continuing controversy about the role of augmented feedback in terms of whether it should emphasize errors made or aspects of performance that are correct. Magill (1998) writes that augmented feedback (as error information) functions in an informational role that is related to facilitating skill improvement. Augmented feedback about what the person did correctly has a more motivating role but may not be sufficient to produce optimal learning, particularly in the early phase (Magill 2001).

If practice conditions create a dependency on augmented feedback, the individual may rely on it with the result that performance deteriorates and learning is impeded when it is removed (Magill 2001). Individuals may learn to depend on the therapist or the instrumentation for guidance instead of attending to task-relevant cues (Sidaway et al. 2001). There is evidence in clinical studies of this reliance on instrumented feedback and subsequent deterioration of performance when feedback is removed (Engardt 1994, Fowler and Carr 1996). The equivocal results of many clinical studies on instrumented feedback may be largely due to this problem of withdrawal. Overreliance on feedback may be avoided if the patient is assisted to replace augmented feedback by attending more to the action itself, i.e. was the goal achieved easily and quickly? If not, then what was the reason?

Reducing the number of trials for which feedback is given is likely to result in better learning than feedback after every trial. There is some evidence that providing feedback after each attempt may not be as useful as encouraging the patient to ask for feedback whenever they think it might be beneficial (Janelle et al. 1997). The active role of the learner has been neglected in the study of feedback until recently. Giving the learner some responsibility in and control over the learning situation may encourage the individual to engage in more effective learning strategies and increase confidence and motivation (Janelle et al. 1997).

In a recent study, Talvitie (2000) videotaped and systematically observed physiotherapist–patient interactions during treatment and noted the way in which feedback was given. The author reported that therapists did most of the talking, patients were rarely involved in the dialogue, information feedback appeared very seldom, and verbal and physical guidance were given more than visual cues. The methodology of this study provides a useful way for therapists to get feedback about their own interactions with patients. Therapeutic relationships may be based on the physiotherapist as authority figure or on a more equal footing with the patient. The latter based on dialogue helps to create the opportunity for more positive relationships (Lundvik et al. 1999).

Vision plays a key role in motor learning and is probably the most widely used source of information feedback in performing motor tasks. Vision provides powerful intrinsic feedback, information about environmental conditions, and exproprioceptive information for determining the individual's relative position within the environment (Lee and Aronson 1974).

Early after stroke, patients typically have difficulty directing their visual attention to environmental cues and the therapist may need to direct vision to the appropriate cue. When reaching for an object, a reminder is given to look at the object; when walking in a busy corridor, vision is directed well ahead, not at feet or floor. As skill progresses, the individual learns to direct their own vision and to pay attention to the critical features in the environment which provide the most useful information for achieving the goal, and enable prediction of potential hazards in order to take appropriate avoidance action.

Transfer of learning

Early rehabilitation typically takes place almost entirely within the rehabilitation setting itself. The purpose of both strength training and task practice in rehabilitation is, however, to increase the patient's ability to perform the action in situations where it is needed, in both everyday and novel contexts. A major goal of the therapist as facilitator and teacher is, therefore, to assist the patient to transfer training (learning) from the practice environment (the rehabilitation setting) to these other environments.

Transfer of learning from one performance situation to another is an integral part of skill learning (Magill 2001). This concept lies at the heart of understanding motor learning, acknowledging that an action cannot be separated from the environment in which it is carried out. How we move is the sum of the task undertaken and the environment in which it is performed. Gentile's (1987) *taxonomy of motor skills* is a framework for encouraging transfer of a particular motor task into different environments. The taxonomy differentiates motor skills depending on the environmental context. A closed motor skill is one in which the environment is stable. If the environment is changeable, skills are categorized as open. Regulatory conditions during performance are either stationary (walking up a flight of stairs) or in motion (walking through automatic doors); intertrial variability is either absent (walking in an uncluttered room) or present (catching a ball). Constraints from the environment alter the biomechanics of an action and the amount of information to be processed. When performance depends on external timing, the demand on information processing increases because success depends on predicting future events. For example, consider the demands of crossing a road, even at traffic lights. Performance also varies according to spatial relationships. Walking differs depending on whether one is walking on a flat surface, a slippery surface or approaching a kerb.

A patient may learn to walk in the closed environment of the physiotherapy area but not be able to walk outside it unless given the opportunity to practise in open and more complex situations. Categorization of motor skills provides the therapist with a basis on which to set up practice conditions that provide a variety of relevant situations and challenges for training that prepare the individual for the real world. When practice is varied by changing aspects of the environmental context, the motor skill that develops is flexible and generative, facilitating a kind of motor problem-solving ability. Huxham et al. (2001) provide some clear examples of assessing and training balance in relation to function and the physical environment using Gentile's taxonomy.

Also of interest is the issue of *transfer from strength training to the performance of a specific action*. Some years ago, Thorndike suggested that transfer was the result of identical elements being transferred from one task to another. Since then the motor learning and exercise science literature on able-bodied people has provided evidence that a transfer can occur to tasks with similar dynamic characteristics (Oxendine 1984, Gottlieb et al. 1988). Clinical literature suggests that this also occurs in disabled populations (Nugent et al. 1994, Sherrington and Lord 1997). This issue is discussed in Chapter 7.

Practice

From the literature on motor learning it is clear that, as a general rule, the action to be acquired should be practised in its entirety (*task-specific practice*), since one component of the action is to a large extent dependent on preceding components. Several studies of gait have demonstrated that power generation in the ankle plantarflexors for push-off at the end of stance phase is critical to the subsequent swing phase in terms of step length. Power generation in the ankle plantarflexors, as part of the gait cycle, also affects walking speed and can ensure an effective pattern of energy exchange (Winter 1983, Olney et al. 1986). These mechanisms can only be optimized through the practice of walking itself. The strength training literature is also clear that, above a certain activity-specific threshold of strength, exercises should resemble as closely as possible the action being trained.

There are many reasons why functional improvement in performance of an action depends on practice of the action itself. Nevertheless, in rehabilitation it may be necessary for the patient to spend time in part practice, i.e. *practising a sub-task*. An important question is determining which component part of the action to practise separately. If a patient cannot activate plantarflexor muscles with the necessary force and at the appropriate time for push-off, repetitive, resisted exercises are necessary to strengthen (and actively stretch) these muscles. Practice of this sub-task is then incorporated into walking during training.

When an individual has difficulty performing an action due to muscle weakness, and can only practise that action using grossly ineffective compensations, *modifying the task or environment* is a way of reducing task difficulty. Such modifications enable practice of a simplified form of the action. Raising seat height decreases lower limb muscle force demands and may enable a person to practise standing up and sitting down with some weight through the affected lower limb or more evenly distributed between the two lower limbs; walking on a treadmill with partial body weight support enables early walking practice even in a very weak patient provided assistance is given to the swing phase; constraining mechanically inappropriate movement with a splint or strapping enables practice of limb loading exercises without loss of control into hyperextension (Fig. 1.6).

| FIGURE 1.6 | *(a) A tendency for the knee to collapse into hyperextension is prevented by strapping across the back of the joint. (b) This enables the limb to be loaded with thigh and shank segments in an alignment which may encourage activation of lower limb extensor muscles.* |

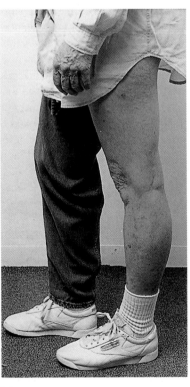 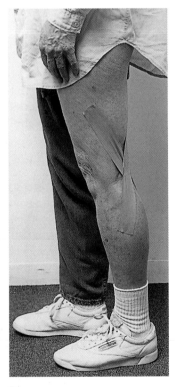

(a)   (b)

In both strength training and skill development, *repetition* is an important aspect of practice. Repetitive exercise and practice of an action facilitates the contraction of the muscles involved and improves performance in both able-bodied and disabled individuals (Asanuma and Keller 1991, Butefisch et al. 1995, Dean and Shepherd 1997). Thousands of repetitions of an action may be necessary for the patient to develop an optimal way of performing the action (Bernstein in Latash and Latash 1994). Traditional physiotherapy neglects the repetitive element of skill acquisition that probably forms an essential prerequisite in motor rehabilitation (Butefisch et al. 1995).

In the early stages of rehabilitation, repetitive practice of an exercise or part of an action is necessary to increase muscle strength and train coordination of the muscular synergies that move the segmental linkage. The therapist should sustain the patient's motivation during repetitive practice, for example, by counting repetitions (or providing a counter), and by providing concrete feedback of the effects of practice in terms of increases in strength or in speed. It may be useful to explain to the patient that learning continues even though performance may deteriorate due to muscle fatigue. After a rest period or a change to a less demanding or different activity, an improvement in performance is usually evident.

Acquiring skill does not only mean to repeat and consolidate but also to invent and to progress (Whiting 1980), i.e. a particular type of 'repetition without repetition' (Bernstein 1967). Thus skill acquisition involves the ability to solve motor problems posed by the environment. Patients need the opportunity to practise motor actions in different task and environmental contexts in order to develop this flexibility.

Practice can be considered as a continuum from overt physical practice at one end of the spectrum to covert or mental practice at the other. *Mental practice* is a technique that uses imagery to mentally rehearse a physical action without overt movement of the body or limbs. A meta-analysis of research into the effect of mental practice in able-bodied subjects found that, in general, mental practice is more effective than no practice, although the effects reported have been inconsistent (Feltz et al. 1988). Mental practice is likely to be most effective once the individual has developed a basic understanding of the movement's topology and when combined with physical practice. There is some empirical evidence in healthy subjects that mental practice activates the appropriate muscles and neural networks and helps establish and reinforce appropriate coordination patterns (Magill 2001).

Mental practice in rehabilitation may only be suitable for patients who do not have communication or perceptual problems and who understand the idea. Time should be taken to ensure that the patient understands the details of the movement to be rehearsed mentally. Observing a demonstration of the action can help the person develop a mental picture of the action to be performed. The patient can repeat back what he/she is imaging and have a photograph or drawing of the action for reference. A list and/or audiotape of the steps to remember should also be provided. Mental practice may have a role to play in motor training when the patient has very little muscle activity. It may also provide a means of maximizing the time spent practising outside structured exercise sessions (Van Leeuwen and Inglis 1998, Page et al. 2001).

In summary, given the evidence that experience and use-dependent training drive brain reorganization either positively or negatively, a rehabilitation unit should provide:

- a stimulating and challenging environment to facilitate social interaction and active participation
- facilities for intensive task- and context-specific exercise and training to optimize motor performance and skill
- a varied delivery of intervention, i.e. in groups and in circuit training, using exercise equipment and electronic aids.

The reader is referred to reviews of motor learning theory and research for more detail (e.g. Gentile 2000, Magill 2001).

MEASUREMENT

Rehabilitation of patients after stroke remains a major challenge to the health-care system. The cost–benefit relationship of stroke rehabilitation as much or more than humanitarian concerns has increased the need for the health-care community to be accountable for the services they provide (Keith 1995).

There is a continuing discussion about the value of focused stroke rehabilitation and no clear indication that patients in these programmes do better than those in general programmes. All those involved in this controversy agree that there is not only a need for a more scientific foundation of therapeutic intervention but also for better documentation of the benefits of stroke rehabilitation (Mauritz 1990).

Major problems in clinical rehabilitation research are the lack of consistency in measures used and the amount of heterogeneity in both patient groups and interventions. It can be difficult to make useful comparisons of data from different studies, centres and countries. A consensus on a few well-grounded outcome measures would help in examining the value of stroke rehabilitation and texts already exist that identify valid and reliable measures. The usefulness of rehabilitation research depends also on the inclusion of details of interventions given and patient population in order to make a link between the methods used in rehabilitation and the functional outcomes.

Evidence-based practice (for discussion see Herbert et al. 2001) is an important strategy for 'meeting the ethical imperative of providing the best possible care for our patients' (Sherrington et al. 2001). Qualitative and quantitative research, in which measurement plays a critical part, makes a major contribution to the development of evidence-based clinical practice. The best evidence of the effects of intervention is provided by randomized controlled trials and systematic reviews[†]. The Physiotherapy Evidence Database[*] is an internet-based

[†]www.cochranelibrary.net; [*]ptwww.fhs.usyd.edu.au/pedro

database of all randomized controlled trials and systematic reviews relevant to physiotherapy. We agree with Sherrington and colleagues (2001) who point out that it is of vital importance that physiotherapy clinicians ensure that evidence is translated into practice. A further responsibility for clinicians is the collection of objective data. Since physiotherapy is concerned principally with training the individual to improve performance of motor actions, motor performance is the focus of measurement.

Measures of motor performance

It is essential in everyday clinical practice that there is a systematic examination of the effects of interventions in order to document patient progress and improve outcomes. Anecdotal evidence suggests that many physiotherapists do not systematically evaluate their treatment methods and therefore do not obtain any objective feedback about their work.

Interesting insights come from a recent follow-up survey of Canadian physiotherapists (Kay et al. 2001). Following a deliberate focus in continuing education on methods of measurement, therapists surveyed were more aware of the complexities of outcome measurement than they were in the previous survey (1992). However, they reported that they lacked confidence and the skills necessary to measure their clinical practice. There is some evidence from the medical literature that skill training in addition to confidence building is a major determinant of whether clinicians attempt new behaviours and persist in the face of obstacles. It may not be well understood that carrying out standardized measurement procedures requires training and practice.

The collection of accurate and objective (i.e. measurement-generated) data about an individual's motor performance in critical everyday actions and documentation of the specifics of intervention makes a critical contribution to developing best possible practice. The measurement of outcome without documentation of intervention details has, however, limited relevance.

Objective information is critical to the design and ongoing modification and variation of a training program. The information collected provides the knowledge necessary to plan appropriate exercise and practice, and can be used to collate data on particular patient groups within a centre and between centres or countries. Collecting such information is not only an important means of establishing best possible practice but also of making changes to practice as more effective methods of intervention are developed.

Measures used may involve both functional and laboratory tests depending on the questions to be answered and the availability of equipment and technical expertise. Data are collected on the individual's entry to physiotherapy, at regular intervals during rehabilitation, and on discharge and follow-up. Follow-up measurements are necessary to provide information about real outcomes, such as retention of gains after discharge from rehabilitation and how an individual functions at home and in the community. Some suitable measures of health needs and status are described below.

Many valid and reliable measures exist for evaluating change in functional performance. These are listed in each chapter after the guidelines. Tests for sensation, muscle strength, cardiovascular responses and range of motion are also included. Standardized protocols describing how the test is administered must be observed during initial testing and repeated on subsequent testing. The examination of similarities in test characteristics, and on ceiling and floor effects will assist the future selection of a core group of clinically useful measures to monitor change in motor performance (e.g. Bernhardt et al. 1998).

Functional outcomes

Global instruments

Functional outcomes are commonly measured with global instruments such as the *Barthel Index* (Mahoney and Barthel 1965, Wade 1992) or the *Functional Independence Measure* (FIM) (Granger et al. 1986). These instruments mainly focus on dependence (i.e. assistance required) and do not include social and emotional aspects or the patient's perceived quality of life. These factors have tended to be neglected areas of research.

Quality of life

The Sickness Impact Profile (SIP) (Bergner et al. 1981) is one of the most widely used measures to assess quality of life (QoL). The original form included 136 items. A short, stroke-adapted, 30-item version (SA-SIP30) has more recently been developed and found to be a feasible and valid clinical measure to assess patient-centred outcomes after stroke (van Straten et al. 1997). Sub-sections included are: Body Care and Movement, Social Interaction, Mobility, Communication, Emotional Behavior, Household Management, Alertness Behavior, Ambulation. The *Nottingham Health Profile* is another short and simple measure of health needs and outcomes (Hunt et al. 1985).

The *Human Activity Profile* (HAP) samples 94 activities across a broad range of energy requirements (e.g. getting in and out of a chair or bed without assistance) to higher activity levels (e.g. vacuuming carpets for 5 minutes with rest periods; walking for 2 miles non-stop). The items are based on estimated metabolic equivalents that allow quick and meaningful measurement of changes in activity levels. Respondents answer each item with one of three responses 'Still doing activity', 'Have stopped doing this activity', 'Never did this activity' (Fix and Daughton 1988).

Self-efficacy

Patient satisfaction (self-efficacy) has also received little attention in rehabilitation. Input from patients can be sought about such issues as their expectations and experiences during rehabilitation. Questionnaires completed anonymously provide an indication of the individual's perception of the value of aspects of rehabilitation such as their exercise and training programme. Although patients are seldom asked to evaluate their experiences during rehabilitation, there are several insightful publications written by individuals who have survived a stroke (e.g. Brodal 1973, Hewson 1996, McCrum 1998, Smits and Smits-Boone 2000).

In conclusion, there should be great satisfaction among clinicians knowing that they are up-to-date in what is considered best possible practice and that they have an ongoing commitment to pushing the limits of what patients can achieve. All of this depends on an organized systematic plan for intervention and on the collection of objective data, the results of which are more informative and satisfying than observations that are subjective and open to bias. It is encouraging to see a growing number of clinical investigations that record quantitative change in movement parameters together with content, frequency, dosage and intensity of physiotherapy intervention.

CIRCUIT TRAINING: EXAMPLE OF ORGANIZATION

Figure 1.7 shows an outpatient circuit class in progress for the lower limbs in the Physiotherapy Department at a New South Wales Hospital. Work stations illustrated include walking sideways, standing balance, step-ups and stair walking. In Figures 1.8–1.10 individuals are working at specific stations. They attend the class for 6 weeks and functional performance is measured at the beginning and completion of the programme with 6- and 12-month follow-up testing (Fig. 1.11). A booklet is given to participants with details about the class (Fig. 1.12) as well as a folder with instructions and diagrams of exercises to practise at home and how often, with a form on which to record what they have done. Photographs were taken by courtesy of F. Mackey and colleagues, Illawarra Area Health Service.

FIGURE 1.7	Overview of lower limb circuit class.

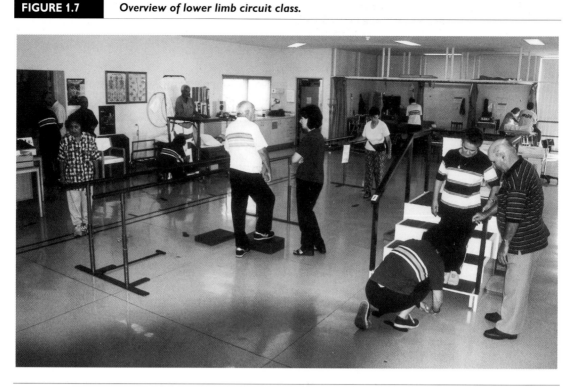

FIGURE 1.8	(a) Sit-to-stand station. Holding a glass of water reinforces the need to balance. (b) The line drawing illustrates the action and the number of repetitions to be performed.

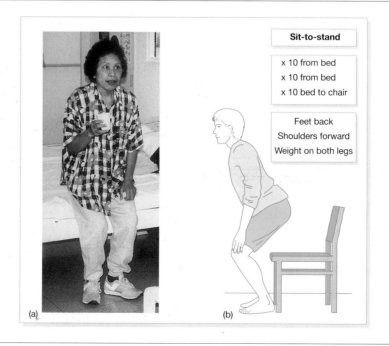

Sit-to-stand

x 10 from bed
x 10 from bed
x 10 bed to chair

Feet back
Shoulders forward
Weight on both legs

(a)   (b)

FIGURE 1.9   *Two other stations. Left: heels raise and lower with back against the wall. Right: modified squats against the wall.*

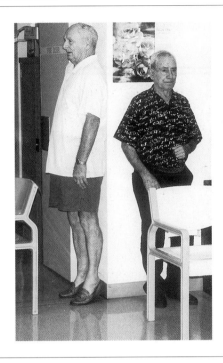

FIGURE 1.10   *Participant's husband supervises practice at stairwalking station.*

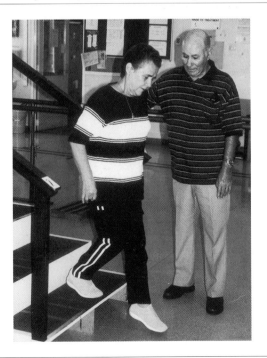

FIGURE 1.11 *The form for data collection. (Courtesy of F Mackey, Physiotherapy Department.)*

Lower Limb Circuit Class – Assessment

Date	MRN

1. Diagnosis	
2. Date of incident	1st CVA Y N
3. Medications	
4. Relevant medical history/precautions	
5. Date of birth	
6. Sex	
7. Nationality	Interpreter required Y N
8. Address/postcode	
9. General practitioner	
10. 10 m walk (with aid)	(no aid)
11. Timed Up and Go test	
12. 10 steps – up	
– down	
13. 6 minute walk	
14. Step test (L)	(R)
Signed	
Print name	

Lower Limb Circuit Class – Reassessment

Date	No. of sessions

1. 10 m walk (with aid)	(no aid)
2. Timed Up and Go test	
3. 10 steps – up	
– down	
4. 6 minute walk	
5. Step test (L)	(R)
6 month follow-up	12 month follow-up
Signed	
Print name	

FIGURE 1.12 *Explanatory six page booklet. Read from left to right, top then bottom. (Courtesy of F Mackey, Physiotherapy Department.)*

What is the Lower Circuit Class?

This is an exercise class which aims to
  a) improve your ability to stand-up, balance and walk
  b) improve your ability to walk up and down stairs and
  c) improve your fitness and your ability to walk long distances

What will I do?

- a warm-up where you will walk at a comfortable pace for 5 to 6 minutes.
- stretches for your calf muscles.
- a series of 8 workstations or exercises. You will exercise at 1 workstation for 3 to 5 minutes then move onto the next workstation until you have completed all 8 workstations.

- and lastly, walking inside or walking outside or on slopes, stairs and grass

When does the class run?

The class is run on a Monday and Thursday at 9.00 am for six weeks

How many people will be in the class?

There will be somewhere between 4 to 8 participants in each class with 2 staff members to supervise the group.

Do I exercise on my own?

Yes. The 2 therapy staff will advise you what to do and there will be diagrams advising you what to do at each station, then you will spend time at each workstation exercising with as well as without the therapist. We feel this semi-supervised practice is vital to help you learn how to keep practicing at home.

Can my partner attend with me?

Yes. We welcome any person who is interested in attending to assist you in completing each station. This may also help you when you are practicing at home. There may be some occasions when we will practice without partners present.

Will I be disadvantaged if my partner cannot attend?

No. We will endeavour to ensure that you understand what to do at each workstation and that you are able to practice safely at home.

What should I wear?

You will need to wear comfortable clothing and shoes. We usually recommend shorts or trackpants, a T-shirt, walking shoes and a warm top for occasions when we are outside.

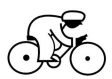

Can the hospital provide me with transport?

The hospital is able to provide a limited number of people transport on our bus. On most occasions we will endeavour to find alternative transport where possible.

Will I need to practice at home?

Yes. To maximize your recovery you will need to practice at home. The therapist will discuss with you what exercises you are safe to continue with at home. It is important to continue the exercises you have been given for home even when the class has finished.

Are interpreters for available?

Yes. Interpreters are available for people from most non-English speaking backgrounds.

Physiotherapy Requirements

1. You are expected to arrive for appointments on time.
2. If you are having difficulties arriving for your appointment on time, or are unable to attend, please notify the Physiotherapy Department. (Telephone 42238211) Failure to attend on 2 occasions will lead to automatic discharge and your referring doctor will be notified.

Should you have any problems with any part of your program, please discuss this with the therapist.

2 Training guidelines

SECTION CONTENTS

2	**Balance**	**35**
3	**Walking**	**76**
4	**Standing up and sitting down**	**129**
5	**Reaching and manipulation**	**159**

2 | *Balance*

CHAPTER CONTENTS

- **Introduction**
- **Biomechanical description**
  Balancing during motor actions in standing
  Balancing during motor actions in sitting
  Balancing during body transport
- **Age-related changes**
- **Analysis of motor performance in sitting and standing**
  Research findings
  Observational analysis
- **Guidelines for training**
  Sitting balance
  Standing balance
  Soft tissue stretching
  Strength training
- **Measurement**
  Functional tests
  Biomechanical tests

INTRODUCTION

Balance dysfunction, particularly in standing, is a devastating sequel of stroke since the ability to balance the body mass over the base of support under different task and environmental conditions is one of the most critical motor control factors in daily life. Training balanced movement may be the most significant part of rehabilitation.

Balance involves the regulation of movement of linked body segments over supporting joints and base of support (MacKinnon and Winter 1993). It is the ability to balance the body mass relative to the base of support that enables us to perform everyday actions effectively and efficiently. Many of these actions involve the lower limbs supporting and moving the body mass over the feet in standing or in sitting during reaching and manipulative tasks, raising and lowering the body mass to stand up, or transporting the body from place to place as in walking. Sometimes we just stand still. However, even simple actions such as breathing and turning the head are characterized by oscillations in the line of gravity which are countered by muscle activity and small, barely detectable movements, usually at ankles and hips (Bouisset and Duchenne 1994, Vandervoort 1999). The ability to balance and maintain a stable posture is integral to the execution of motor skills and cannot be separated from the action being performed or the environment in which it is being carried out (Carr and Shepherd 1998). The regulation of the dynamic interactions between linked segments as they move one upon the other therefore plays an important role in balance control (Nashner and McCollum 1985, Yang et al. 1990).

The mechanical problem of remaining balanced as we move around is a particular challenge to the central nervous system (CNS). Ghez (1991) refers to a family of adjustments needed to maintain a posture and to move which has three goals:

- to support the body against gravity and other external forces
- to maintain the centre of body mass aligned and balanced over the base of support
- to stabilize parts of the body while moving other parts.

These postural adjustments to preserve or regain balance are brought about by muscle activations and movements of segments. They are the consequences both of internal mechanisms (e.g. muscle strength, visual, tactile, proprioceptive, vestibular sensory inputs) and of the environment in which action takes place (Slobounov and Newell 1993). In standing, the CNS functions to keep the centre of body mass (CBM) within the limits of stability, which is the perimeter of the base of support beyond which we cannot preserve balance without making a new base of support (e.g. taking a step) or falling. Whether or not we take a step appears to be governed not only by the position of the CBM relative to the base of support but also the horizontal velocity of the CBM as the body moves about over the base of support (Pai and Patton 1997). Our perceived limit of stability may differ if we anticipate or sense a threat to balance, misinterpret visual inputs or experience fear or apprehension.

The roles of sensory inputs are controversial but it is apparent that the inputs critical to the events unfolding are coordinated in an action- and environment-specific manner. Redundancy in the sensory system allows for compensation when one system is dysfunctional (Winter et al. 1990). Visual inputs, however, appear particularly important in balance control, providing information about where we are in relation to our surroundings and enabling us to predict upcoming perturbations. For example, vision enables us to judge when we will arrive at the kerb so we can time our stride for appropriate foot placement (Patla 1997). It assists us to orient ourselves vertically, and seems particularly critical with a small support base or a low level of skill (Slobounov and Newell 1993). Cutaneous inputs from the soles of the feet may be critical to our ability to balance in standing and for the control of stepping (Do et al. 1990). Paying attention to the relevant information is also important, particularly so when balance presents a challenge (Gentile 2000). If attention is divided between two tasks this may present a problem to an elderly person (Chen et al. 1996) and to someone with poor balance after a stroke. The ability to sustain attention to a task and avoid distraction appears to be related to the ability to balance after stroke (Stapleton et al. 2001).

As we go about our daily activities, the postural system must meet three principal challenges: maintain a steady posture, generate postural adjustments that anticipate goal-directed movements and are adaptive as movements unfold, and react swiftly and appropriately when we predict a threat to balance or when an unexpected event perturbs our balance. The functional actions we engage in during daily life make different ongoing mechanical and functional demands on the segmental linkage according to the position we are in (body alignment) and the requirements of the task. Reacting to externally imposed destabilizing forces (standing on a moving walkway, being pushed in a crowd) and transporting our body mass from one position to another (walking, standing up) make different demands. Hence the patterns of muscle activity and segmental movement (what joint movement occurs, what muscles act as prime movers or synergists) differ also. In other words, postural adjustments are both task and context specific, a finding which is replicated in many laboratory and clinical studies (Dietz et al. 1984, Horak and Nashner 1986, Do et al. 1990, Eng et al. 1992).

Throughout all the actions in which we are skilled we therefore preserve balance as part of that skill. We fall only when an unexpected event occurs and we fail to respond quickly enough when tripped up by an unseen or misjudged obstacle, or when we stretch ourselves to the limits of performance capability and 'over-balance'. The likelihood of falling increases in the weak or frail, or in the presence of an impairment affecting the neuromuscular or sensory systems, since under these conditions actions which are normally performed skilfully can no longer be performed effectively.

Major requirements for good balance are an accurate sense of being balanced, the ability of muscles, particularly of the lower limbs, to produce force rapidly and at the appropriate time, and muscles which are extensible, i.e. not stiff or short. The systems involved need to be adaptive, since balance control requires the ability to adapt our movements to changes occurring both internally and in our external environment.

The adjustments we make to preserve balance are flexible and varied. It is therefore clear that the terms 'equilibrium reactions', 'balance reactions' and 'postural reflexes', introduced into physiotherapy from the scientific literature half a century ago and still in use for the testing of balance and as a goal of therapy (de Weerdt and Spaepen 1999), do not account for balance control during skilled, purposeful movements. These terms, which reflect an older view that balance is essentially reflexive or reactive, can divert attention in physiotherapy away from the specificity of postural (balance) adjustments and the fact that they occur in anticipation of and during voluntary motor actions as well as in response to a perturbation. Patients need to acquire again considerable skill in preserving balance under conditions encountered in daily life, a large proportion of which involve intentional movement of the limbs and the body mass.

Regaining the ability to perform any functional action following a neural lesion is almost entirely a matter of learning to balance body segments over the base of support, yet intensive and varied balance training is not always the major priority in clinical practice that it should be. It is highly likely from the evidence so far that patients will only improve if they practise a range of actions under the conditions occurring in daily life and if they are challenged to extend the limits of their stability. From the research evidence so far, it is also critical that, when lower limb muscles are too weak to support the body mass and to regulate movements of the body mass, training also involves intensive muscle strengthening exercises for the lower limbs.

BIOMECHANICAL DESCRIPTION

Forces which disturb balance derive from the effects of gravity (gravitational forces) and from the interactions between segments which are generated as we move (reactive, interactive forces). Hence, gravitational and acceleration forces must be controlled for posture and equilibrium to be maintained. Below is a brief description of the principal findings from investigations of balance in standing and sitting, and during walking, standing up and sitting down.

Balancing during motor actions in standing

In quiet stance, small movements of the body mass occur, making up what is called postural sway. The extent and direction of sway is measured at the support surface by calculating the movement of forces under the feet, indicating the centre of pressure (COP). The amount of body sway in quiet stance is affected by such factors as foot position and the width of base of support (Kirby et al. 1987, Day et al. 1998, Gatev et al. 1999).

The measurement of postural sway gives no information about the movements occurring within the segmental linkage above the base of support (Kuo and Zajac 1993). Although postural sway is sometimes used as a measure of balance in clinical trials, it should be noted that the extent of postural sway is not a sufficient measure of functional postural stability (Horak 1997). Able-bodied individuals, including ballet dancers and athletes, may have a relatively large extent of sway (Horak 1987, Massion 1992), while highly skilled pistol shooters (Arutyunyan et al. 1969) have a minimal degree of sway as they prepare to pull the trigger.

Effects of task and environment on balance mechanisms

Studies of self-initiated movements of the arm performed in standing show that postural adjustments occur before the action as well as during the movement (Eng et al. 1992). These anticipatory or proactive postural adjustments (noted from electromyography, force plate and motion analysis) minimize the anticipated destabilization of the body caused by the action being performed (Zattara and Bouisset 1988). Anticipatory and ongoing postural adjustments ensure the body's centre of mass remains within the base of support. It is of particular note that in arm raising tasks the potentially destabilizing effects on the CBM caused by the arm flexing forward are counterbalanced by appropriate leg muscle action (Belenkii et al. 1967, Lee 1980, Cordo and Nashner 1982, Horak et al. 1984, Nardone and Schieppati 1988). These findings illustrate the interactive effects that occur in a segmental linkage.

Postural adjustments are an integral part of an action since they are highly specific to such factors as initial body position (Cordo and Nashner 1982), conditions of support (Nashner 1982), speed and amplitude of movement (Horak et al. 1984, Aruin and Latash 1996). The experiments illustrated in Figure 2.1 clarify the specificity of muscle activity and illustrate the potent effects of external support. Subjects interacted with a handle in four different ways (Nashner

FIGURE 2.1

Task- and context-specific coordination of arm (biceps brachii) and leg (gastrocnemius) muscles with different tasks performed in standing with subject holding a handle. (A) Subject pulls on handle. (B) Unexpected movement of the handle away from the subject, with chest support. (C) As in B but subject free standing. (D) Unexpected platform movement forward. (Adapted from Nashner 1983, with permission.)

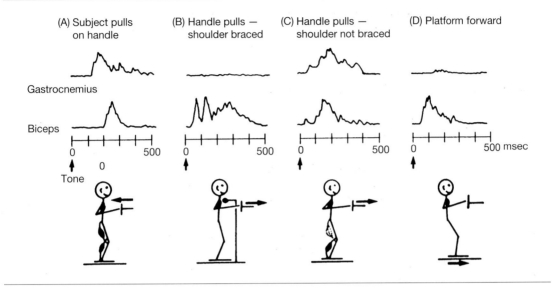

1982): (A) Unsupported in standing, the subject pulled on the handle. This challenge to balance resulted in activation of a postural leg muscle (gastrocnemius) prior to the pull and before the activation of the arm muscle (biceps brachii). (B) With support provided at chest height, when the handle was unexpectedly pulled away from the subject, minimal leg muscle activity occurred since maintaining a balanced position actively was not necessary. (C) When this support was removed, however, calf muscle activity was again evident.

It is not always lower limb muscles that play a balance preservation role in standing. When subjects held the fixed and stable handle and the support surface was unexpectedly moved forward (D), the arm muscle turned on before a small contraction of the leg muscle. That is, arm muscle activation was crucial in preventing balance from being lost since the hand was grasping the only object that provided stability. It was noted that the amplitude of leg muscle activity was also markedly reduced when subjects touched a rail with one finger. A similar result was reported in the study of rising on toes (Nardone and Schieppati 1988), with a reduction in leg muscle activity when subjects held on to two handles.

A group of actions has been studied in which the body mass is shifted in order to free one leg from support. From the evidence, these actions appear to share similar biomechanical characteristics. They all involve raising one leg in standing and include studies of single leg raising (Rogers and Pai 1990), gait initiation (Kirker et al. 2000) and lifting one foot on to a step (Mercer and Sahrmann 1999). In these actions, the CBM is displaced laterally over the stance limb, allowing the other foot to be lifted. This frontal plane movement is itself complex. The data show that the centre of foot pressure is shifted toward the leg to be raised milliseconds before the CBM is shifted toward the single support leg (Fig. 2.2a). This shows that weight is shifted to the support limb partly by muscle activity of the opposite leg (Fig. 2.2b). The point to be noted is that both lower limbs are involved in any shift of body mass in a lateral direction (Jenner et al. 1997, Holt et al. 2000). This action requires both propulsive force to move the body mass sideways and braking force to ensure it does not move beyond the limit of stability (Rogers et al. 1993). Postural adjustments involved in lateral movements of the body mass occur principally at shank–foot (invertors, evertors) and thigh–pelvis (abductors, adductors) linkages (Winter 1995). Figure 2.2b illustrates the action of hip abductor and adductor muscles in stepping with the left leg (Kirker et al. 2000).

Muscle activation plays balance as well as primary movement generation roles. Such is the task- and context-specific nature of movement control, these roles merge into one another when movement is well controlled. Another group of studies investigating functional tasks performed in standing demonstrate the complexity of this control. Studies of forward and backward trunk bending (Thorstensson et al. 1985, Crenna et al. 1987), rising on to toes (Lipshits et al.

| FIGURE 2.2 | *(a) Subject standing on force-plate, raises R leg sideways. The centre of pressure (COP) first moves toward the R (upper peak) in order to move the centre of gravity (COG) to the L over the supporting leg. The COP then moves to the L (lower peak) under the supporting foot. Note that when the COP completes its movement to the L (at T_2), the ankle is raised sideways. (Adapted from Lee et al. 1995, with permission.) (b) Averaged EMG for an able-bodied subject stepping with the L leg for gait initiation. Before stepping with the L leg, weight is moved to the R by L GM and R ADD. As weight is transferred to the R leg, R GM and L ADD activity peaks (ADD, adductor; GM, gluteus medius). (Adapted from Kirker et al. 2000, with permission.)* |

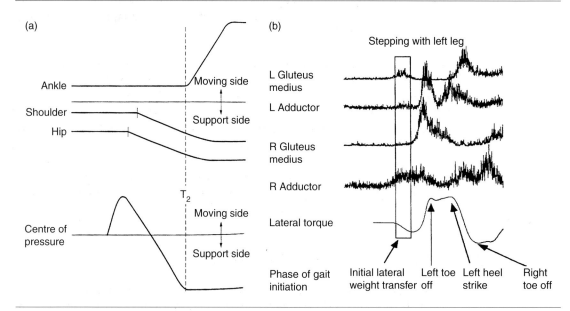

1981, Nardone and Schieppati 1988) and bending down to pick up boxes of different weights (Commissaris et al. 2001) found anticipatory postural adjustments which served to reposition and stabilize the CBM prior to the primary action and were clearly part of the action itself.

Investigations of rising on to toes in standing (Lipshits et al. 1981, Nardone and Schieppati 1988) have shown preparatory activation of tibialis anterior prior to the heel raise associated with forward displacement of the body mass, followed by soleus, gastrocnemius and quadriceps contraction. Contraction of calf muscles raises the heel. Contraction of quadriceps counteracts the flexing force applied at the knee by the two-joint gastrocnemius, and maintains the knee in extension. These studies illustrate the complexity of synergistic muscle activations in what appears to be a rather simple action.

When subjects flex their lower limbs to lift a box from the floor, examination of anteroposterior ground reaction forces (GRFs) has shown that anticipatory adjustments occurring prior to the lift were adjusted to take account of the weight to be lifted and to optimize the lifting phase (Commissaris et al. 2001). Findings such as these show how the different constraints imposed by task and context are adjusted for by the motor control system and point out the need to include a variety of actions with differing constraints in training protocols.

Postural responses to unexpected perturbations

These have been studied principally in regard to support surface perturbations, an environmental condition increasingly encountered in modern life. Studies such as these, and others which have examined stumbling during walking, provide information about the mechanisms of reactive balance responses which form the emergency back-up system when our predictive mechanisms fail (Patla 1995, Huxham et al. 2001). Findings have demonstrated rapid responses to unexpected platform movement which were directionally specific and focused on distal musculature linking shank and foot. Even these rapid responses were adaptive to context.

Putting out one or both hands is a typical reaction to loss of balance. However, in standing, taking a step is used as a means of ensuring stability when we perceive a risk of falling (Maki and McIlroy 1997). This compensatory stepping appears to occur not only in response to loss of balance, but as a preferred strategy, even when perturbations are relatively small (Maki and McIlroy 1998). Stepping is initiated very rapidly, and inability to step accurately and quickly enough may be a major cause of loss of balance confidence and of falls in at-risk individuals. A recent study of older individuals reports that slow speed of stepping plus delayed gluteus medius muscle onset in the stance limb may predict the likelihood of falls (Brauer et al. 2000).

Balancing during motor actions in sitting

In sitting, the CBM is closer to the base of support which is relatively large compared to standing. Effective performance of actions such as reaching for an object involves not only the ability to maintain the seated position on seats of various dimensions, but also to balance the body mass over the lower limbs while performing a variety of actions in the frontal and sagittal planes, often at more than arm's length. The lower limbs play an important role in stabilizing the trunk and pelvis (Son et al. 1988). Although there has been relatively little investigation of sitting balance, it is clear that, as in standing, postural adjustments (balance mechanisms) are highly specific to task and environmental conditions.

The major role of the lower limbs in supporting and balancing the body mass in sitting is evident from experimental studies of reaching beyond arm's length, both at fast and slow speeds (Crosbie et al. 1995, Dean et al. 1999a,b). Lower limb muscles are involved in anticipatory, ongoing and reactive postural adjustments. Tibialis anterior is activated and ground reaction forces through the feet occur in advance of and during fast arm movement. Calf (soleus) and knee muscle activity (vastus lateralis, biceps femoris) brakes the forward movement of the body mass towards the end of a reach (Crosbie et al. 1995) (Fig. 2.3). The shank and thigh muscles play a less active role when reaching is self-paced and within arm's length (Dean et al. 1999a,b).

In general, trunk muscles act as postural stabilizers during movements in sitting that involve the upper limbs. However, when an action such as reaching involves moving beyond arm's length in order to transport the hand to the target, the trunk also plays a role in extending the distance that can be reached. That is, movement of the trunk by flexion and extension at the hips is an integral part of the reaching movement (Kaminski et al. 1995, Dean et al. 1999a,b). The distance we can reach is also affected by the extent of thigh support (Dean et al. 1999b).

Reaching sideways in the frontal plane would be expected to be more destabilizing than reaching forward in the sagittal plane since the perimeter of the base of support is reached earlier. However, no investigations of movements in this direction were found.

The upper body can move about much less when the feet are hanging free, such as over the side of the bed, compared to when they are on the floor; i.e. the limit of stability is reached much sooner with feet unsupported than with feet supported. Hence there is less possibility for vigorous action (e.g. reaching beyond arm's length) when the feet are unsupported (Chari and Kirby 1986). In this position, muscles linking thighs to the pelvis (e.g. iliopsoas, rectus femoris, gluteus maximus) would be critical. Whether or not the feet are on the floor, muscles linking pelvis and trunk (e.g. spinal flexors and extensors) ensure appropriate alignment and stability of the trunk and head during activities performed in sitting.

Balancing during body transport

Walking

Variations in task and environmental context affect balance mechanisms during gait. For example, balance is more challenged when walking in a dark

| FIGURE 2.3 | *Fast reaching to a target with the R arm. Trial from one subject showing typical EMG traces from ipsilateral vastus lateralis (VL), biceps femoris (BF), tibialis anterior (TA), soleus (Sol) and anterior deltoid (AD) in a forward reach.* |

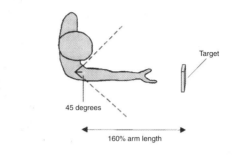

Target

45 degrees

160% arm length

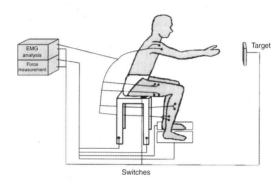

EMG analysis

Force measurement

Target

Switches

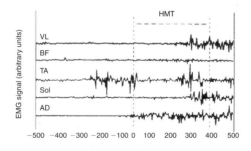

HMT

VL

BF

TA

Sol

AD

EMG signal (arbitrary units)

−500 −400 −300 −200 −100 0 100 200 300 400 500

room or crossing a street (Huxham et al. 2001); balance has to be preserved when walking on sand, on ice, and on a moving surface. Vision plays a particularly critical role in providing inputs about environmental features, including changes occurring within the environment which are essential to the formulation of predictive adjustments and avoidance strategies.

Given the specificity of postural adjustments, it is not surprising that control of balance while walking differs from control of balance in standing. Although in standing the goal is to maintain the centre of gravity (COG) within the base of support, walking is essentially controlled instability. The COG moves forward along the medial borders of each foot, oscillating less than 2 cm to either side, resulting in the body being in a constant state of 'imbalance' throughout single support (MacKinnon and Winter 1993) (Fig. 3.1). Stance in double support phase is not particularly stable since neither foot is flat on the ground (Winter et al. 1990). It is evident that control of foot position after foot placement is critical for stability (MacKinnon and Winter 1993).

The regulation of dynamic balance of the upper body during stance and the safe transit of the foot during swing phase (toe clearance and foot landing) present a particular challenge to the CNS. The large upper body mass (head, arms, trunk) consists of two-thirds of the total body mass and the CBM is located about two-thirds of body height above ground level. Walking therefore requires complex control of the movement of the total body mass over the supporting feet. Balance is particularly challenged in stepping over obstacles, since the clearance of both lead and trail limbs has to be greater than in unimpaired walking.

Since the base of support during single support phase is narrow, frontal plane balance in particular requires precise control (MacKinnon and Winter 1993). Balance of the upper body over the weightbearing hip appears to depend largely on control of the pelvic segment at the hips, particularly by abductor movements at the hip acting on the pelvis (MacKinnon and Winter 1993), and also requires coordination between pelvis and trunk. In the sagittal plane, tight coupling between hip flexors and extensors and knee muscles during single and double support help balance the upper body over the lower limbs. As well as the requirements of balance, the lower limbs must also be able to support the body weight. Therefore, due to the effects of gravity, there is always net extensor activity in supporting limbs in order to prevent collapse, even when one or two joints are flexing (Winter 1995).

Loss of balance may occur due to such factors as stumbling, tripping or slipping while taking a step, staggering while turning (Tinetti et al. 1986), and when increasing speed. Precise control of the swinging foot, with toe clearance of around 1–2 cm, plus control of all the segments involved in the stance and swing of legs ensures we seldom trip. The process of turning consists of decelerating forward motion, rotating the body (either by spinning on one foot or taking a step) and striding out into a new direction, movements which can cause staggering if balance is not controlled (Hase and Stein 1999).

Standing up (STS) and sitting down

In STS, the control of linear momentum of the body mass, particularly in a horizontal direction, plays a critical role in dynamic stability and requires complex interactions between accelerating and decelerating muscle activations. There is evidence that healthy elderly individuals may decrease the speed of standing up in order to decrease the demands made by momentum on weak muscles and on balance control. Important muscle groups for controlling horizontal momentum of the body mass include quadriceps and in particular gastrocnemius–soleus since their activity on the shank has a braking effect on forward movement (Crosbie et al. 1995, Scarborough et al. 1999).

Falls due to loss of balance are reported to be common in elderly individuals during standing up and sitting down (Tinetti et al. 1988), actions which require complex coordination of body segments to transport the body mass from over one base of support to another while preserving balance. Patients with weakness of lower limb extensor muscles and dysfunctional motor control experience difficulties with balance throughout STS, for example, controlling both horizontal momentum of the body mass prior to thighs-off and while sitting down.

In conclusion, it is clear from the scientific evidence so far that postural adjustments are specific to task (reaching for an object, walking across the room, standing up), and context (body position, environmental features). Even rather small changes in task and conditions can produce marked changes in patterns of muscle activity (Mercer and Sahrmann 1999). This specificity underlies the apparent lack of transferability from balance training in one task to performance of another, mechanically different task. For example, training to improve lateral weight shift in standing does not necessarily transfer into improved ability to walk (Winstein et al. 1989).

Stroke results in impairments which affect the force-generating capacity of muscles, the control of movement and therefore the performance of a range of different actions. From the scientific research so far we can assume that an acceptable degree of skill will only be regained by functionally specific strengthening exercise for the lower limbs and motor training of actions in their usual environments. The ability to balance is trained as an integral part of each action and it is the practice of balancing the body mass throughout performance of the action that enables the individual to optimize performance and regain skill.

AGE-RELATED CHANGES

The effect of the ageing process upon balance is complex and unclear. The results of studies of elderly people can be confusing if they include individuals with CNS and/or musculoskeletal problems. Elderly individuals are at greater risk of falling and it can be assumed that balance deficiencies are a significant cause. Postural instability in the elderly and a tendency to fall is associated with reduced vision, including loss of sensitivity in peripheral visual field, reduced peripheral sensation, vestibular dysfunction and slowing of muscle reaction time (Stelmach and Worringham 1985, Woollacott et al. 1988, Lord et al. 1991), the latter reported for both tibialis anterior (Woollacott et al. 1986) and gluteus medius (Brauer et al. 2000). Woollacott and colleagues (1988) reported increased co-contraction to stiffen lower limb joints in older compared to younger adults which may be an adaptation to deficiencies in balance. In addition, elderly individuals are at risk of developing pathologies which accelerate degeneration in neuromusculoskeletal systems (Horak et al. 1989).

Postural stability is constrained by biomechanical factors associated with decreased musculoskeletal flexibility and muscle strength. Leg muscle strength has been reported to decrease by 40% and arm strength by 30% from 30 to 80 years of age (Asmussen 1980). At ages higher than 70 years, muscle atrophy appears to accelerate (Danneskiold-Samsoe et al. 1984). Such declines in strength impact negatively on balance in standing and during walking, stair climbing and standing up. Risk factors for falling most commonly identified are loss of muscle strength and flexibility (Gehlsen and Whaley 1990), particularly loss of quadriceps strength (Scarborough et al. 1999). An association has been found between a history of falls and weakness of ankle dorsiflexors and plantarflexors (Whipple et al. 1987), which may illustrate the critical role of muscles that link the shank segment to the base of support, i.e. the foot. Individuals with a history of falls have shown significantly decreased ability to maintain one leg stance with and without eyes open (Johansson and Jarnlo 1991), and significantly weaker lower limb extensor muscles compared to non-fallers (Gehlsen and Whaley 1990, Scarborough et al. 1999).

Limited ankle joint mobility may provoke tripping and falling. Decreased mobility may be due to increased passive resistance of the elastic component in soft tissues (Vandervoort 1999) and muscle shortening (Mecagni et al. 2000). A study of elderly individuals found loss of ankle mobility, particularly evident in women, associated with stiffer connective tissue and reduced strength of dorsi- and plantarflexors (Vandervoort et al. 1992). Stretching and exercise programmes have shown beneficial effects on ankle flexibility, with increases in strength and decreases in stiffness (Vandervoort 1999).

Increased amplitude of body sway in quiet standing in older adults has been commonly reported but the functional relevance of this is unclear. Tests of sway in standing are not a direct measure of functional postural stability (Horak 1997). However, the results of one study of postural sway suggest that elderly individuals may have difficulty preserving balance in standing when they turn their head (Fig. 2.4) (Koceja et al. 1999). Very elderly individuals hospitalized for various reasons and who had poor balance in standing were reported to

FIGURE 2.4   *Postural sway (mean sway in a sagittal direction) in quiet standing and during a volitional head turn with eyes open in a group of elderly compared to young individuals. (Adapted from Koceja et al. 1999, with permission.)*

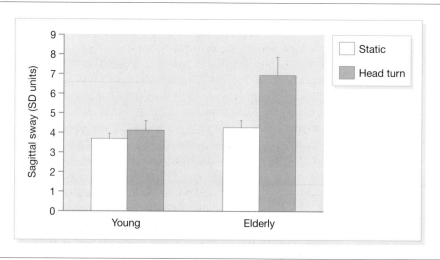

consistently lose their balance in a posterior direction (Bohannon 1999). This is a common observation in elderly people after a period of bedrest and seems to reflect a perceptual bias away from the erect position which may be provoked by the supine position. Older people seem also to have difficulty controlling lateral stability, noticeable during stepping to regain balance, which is a particular risk in the elderly as it is associated with hip fracture (Maki and McIlroy 1997, 1998).

There is evidence that a programme of lower limb strengthening exercises can have a positive effect in the elderly on muscle strength, balance and gait (Fiatarone et al. 1990, 1994, Johansson and Jarnlo 1991, Lord and Castell 1994, Means et al. 1996, Campbell et al. 1997, Krebs et al. 1998, Hortobagyi et al. 2001). There is also evidence that a strength and balance exercise programme can improve other motor functions involving balance and result in a reduction of falls in the very elderly (Shumway-Cook et al. 1997). One study of women (Campbell et al. 1997), that consisted of open chain (with ankle cuff weights) lower limb strengthening exercises plus balance exercises, showed that at 6 months the women had significantly improved their balance and their ability to stand up compared to the control group. The exercises were done for 30 minutes, at least three times a week, and the programme included practice of tandem standing and walking, walking on toes and heels, walking backward, sideways and turning around, stepping over an object, bending to pick up an object, stair climbing and knee squats. After 1 year the exercise group had a lower rate of falls than the control group, 42% of them were still doing the exercise programme more than three times a week, whereas the control group had become less active and their fear of falling had increased.

Frequent, intensive, stimulating and enjoyable strength and balance training classes may help elderly stroke patients develop confidence and an understanding of the need to keep active. From the evidence so far, it seems clear that exercise programmes need to go on for several weeks and that individuals will need to continue exercising in order to maintain the gains achieved (Vandervoort 1999).

Other exercise programmes emphasizing sensory function (Telian et al. 1990, Ledin et al. 1991, Hu and Woollacott 1994) have been successful in improving aspects of balance such as the ability to stand on one leg. Tai Chi Chuan training, which emphasizes control over large movements of the CBM, has also been found to have positive effects on functional balance, decreasing fear of falling and frequency of falling (Tse and Bailey 1991, Wolf et al. 1997, Wong et al. 2001). This training combines slow and gentle movements which flow into each other, and includes stepping from one leg to the other with slow and deliberate foot placement (Kirsteins et al. 1991).

It is evident from the research available that the consequences of physical inactivity can be very serious in elderly individuals, with sequelae that include loss of strength, stability, cardiovascular fitness and joint flexibility. A major challenge for those responsible for physiotherapy after stroke is to ensure that disuse effects do not compound the functional problems resulting from an individual's stroke. Many people who have a stroke, and it is highly probable that this applies to frail elderly women in particular, may have, before their stroke, developed musculoskeletal disuse effects, poor balance, loss of self-confidence and fear of falling (Tinetti et al. 1994).

ANALYSIS OF MOTOR PERFORMANCE IN SITTING AND STANDING

The sensory and motor impairments after stroke which impact upon balance may include muscle weakness, decreased soft tissue flexibility, impaired motor control and sensory impairments. The functional results of the motor control impairments are loss of coordination, loss of an accurate sense of being balanced, and therefore an increased risk of falling. In addition to abnormalities of balance, posture (the ability to take up and maintain a specific segmental relationship) may also be affected in some individuals. Difficulty achieving and sustaining an appropriate posture (segmental alignment) may be noticeable in the patient's initial attempts to get into and maintain the sitting or standing position and in those individuals with an impaired sense of their body position in relation to the vertical.

Reduced muscle function, in the lower limbs in particular, affects the ability to support, shift and balance the body mass. However, it is not only the inability to generate appropriate force but also difficulty initiating, timing and sequencing muscle forces, sustaining force, and generating force fast enough which affect the ability to balance (di Fabio 1997). These elements of dysfunction affect anticipatory as well as ongoing postural muscle activity, with muscles activated later than in the able-bodied (Viallet et al. 1992, Diener et al. 1993). Delay in initiating muscle activity and slowness to build up force affect both the preparation for an impending disturbance to stability and the speed of response to loss of balance. Consider, for example, the destabilizing effects of raising the arm in standing if preparatory muscle activity and joint movement do not take place prior to the destabilization. A particular difficulty for many patients is a decreased capacity to take a step when in danger of falling in standing or in walking.

Secondary muscle adaptations, such as length and stiffness changes, also have a significant impact on muscle activation and balance. Decreased soft tissue elasticity and muscle shortening limiting ankle joint mobility may have a particularly strong effect following stroke as they do in the elderly (Vandervoort 1999). Sensory system and perceptuo-cognitive dysfunction also impact negatively on balance in sitting and standing, particularly in the early stage after stroke, and may include disordered somatosensory, labyrinthine, visual function and perceptuo-cognitive deficits such as unilateral spatial neglect. One cause of difficulty in stepping out for older individuals is loss of cutaneous sensation from the plantar surface of the foot.

Falling has been reported as a frequent occurrence in individuals following stroke and after their discharge from hospital, particularly those who are

60 years of age or over. One study reported that 73% of the 108 individuals studied had a fall in the 6 months following discharge. Of the 108 individuals, 21% reported having fallen prior to their stroke. Most falls occurred while performing everyday activities such as walking, standing up and extreme reaching, activities which in particular challenge an unbalanced system. Most individuals had difficulty getting up from the floor when they fell, including those who had been trained by a physiotherapist in how to do so. Individuals who had fallen at least twice were depressed and less active socially (Forster and Young 1995).

Research findings

Some biomechanical analyses of balance dysfunction in standing following stroke have focused on laboratory investigations of responses to unexpected perturbations, such as support surface movements or lateral pushes. Studies of support surface movement have shown abnormal coordination of postural responses (Horak et al. 1984, di Fabio and Badke 1990, di Fabio 1997), with latency of postural muscle response favouring the non-paretic limb, reductions in magnitude of response, including absence of any response from some muscles, and agonist–antagonist coordination deficits.

Studies of the ability of stroke patients to withstand a force applied laterally to the hip region to either side have demonstrated slowness in muscle activation, difficulty with sustaining muscle force to resist displacement and also in coping with the release of the applied force (Lee et al. 1988, Wing et al. 1993, Holt et al. 2000, Kirker et al. 2000). These studies demonstrate ways in which individuals adapt to severe muscle weakness by using stronger muscles. For example, during sideways pushes in standing, activity in adductor muscles of the stronger leg increased to compensate for diminished and delayed recruitment of hemiparetic abductor muscles (Jenner et al. 1997).

Force platform studies of postural sway during quiet standing following stroke have demonstrated both increased and decreased sway (Mizrahi et al. 1989). The relevance of such results is not clear. Measures of postural sway are not necessarily correlated with tendency to fall or with an individual's perception of stability (Horak 1997), postural sway is poorly related to dynamic actions such as walking (Gill-Body and Krebs 1994, Colle 1995), and limiting body sway does not necessarily lead to improved stability.

In outcome studies of individuals with brain lesion, no relationship has been found between decreased postural sway and functional scores or scores on other balance tests (Fishman et al. 1997). Holding the body stiffly is a commonly observed adaptation to poor balance and fear of falling after a brain lesion (Carr and Shepherd 1998), and, therefore, elderly individuals and those with neurological impairments who have minimal postural sway may not be stable and are likely to fall. As several authors have pointed out (Horak 1997), immobility (i.e. decreased sway) should not be confused with stability. In clinical interventions, the focus should not be on postural sway but on regaining the ability to move freely without losing balance.

Force platform investigations of weightbearing characteristics confirm the clinical observation that less weight is taken through the affected lower limb in standing and that there may be minimal movement towards that leg (Dickstein et al. 1984, Goldie et al. 1996a). Studies of the ability of patients to deliberately redistribute their weight in different directions have shown a restriction in the excursion of the COP laterally in both directions, backward and forward, with extraneous balance activity biased toward the non-paretic lower limb (Dettman et al. 1987, di Fabio and Badke 1990, Goldie et al. 1996b, Turnbull et al. 1996).

Difficulty shifting weight from one leg to another is particularly evident in studies of taking a step or raising one leg. The findings typically show a reduced and inappropriate displacement of the body weight to *both* sides, whether moving at average or fast speeds (Rogers et al. 1993, Pai et al. 1994, Laufer et al. 2000). For example, in making fast single leg raises, a delay in initiating ground reaction force changes under the paretic limb was evident with a reduction in the proportion of actively generated horizontal force for propelling the body mass laterally (Rogers et al. 1993). Studies of obstacle crossing show the difficulties patients have with balancing on one leg while stepping over an obstacle (Said et al. 1999).

Difficulty balancing in sitting has been shown to be associated with poor functional outcome after stroke (Loewen and Anderson 1990, Sandin and Smith 1990). A study of individuals more than 1 year post-stroke has illustrated that the inability to use the affected lower limb for balancing limits the distance which can be reached and the speed of the reaching movement (Dean and Shepherd 1997). Figure 2.5 illustrates the changes that took place in vertical ground reaction forces after a period of training.

Conclusion

Following stroke, patients with muscle weakness and poor control lack effective anticipatory, ongoing and reactive postural adjustments and therefore experience difficulty performing actions which involve:

- supporting the body mass over the paretic lower limb
- voluntarily moving the body mass from one lower limb to the other and one position to another
- responding rapidly to predicted and unpredicted threats to balance.

As a result, in actions carried out in sitting and standing, and others including walking, standing up and sitting down, the patient favours the stronger, better coordinated and more rapidly responsive leg, and the ability to carry out even simple tasks is seriously limited. Additional factors that are likely to impact on stability include abnormal perception of verticality and other disorders of visuospatial perception (Dieterich and Brandt 1992) and somatosensory perception (Niam et al. 1999).

Observational analysis

There is a clear distinction between measurement, i.e. the collection of objective data, and observational assessment which is non-standardized and subjective.

FIGURE 2.5   *Patterns of vertical ground reaction forces (GFR) (% body weight) of one stroke subject, reaching in three different directions, pre- and post-training. Heavy line, paretic leg; light line, non-paretic leg. Lower trace shows a healthy elderly subject reaching with the R hand for comparison. Heavy line, L leg; light line, R leg. Dotted vertical lines indicate onset and end of hand movement. (Reproduced from Dean and Shepherd 1997, with permission.)*

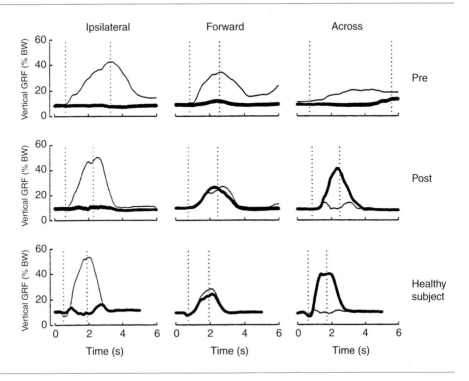

Although it is not at present possible for biomechanical tests to be performed in most clinics, there are many reliable and valid tests which give objective and functionally relevant data about progress and outcome. Using these tests, each patient is measured at the start of intervention, at intervals during rehabilitation, before discharge and at follow-up some time after discharge, in order to obtain data about progress and final outcome.

Therapists must rely on visual observation for ongoing analysis and as a guide to intervention. However, observational analysis has some major drawbacks. For example, the validity of the observations and subsequent analysis are dependent on the clinician's knowledge of normative biomechanics and skill in interpretation. In addition, although such kinematic characteristics as segmental alignment are observable, critical kinetic characteristics, such as ground reaction forces and muscle forces, are not.

Biomechanical research is providing an increasingly large body of knowledge about balance mechanisms, the findings of which assist the clinician in making informed observations as the patient attempts to carry out tasks which range from simple to complex depending on the patient's abilities. From these observations, a skilled observer can make inferences about the effects of lower limb muscle weakness, reduction in speed of muscle response, and lack of extensibility of soft tissues on posture and movement under specific conditions.

The taxonomy proposed by Gentile (1987) also assists the therapist's evaluation. It provides a clear picture of the varied conditions in which balance is required (see Huxham et al. 2001), reflects the environmental contexts in which we perform daily actions, and makes clear the inseparability of balance and movement in a gravitational environment. A person's movements need to conform to the specific environmental features (the context) (Fig. 2.6) if they are to be successful in achieving the goal (Magill 1998).

Given the variability of postural adjustments according to task and context, it is not possible to provide detailed and critical biomechanical features of postural adjustments in isolation from the tasks themselves. Balance control involves bilateral interlimb and limb–upperbody–head coordination, with head position being relevant to visual and vestibular inputs. In the clinic, the directly observable characteristics indicative of balance in sitting and standing are the relative alignment of body segments and such spatiotemporal adaptations as speed of movement, step length, and width of base of support. It is possible, therefore, to identify the inability of an individual to sustain the necessary *body alignment* for stability and the *spatiotemporal adaptations* which are invariably

FIGURE 2.6	*Reaching to pick up a glass involves limb and upper body movement including postural adjustments that are specific to the shape of the object, its position and what is to be done with it.*

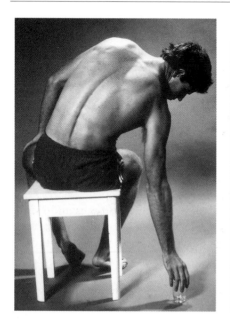
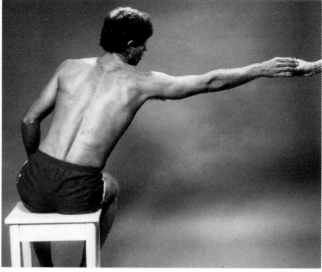

made in response to fear of losing balance. These are clearly observable and form the basis of the therapist's analysis during training as the patient attempts various tasks.

Body alignment

Inability to take up and maintain a specific segmental alignment (posture) in sitting or standing may be evident when the person first attempts to sit or stand. Normally when we are about to carry out an action we make certain preparations to ensure effective performance. For example, we move to a position of postural (segmental) alignment that is more suited to the action, particularly to the organization of supporting balance activity (Magill 1998). This postural alignment is one which favours the necessary muscle activity and feels comfortable. When training patients, it is not 'sitting up or standing up straight' that is important, but the taking up of a position which optimizes performance and maximizes success. Body alignment appropriate to quiet standing and sitting is outlined in Box 2.1.

Box 2.1 Body alignment appropriate to quiet standing and sitting

Standing alignment	Sitting alignment
Head balanced on level shoulders	Head balanced on level shoulders
Upper body erect, shoulders over hips	Upper body erect
Hips in front of ankles	Shoulders over hips
Feet a few cm (10 cm) apart	Feet and knees a few cm apart

Spatiotemporal adaptations

These include:

- *Changing the base of support*
  - wide base of support (legs/feet apart, externally rotated)
  - shuffling feet with inappropriate stepping
  - shifting on to stronger leg (Fig. 2.7a,b).
- *Restricting movement of body mass*
  - stiffening the body with altered segmental alignment (Fig 2.7a)
  - moving slowly
  - changing segmental alignment to avoid large shifts in COG
    standing reaching forward – flexing at hips instead of dorsiflexing ankles (Fig. 2.7c)
    standing reaching sideways – flexing trunk sideways instead of moving body laterally at hips and feet (Fig. 2.7a,b)
    sitting reaching sideways – flexing forward instead of to the side (see Fig. 2.9a)
    in standing – not taking a step when necessary.
- *Using hands for support*
  - holding on to support
  - grabbing.

FIGURE 2.7   *Adaptations made to avoid supporting and balancing body mass over the paretic lower limb. (a,b) It is possible to reach sideways beyond arm's length by lateral movement of the spine and increased shoulder girdle protraction. (c) In reaching forward, reach distance can be increased by flexion at the hips and protraction of the shoulder girdle. In both directions, however, the distance to be reached is limited.*

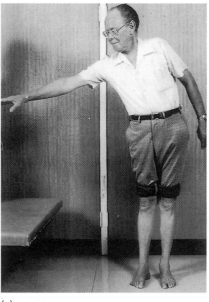
(a)

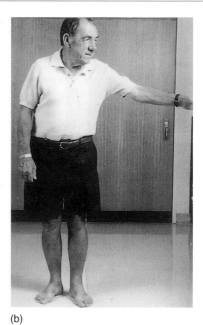
(b)

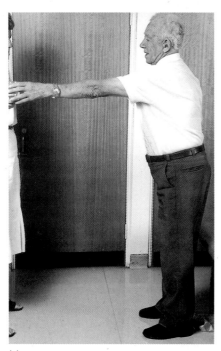
(c)

GUIDELINES FOR TRAINING

Balance cannot be trained in isolation from the actions which must be relearned. In training walking, standing up and sitting down, reaching and manipulation, postural adjustments are also trained, since acquiring skill involves in large part the fine tuning of postural and balance control. Postural adjustments are specific to each action and the conditions under which it occurs. It cannot be assumed that practice of one action will transfer automatically into improved performance in another. For example, balancing exercises in sitting on an inflated ball, advocated in some texts, focus on trunk and hip flexor muscles since the feet are not on the floor. Transfer into improved sitting balance under different conditions and for different tasks cannot be inferred. Exercises on a ball are difficult and strenuous, and, since the patient may require considerable physical support from the therapist, there may actually be little training effect.

Emphasis in the guidelines below is on performing tasks which require voluntary movements of the body mass in sitting and standing. The availability of harness support makes it possible for people to practise simple balancing tasks in standing very early after stroke. It should be noted that an overhead harness does not appear to interfere with responses to loss of balance according to a test of able-bodied subjects (Hill et al. 1994). Progressive complexity is added by increasing the difficulty under which goals must be achieved, keeping in mind the various complex situations in which the patients will find themselves in the environment in which they live, both inside and outside their homes, and the precarious nature of balance. As control over balance and confidence improves, tasks are introduced which require a stepping response, and responses to external constraints such as catching a thrown object and standing on a moving support surface (e.g. moving footway).

The conditions under which balance control is necessary in daily life can be broadly categorized as occurring:

- during performance of a self-initiated action
- when predicting destabilization and taking avoiding action
- when making a reactive response as a last resort in an attempt to avoid a fall.

The above categorization is a simplification. However, it provides a framework for the development of training protocols, with balance trained as an integral part of actions in the above categories. Practice is designed to enable the individual to learn again, with a disordered system, how to control movements of the body mass over the base of support and learn the 'rules' of preserving stability as part of acquiring skill.

Intervention aims to optimize balance by training:

- balance of the body mass during voluntary actions in sitting, standing and during body transport
- quick responses to predicted and unpredicted destabilization.

For training to be effective given the impairments and adaptations following stroke, it is also necessary to:

- prevent adaptive shortening of lower limb soft tissues
- increase lower limb extensor muscle strength and coordination (for support of body mass).

Sitting balance

The ability to balance in sitting while reaching for objects both within and beyond arm's length is critical to independent living. In the acute stage post-stroke, major goals are to prevent medical complications associated with the supine position and bed rest and to train balance in sitting. Re-establishing sitting balance early is critical since it impacts positively on many functions. It provides greater stimulus for gaseous interchange and facilitates coughing, enables more effective swallowing, encourages eye contact and focusing attention, communication and more positive attitudes, stimulates arousal mechanisms, and discourages learned 'sick role' behaviour. In contrast, mobility exercises performed in supine, such as rolling and bridging, are often given excessive emphasis in early rehabilitation, taking up time which should be spent with the patient upright and active.

The first exercises may be useful for patients who, early post-stroke, are frightened of moving. The exercises take attention away from the need to balance by focusing the patient's efforts on achieving a concrete goal. Practising simple actions that involve small shifts of the body mass initially enables patients to regain a sense of balance and confidence that they can move independently. Actions are practised repetitively with no pause.

Head and trunk movements

Sitting on a firm surface, hands in lap, feet and knees approximately 15 cm apart, feet on floor.

(i) Turning head and trunk to look over the shoulder, returning to mid position and repeating to other side.

Check
- Ensure patient rotates the trunk and head, with trunk erect, and remains flexed at the hips.
- Provide visual targets, increasing the distance to be turned.
- Stabilize the affected foot and prevent external rotation and abduction at the hip if necessary.
- Ensure hands are not used for support and that feet do not move.

(ii) Looking up at the ceiling and returning to upright.

Check
- Patient may overbalance backward and is warned to keep upper body forward over the hips.

Note

- These exercises can also be done sitting over the side of the bed with feet on a firm surface. A weak patient is assisted to turn on to the side and to sit up over the side of the bed (see Fig. 8.1).

Reaching actions

Sitting, reaching to touch objects with the paretic hand: forward (flexing at the hips), sideways (both sides), backward, returning to mid position (Fig. 2.8). Very weak patients can practise reaching forward with arms resting on a high table (see Fig. 8.4b).

When patient achieves a sense of balance, reaching with non-paretic arm across body to load the paretic foot.

Check

- Reaching distance should be more than arm's length, involving movement of the whole body, and as close to the limits of stability as possible.

FIGURE 2.8 *Some exercises to train the ability to perform simple actions in sitting that require small amounts of body movement: (a,b) Practising using the paretic L leg for support and balance while reaching forward and sideways. (c) Moving the feet back emphasizes the feet as an active part of the base of support and increases the load through the paretic leg. The legs also play a part in moving back to upright which involves lower limb extensor muscle forces and ground reaction forces, particularly during faster movement. (d) At the first attempt at reaching (left) the person may be reluctant to move to the paretic side; some improvement is evident (right) after a few repetitions.*

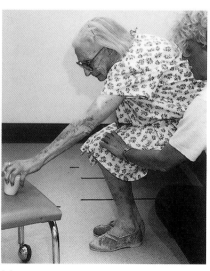
(a)

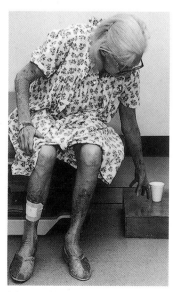
(b)

FIGURE 2.8 *(Continued)*

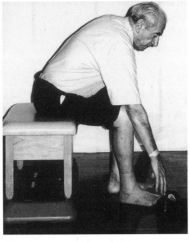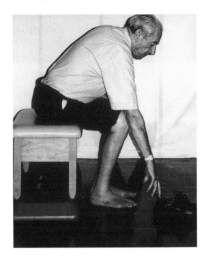

(c)

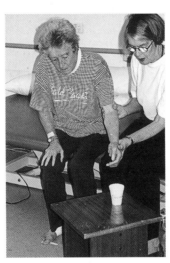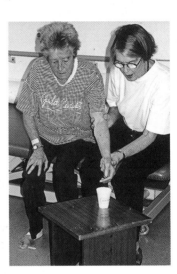

(d)

- In reaches toward the ipsilateral side, emphasis is on weightbearing through the paretic foot since lower limb muscle activity is critical to balancing in sitting.
- Discourage unnecessary activity of non-paretic upper limb (e.g. raising shoulder, grabbing for support).
- Therapist can support affected arm during reaches to that side. Do not pull on the arm.

Note
- If patient falls persistently toward the affected side, it may help the regaining of a sense of balance if the patient is encouraged to reach toward that side and return to mid position. The therapist can provide

FIGURE 2.9   *Reaching sideways in sitting. The task has been modified by setting up the environment to require less lateral movement of the body mass (centre) since he cannot reach down to the floor (left). Weakness of the L lower limb muscles makes it difficult to stabilize the leg. Reaching to the L gives him practice of loading that leg and using it to shift his body mass back to upright sitting.*

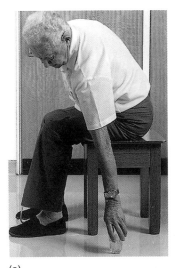 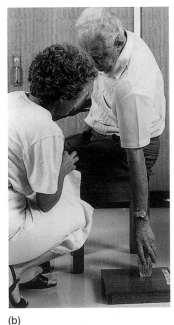 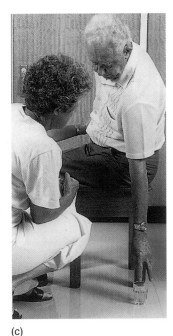

(a)   (b)   (c)

some stability by anchoring the paretic foot on the floor. The effectiveness of this strategy may result from the patient getting the idea of actively controlling movement toward the affected side and back to the midline, rather than compensating for the tendency to fall by keeping the weight on the intact side.

- This training can also be useful for patients with a misperception of the true midline (the true vertical). The therapist should avoid pushing the patient passively toward the midline.

Reaching to pick up objects from the floor, forward and sideways, one and two hands. This can be made easier by placing the object on a box (Fig. 2.9).

Note
- A patient who lacks sufficient control of manipulation can reach to touch the object.
- If necessary, therapist can support affected arm. Do not pull on the arm.

Maximizing skill

The majority of patients trained with repetitive practice of these simple exercises regain a degree of sitting balance within a relatively short period.

FIGURE 2.10　　*The task to practise is lifting the tray without spilling water or dislodging the utensils.*

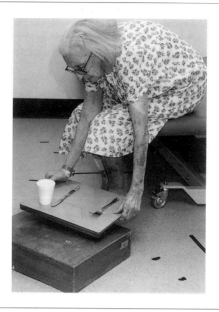

Varying practice to increase skill includes:

- increasing distance to be reached
- varying speed
- reducing thigh support
- increasing object weight and size to involve both upper limbs (Fig. 2.10)
- adding an external timing constraint such as catching or bouncing a ball.

Standing balance

Learning to balance in standing requires the opportunity to practise voluntary actions in this position early in the acute stage. Standing balance is not the static maintenance of a position. However, supporting the body mass over the feet requires the ability to generate sufficient muscle force in the extensors of the paretic lower limb to prevent the knee from collapsing.

Opportunity to load the lower limb seems critical for promoting muscle activity in that limb. Receptors sensitive to load have been shown to activate leg extensor muscles during locomotion in cats. Sensitivity to load has also been observed in humans, with a high correlation between degree of leg extensor activity and percentage of body weight loading of that limb.

Given that it is critical for the person to practise in standing, if the lower limb tends to collapse, there are several ways of enabling balance practice.

FIGURE 2.11	*(a) The knee support enables him to load the R leg without the knee collapsing while he practises stepping forward. (b) The harness enables practice of actions in standing which involve balancing the body mass without fear of falling.*

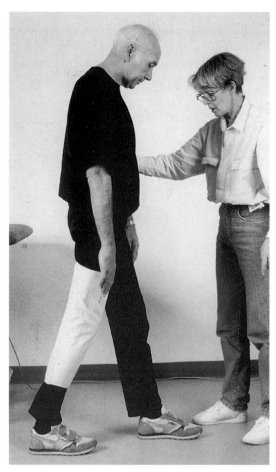 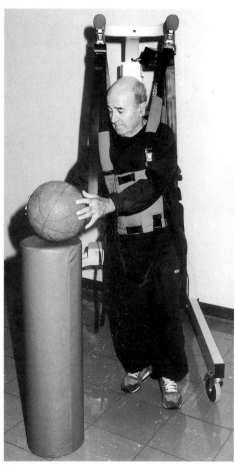

(a)   (b)

For example, a light splint prevents collapse at the knee, and a harness can reduce body weight through the lower limbs. In standing, the patient practises small movements of the centre of body mass. In addition, a programme of exercises, with methods of eliciting muscle activity, increasing strength and preserving length in critical lower limb muscle groups is instituted.

Asymmetrical standing is often a focus of the therapist's intervention. Favouring one leg in standing is primarily due to inability to generate and control supportive forces in the paretic limb and is an adaptation to the problem of an unreliable or collapsing lower limb. Improving support through the limb by strengthening exercises, and training in standing with knee support or harness, should be a major focus in intervention (Fig. 2.11).

The exercises below include movements of the body mass ranging from small displacements when patients are weak and apprehensive, progressing to larger displacements performed faster. Focus is on actions such as turning to see who is coming through the door or reaching to take an object. These activities take the person's attention away from the need to balance by directing it toward a concrete non-balance goal. This can be particularly useful for a person early after stroke who is frightened of moving. Emphasis from the start of training is on reaching beyond arm's length, varying object placement and therefore direction and extent of reach, increasing repetitions and complexity.

Head and body movements

Standing with feet a few cm apart, look up at ceiling and return to upright (Fig. 2.12a).

Check
- Correct tendency to fall back by a reminder to bring hips forward (hip extension beyond neutral) *before* looking up.
- Disallow foot movement.

Standing with feet a few cm apart, turn head and body mass and look behind, return to mid position, repeat to other side (Fig. 2.12b).

Check
- Ensure standing alignment is preserved, with hips extended while body rotates.
- Disallow foot movement. If necessary put your foot against patient's foot to stop movement.

Note
- Provide visual targets.

Reaching actions

Standing, reaching to take object forward, sideways (both sides), backward.

One hand, both hands. Variety of objects and tasks. Reaches should be beyond arm's length, challenging the patient to extend the limit of stability, and return (Fig. 2.13).

Check
- Ensure movement of body mass takes place at the ankles and hips, not just within the trunk.
- Discourage a stiff posture and breath holding – encourage relaxed movement.

FIGURE 2.12   *Some exercises to train the ability to perform actions in standing that require small amounts of body movement. (a) On her first attempt at standing, she practises looking up at the ceiling to locate a target. She needs reminding to keep her body mass (hips) forward. (b) Looking around to locate a target on the wall to the side.*

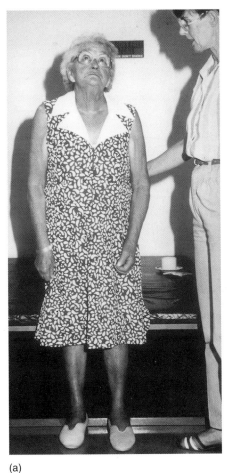

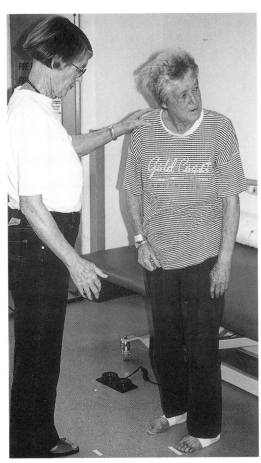

(a)   (b)

Note

- When these exercises are practised without a harness, therapist should avoid holding the person as this diminishes the need to make active anticipatory adjustments and corrections. Use of a belt with grab handles (Fig. 2.14) may increase confidence of both patient and therapist.
- Base of support is varied to increase difficulty (e.g. feet together, one foot in front, one foot on a step, tandem standing). The patient learns to control movement by reaching laterally to each side, forward and backward. Attention, however, is focused not on balance itself but on concrete goals.

FIGURE 2.13   *(a) Reaching sideways, attempting to move weight over the paretic leg. (b) Training balanced movement in a harness. Note (left) that he stands with more weight through the R leg. He practises reaching to the L to pick up a cup (centre). Reaching across the body (right) requires a greater shift to the L with some body turning.*

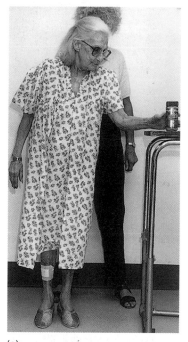

(a)

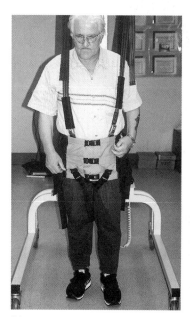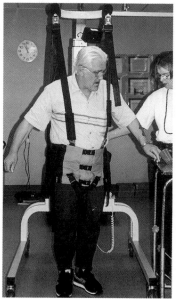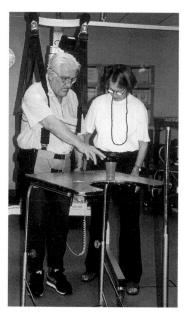

(b)

FIGURE 2.14   *A belt with grab handles gives some reassurance without interfering with the patient's movements. (Handi-Lift/Walk belt, Pelican Manufacturing Pty Ltd, Osborne Park, Western Australia 6017.)*

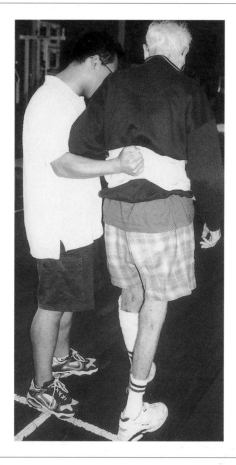

Single leg support (with or without harness or splint)

Stepping forward with non-paretic limb to place foot on a step (Fig. 2.15). Standing with either foot on step, practise reaching tasks.

Check
- Ensure that the stance hip extends. Exercise can be practised initially in a harness.

Note
- Laufer et al. (2000) have shown that stepping forward on to a step of different heights with the non-paretic leg significantly increases weight borne through the paretic limb.
- The exercise directs attention to the concrete goal of raising the leg rather than the more abstract goal of shifting body mass.

FIGURE 2.15 *Training stepping with non-paretic leg in a harness. (a) At first it is difficult for her to keep her R knee extended to support her body mass. The therapist encourages her to 'move her hips forward' (extending her hip) and extend her knee. (b) Stepping with her L leg on to a step. Therapist encourages her to move her body mass forward toward the step, i.e. over the affected leg. (c) She no longer needs to hold on. Note that as soon as she felt more stable she lets go of the handle as she performs a prescribed number of repetitions.*

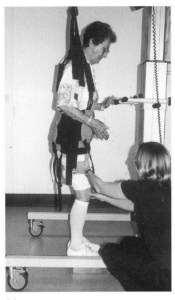 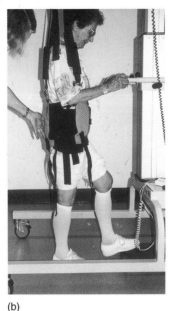 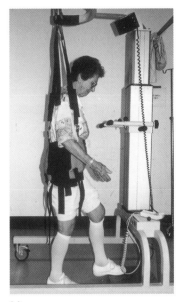

(a)   (b)   (c)

Sideways walking

Walking sideways with hand(s) on wall (Fig. 2.16), or raised bed rail (see Fig. 3.20a).

This exercise enables practice of shifting weight from side to side with hips extended.

Picking up objects

Standing, lowering body mass to pick up or touch object, forward, sideways, backward and return (Fig. 2.17).

Check
- Ensure that hips, knees and ankles flex and extend.
- Start with object on stool to minimize distance to be moved (see Fig. 2.17c).
- Increase flexibility by changing base of support.

FIGURE 2.16 | *Walking sideways with some support. A line on the floor guides her to abduct/adduct her legs without flexing the hip.*

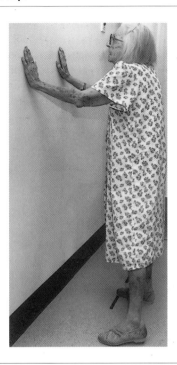

Note

- Overbalancing is prevented by the close proximity of a table, or a therapist, and by well-timed instructions that help the individual make their own segmental adjustment. For example, if observation of body alignment suggests patient is losing balance backward the advice is to 'move your hips forward'.

Computerized feedback training

A computerized footplate system with instrumented platform (e.g. Chattecx*) provides the patient with feedback on position of COP as the possibilities of moving in standing or sitting are explored (Fig. 2.18). An instrumented platform allows the individual to practise moving the body mass voluntarily with visual feedback and responding quickly to unexpected platform shifts. This training may be useful in promoting a sense of control over body mass and an understanding of the mechanical and functional effects of moving the body about over the base of support. Responding to unexpected platform perturbations may train individuals for moving walkways and escalators (Horak et al. 1997).

*Chattecx Corporation, Hinton, TN.

FIGURE 2.17 *(a) This reach involves hip, knee and ankle flexion and extension and weight shift to the L. (b) Moving a stool on wheels introduces the possibility of unexpected movement. (c) At first she is doubtful whether she can pick up the cup but with stand-by reassurance she can practise. Reaching with her R arm across the body moves the body mass toward the L. (d) Practising with the cup on a box develops confidence to reach even lower, (e) and to pick up objects from the floor, a difficult exercise for the weak R limb. (f) He practises taking weight through his affected L leg. His R leg is also weak from a previous injury to hip muscles so he practises to both sides.*

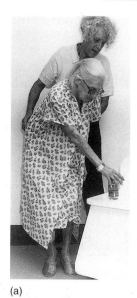
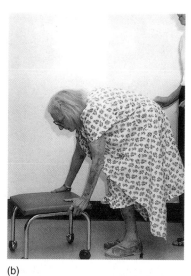

(a)　　　　　　　(b)

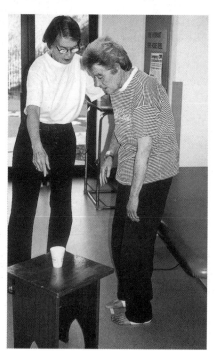
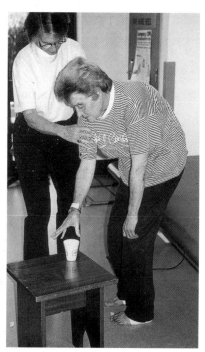

(c)

FIGURE 2.17   *(Continued)*

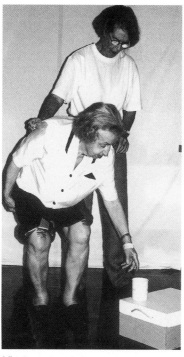

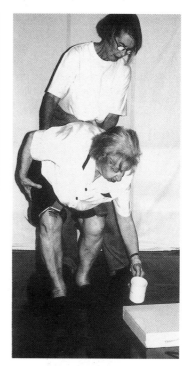

(d)

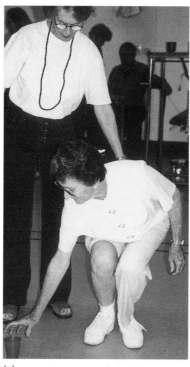

(e)

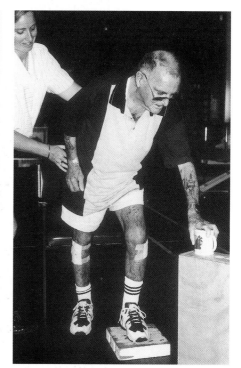

(f)

FIGURE 2.18 *Simple computerized devices can be used to give feedback about body position. (Balance Performance Monitor, courtesy of SMS Technologies.)*

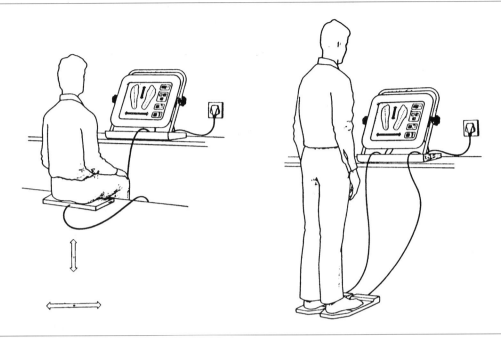

Note
- Patient may practise with minimal supervision.
- A harness may be needed.

There is some evidence that *computer-derived visual feedback* related to weight distribution is effective in gaining symmetrical stance following stroke. However, there is only limited evidence that this training generalizes into improved performance of functional actions (Winstein et al. 1989, Sackley and Lincoln 1997). Given the specificity of exercise and training effects, it is necessary for patients to practise utilizing the visual feedback natural to different environmental conditions.

Maximizing skill

For balance to improve, individuals are challenged with increasingly difficult tasks and more complex contexts in order to extend their abilities to the limits. Flexibility in coping with a variety of real-life tasks and environmental demands is introduced as soon as possible.

- *Reaching and pick-up exercises*
  — place object beyond stability limit so it is necessary to take a step
  — increase weight of object
  — increase size of object to require two hands
  — include unpredictability

— vary speed of movement
— decrease the area of the base of support, e.g. one foot in front of the other (Fig. 2.19a), standing on one leg (Fig. 2.19b), changing compliance of support surface (see Slobounov and Newell 1993).
● *Stepping exercises*
— standing, weight through non-paretic leg (repeat on affected leg) stepping to markers on the floor (Fig. 2.19)
stepping on to high step
foot on ball, move ball about with affected leg.
● *Games to make rapid response time an imperative*
— catching, throwing a ball, bouncing a ball, bat and ball games – involving having to step out.
● *Introduce complexity and uncertainty into the environment*
— playing ball games in a group
— negotiating an obstacle course (see Fig. 3.27).
— stepping over obstacles of different sizes (Fig. 3.28).

Soft tissue stretching

It is critical that contracture and stiffness of calf muscles, particularly soleus, are prevented as these problems restrict the ability to balance and may be a cause of falls in elderly individuals. Short calf muscles interfere with hip extension in standing and walking and a short soleus interferes with initial foot placement backward in standing up. Exercises to prevent these problems are as follows.

● *Sustained passive stretch to calf muscles in standing* (Fig. 3.18a,c)
● *Sustained passive stretch to soleus muscle in sitting* (Fig. 4.13)
● *Active stretch to calf muscles and hip flexors while exercising in standing* (Fig. 3.18d).

Strength training

Lower limb strength training is carried out individually, in a group and as part of circuit training. The goal is for these exercises to transfer into improved performance of actions performed in both sitting and standing and walking. The exercises listed below are described in Chapter 3.

● *Step-up exercises* (Fig. 3.22)
● *Heels raise and lower* (Fig. 3.24)
● *Non-weightbearing exercises* (Fig. 3.26).

Getting up from the floor

Teaching individuals how to get up from the floor after a fall is often a priority in rehabilitation involving elderly individuals, although there is some evidence that it is rarely done (Simpson and Salkin 1993). A major problem is that many people after stroke have difficulty rising from the floor or find

FIGURE 2.19   *(a) One station in a circuit training class involves stepping forward with a narrow base, and practising various tasks such as reaching to pick up an object. (Courtesy F Mackey, Physiotherapy Department, Port Kembla Hospital.) (b) Stepping on to a plastic cup requires careful foot placement and continuous loading of the affected leg. The exercise can also be done with the affected leg to train control. (c) Stepping exercises should be started as soon as possible and practised to both sides. Stepping across the other leg is specifically trained as it is a difficult action for people with poor balance and can cause tripping. (Courtesy of K Schurr and S Dorsch, Physiotherapy Department, Bankstown-Lidcombe Hospital, Sydney.)*

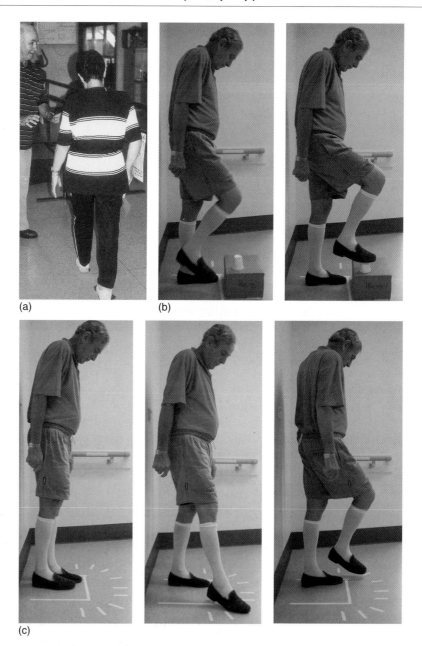

(a)   (b)

(c)

the action impossible unless they have good strength in the lower limb extensors and arm muscles. There is now sufficient evidence to support the need for intensive weight-resisted strengthening programmes for elderly individuals with a history of falls or potential for falling, and in all patients with motor impairments, in addition to balance training. Increasing muscle strength increases the person's range of activities, assists in preventing falls and makes it more likely that the person who falls is able to get up from the floor.

MEASUREMENT

Measurement of balance provides objective information about an individual's progress and is essential in clinical research to determine the effects of intervention. Tests used must be valid and reliable, and strict standardization followed. Choice of test, given that many are available, may be a dilemma for the clinician which can be resolved by considering what information is required. Choice of balance assessment is discussed by several authors (Maki and McIlroy 1997, Carr and Shepherd 1998, Huxham et al. 2001).

Functional tests

The functional tests below measure the ability to balance the body mass during self-initiated actions. They provide measures of different aspects of balance in which the perturbations arise from actions performed in simple and stationary environments. Most measure a single aspect of balance, while the Berg Scale evaluates performance on 14 items common in daily life.

- *Functional Reach Test* (Duncan et al. 1990, Weiner et al. 1993)
- *Step Test* (Hill et al. 1996)
- *Timed 'Up and Go' Test* (Podsialo and Richardson 1991)
- *Berg Balance Scale* (Berg et al. 1989, 1992, Stevenson and Garland 1996)
- *Motor Assessment Scale*: Sitting balance item (Carr et al. 1985)
- *Falls Efficacy Scale* (Tinetti et al. 1993)
- *Activities-Specific Balance Confidence (ABC) Scale* (Powell and Myers 1995, Myers et al. 1998)
- *Obstacle Course Test* (Means et al. 1996)

There is no single test that can measure all aspects of balance, and in general the tests listed above seek specific information. For example:

- The *Functional Reach test* (FR) measures the distance that can be reached in standing in a forward direction. It is therefore an indicator of the extent to which the centre of body mass can be moved in a forward direction toward the limit of stability.
- The *Timed 'Up and Go' test* (TUG) measures the time taken to stand up from a seat, walk off and sit down again. It is an indicator of the ability to balance during body translation from one place to another, the ability to balance being inferred by the time taken to perform the entire sequence. This test is said to be a reliable predictor of the likelihood of falls (Shumway-Cook et al. 2000).

- The *Falls Efficacy scale* measures the degree to which individuals fear falling. The *ABC scale* measures a wider range of mobility-challenging contexts.

The fact that postural adjustments are an inherent part of an action has been shown in many biomechanical studies. It is therefore important to understand the specificity of the many tests, and not to expect the results to reflect changes in aspects of balance not measured. One recent study (Wernick-Robinson et al. 1999) showed no correlation between the score on the FR test and gait velocity – a result which could be expected given that the two actions are dynamically different.

Tests of walking are listed in Chapter 3. Walking tests do not specifically measure balance but data about walking can provide inferences about balance. It has been shown, for example, that stride time variability, measured with force-sensitive insoles, correlates with falling in elderly individuals, with the inference

TABLE 2.1	*Balance: clinical outcome studies*			
Reference	Subjects	Methods	Duration	Results
Sackley and Lincoln 1997	25 Ss 6–31 weeks post-stroke Age range 41–85 yrs	Randomized controlled trial **E**: Visual feedback training on Nottingham Balance Platform (NBP) (e.g. STS, standing, reaching, stepping) + task practice (e.g. gait, climbing stairs) **C**: Placebo programme on NBP + task practice	4 weeks 12 sessions, 1 hour	At week 4, significant* difference between groups on stance symmetry, sway (NBP), gross motor (Rivermead Motor Scale), ADL (Nottingham 10-pt ADL scale) *$p < 0.05$ Difference not retained at 12-week follow-up
Dean and Shepherd 1997	20 Ss >1 year post-stroke Age range 55–83 yrs	Randomized controlled trial **E**: Standardized training programme of reaching beyond arm's length in sitting **C**: Sham training of cognitive-manipulative tasks within arm's length	2 weeks 10 sessions, 30 mins, home-based	**E** reached significantly* further and faster, increased the load through the affected leg in both reaching and STS (force plate), increased activation of leg muscles (EMG) *$p < 0.01$. **C** did not improve
Weiss et al. 2000	7 Ss >1 year post-stroke Age >60 yrs	Time series **1**: Baseline **2**: Supervised high-intensity progressive resistance training for lower limb muscles	12 weeks 2 hours/week	Significant improvements in muscle strength $p < 0.01$, time taken on repetitive sit-to-stands $p < 0.02$, Berg Balance Scale and Motor Assessment Scale (gait) $p < 0.04$, Medical Outcome Survey (physical function) $p < 0.03$. Significant correlations between repeated sit-to-stands and knee extensor strength $p < 0.04$

ADL, activities of daily living; C, control group; COG, centre of gravity; E, experimental group; EMG, electromyography; PT/OT, physiotherapy/occupational therapy; Ss, subjects; STS, sit-to-stand.

that this variable may be a measure of stability during walking (Hausdorff et al. 2001). The Obstacle Course, listed above, provides a complex environment for measuring gait with inferences about walking balance.

Biomechanical tests

Biomechanical and muscle latency testing, including testing of postural responses to externally imposed perturbations and of the sensory contribution to balance, is used in laboratory research to examine the effect of impairments on postural adjustments. These tests are not typically used in the clinic. However, where an instrumented force platform is available, the following tests may be useful in guiding clinical interventions:

- response to support surface movement (Chattecx Balance System*)
- effects of sensory inputs on balance (for the Clinical Test of Sensory Interaction and Balance – CTSIB[†])
- Postural sway (force plate) (Note: functional relevance is unclear).

Evidence of effectiveness of some interventions is provided in Table 2.1. Surprisingly few studies of the effects of interventions on balance after stroke were found. Most investigations have tested the effect of weight-shifting practice or sensory training on symmetry and postural sway. In general, patients improved in the short term in the actions in which they were trained, with little or no carry-over into improved function.

The most encouraging reports so far are from studies of the effects of task-oriented training of functional actions (Dean and Shepherd 1997, Dean et al. 2000) and of lower limb strength training (Sharp and Brouwer 1997, Weiss et al. 2000, Teixeira-Salmela et al. 1999, 2001), both of which have shown positive effects on balance.

*Chattecx Corporation, Hixton, TN.
[†]Neuro Com International, Inc, Clackamas, OR.

3 *Walking*

CHAPTER CONTENTS

- **Introduction**
- **Biomechanical description**
  Kinematics
  Kinetics
  Muscle activity
  Walking in different environments
- **Age-related changes**
- **Analysis of motor performance**
  Research findings
  Observational analysis
  Typical kinematic deviations and adaptations

- **Guidelines for training**
  Walking training
  Soft tissue stretching
  Eliciting muscle activity
  Strength training
  Maximizing skill
- **Measurement**
  Functional tests
  Biomechanical tests
- **Notes**
  Treadmill training
  Electrical stimulation
  Aids and orthoses

INTRODUCTION

The ability to walk independently is a prerequisite for most daily activities. The capacity to walk in a community setting requires the ability to walk at speeds that enable an individual to cross the street in the time allotted by pedestrian lights, to step on and off a moving walkway, in and out of automatic doors, walk around furniture, under and over objects and negotiate kerbs. A walking velocity of 1.1–1.5 m/s is considered to be fast enough to function as a pedestrian in different environmental and social contexts. It has been reported that only 7% of patients discharged from rehabilitation met the criteria for community walking which included the ability to walk 500 m continuously at a speed that would enable them to cross a road safely (Hill et al. 1997).

Walking is a complex, whole-body action that requires the cooperation of both legs and coordination of a large number of muscles and joints to function together. An important question in the study of motor control is how the many structural and physiological elements or components cooperate to produce coordinated walking in a changing physical and social environment. Bernstein (1967) proposed that to perform a coordinated movement the nervous system had to solve what he termed the 'degrees of freedom problem'. The degrees of freedom of any system reflect the number of independent elements to be constrained. Given the large number of joints and muscles and the mechanical complexity inherent in the multisegmental linkage, Bernstein questioned how these elements can be organized to produce effective and efficient walking.

The coordination of a movement, Bernstein wrote, 'is a process of mastering redundant degrees of freedom of the moving organism, that is, its conversion to a controllable system'. Degrees of freedom can be reduced by linking muscles and joints so that they act together as a single unit or synergy, thus simplifying the coordination of movement. Such a linkage is illustrated in gait by the cooperation between muscle forces at hip, knee and ankle to produce an overall support moment of force to ensure the limb does not collapse.

Sensory inputs in general and visual inputs in particular provide information that makes it possible for us to walk in varied, cluttered environments and uneven terrains. Vision provides information almost instantaneously about both static and dynamic features of the near and far environment. This information is used to plan adjustments to the basic walking pattern (Patla 1997).

Avoidance of falls depends to a large extent on the ability to identify, predict and act quickly enough upon potential threats to stability based on past experience. The visual system plays an important role in identifying and avoiding potential threats to balance. Avoidance strategies include adaptation of step length, width and height, increasing ground clearance to avoid hitting an object on the ground, increasing head clearance to avoid hitting an obstacle above ground, changing direction and stopping (Patla 1997). These strategies are adaptive and are implemented to ensure stability of the moving body. Kinesthetic, tactile and vestibular inputs also play an important role, particularly in the reactive control of balance during walking. Reactive control by definition is a last resort or backup in regaining balance and relies upon triggering of reflexive responses (Patla 1993, 1997).

Walking dysfunction is common in neurologically impaired individuals, arising not only from the impairments associated with the lesion but also from secondary cardiovascular and musculoskeletal consequences of disuse and physical inactivity. Muscle weakness and paralysis, poor motor control and soft tissue contracture are major contributors to walking dysfunction after stroke. Functional gait performance, however, also depends on one's level of fitness. Impairments post-stroke frequently impose excessive energy cost (effort) during walking, limiting the type and duration of activities. Stroke patients, particularly those of advanced age, are often unable to maintain their most efficient gait speed comfortably for more than a very short distance, indicating that muscle weakness, elevated energy demands and poor endurance further compromise walking ability (Fisher and Gullikson 1978, Olney et al. 1986). Stroke patients may self-select a speed that requires least energy (Grimby 1983) and may not have the ability to increase this without increasing energy demands beyond their capacity (Holden et al. 1986). Such individuals are constrained to very limited activity in their home environment, and require the opportunity to exercise and increase their walking speed and endurance.

Individuals who are discharged showing improvements in gait are not necessarily functional walkers. For example, the calculation of walking speed over 10 m, a commonly used clinical measure of gait, may overestimate locomotor capacity after stroke. Whereas healthy subjects can walk in excess of their comfortable speed for at least 6 minutes, stroke subjects may not able to maintain their comfortable walking speed over that time (Dean et al. 2001). This would prevent them from being competent community walkers and may lead to increasing handicap. Despite reports that 60–70% of stroke patients have regained independent walking function at rehabilitation discharge (Wade et al. 1987, Dean and Mackey 1992), there is also evidence that only 15% report walking outside the house 2 years later (Skilbeck et al. 1983).

BIOMECHANICAL DESCRIPTION

During human gait the erect moving body is supported first by one leg then by the other. As the moving body passes over the supporting leg, the other leg swings forward for its next supportive phase. The gait cycle includes a stance (approximately 60%) and a swing (approximately 40%) phase. The stance phase can be further subdivided into weight acceptance, mid-stance and push-off, while swing is divided into lift-off (early swing) and reach (late swing) (Winter 1987). There are two brief periods of double support when both feet are in contact with the ground and support of the body is transferred from the back leg to the forward leg. However, the body is supported on one leg for approximately 80% of the gait cycle.

As the individual increases walking speed, the time spent in double support decreases. Conversely, as walking speed slows, the duration of double support increases. Double support phase is critical in transferring weight from one limb to the other and in balancing the upper body. The time taken for each step is similar, as is the distance covered with each step during forward progression.

The balance requirements of gait are complex (see Ch. 2). In quiet standing the projection from the body's centre of mass (COM), the centre of gravity (COG), falls within the area of the feet. Throughout the gait cycle, however, the path of the body's COG rarely passes within the perimeter of the foot (Fig. 3.1). Apart from the brief double support period the body is in a potentially unstable state. Safe foot clearance and foot contact are, therefore, essential to rebalancing the body mass during double support (Winter et al. 1991). Figure 3.1 shows the path of the centre of pressure (COP), which is an indication of weightbearing through the foot, during single limb support. It is notable that the COP stays close to the centre of the foot and does not approach the outer limits of the base of support.

The major requirements for successful walking (Forssberg 1982) are:

- *support* of body mass by lower limbs
- *propulsion* of the body in the intended direction
- the production of a *basic locomotor rhythm*
- dynamic *balance* control of the moving body
- *flexibility*, i.e. the ability to adapt the movement to changing environmental demands and goals.

FIGURE 3.1   *A translational plot showing the body's COG and foot COP for one walking stride. Note: the COG never passes over the foot. HC, heel contact; TO, toe-off. (Reproduced from Winter et al. 1991, with permission.)*

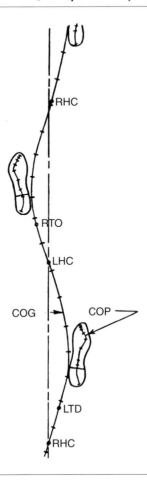

The lower limbs play a significant role in these requirements. In the *stance phase* they are involved in:

- *Support*: the upper body is supported over one or both feet by the action of lower limb extensor muscles and mechanical effects which prevent lower limb collapse.
- *Propulsion* (acceleration of the body in space): generation of mechanical energy to drive the forward motion of the body in a basic locomotor rhythm.
- *Balance*: preservation of upright posture over the changing base of support by postural adjustments occurring in lower limb and limb–trunk segmental linkage.
- *Absorption*: mechanical energy is harnessed for shock absorption and to decrease the body's forward velocity.

In the *swing phase*, in which the foot moves on a smooth path from toe-off to heel contact, the lower limbs are involved in:

- *Toe clearance*: to clear the foot from the ground.
- *Foot trajectory*: to prepare the foot for a safe landing on the support surface.

These are the main functions that must be performed for effective gait (Winter 1987). Simplifying gait in this way not only identifies the major motor control requirements but also clarifies for the clinician the critical requirements of effective and efficient gait and the principal functions on which to concentrate in training.

Gait has been studied more than any other everyday action, resulting in a very large body of literature. Walking has been examined from many perspectives: biomechanical, neural, pathological and developmental. Different types of gait studied include stairwalking, negotiating kerbs and walking over obstacles.

Descriptive research efforts in gait laboratories have focused on quantifying performance in able-bodied subjects as well as examining common functional limitations associated with different pathologies, with a view to developing appropriate intervention strategies to be tested in the clinic. Since differences in such factors as body mass, height, age, gender, cadence and context influence aspects of performance, large databases are required to provide 'normalized' values.

Spatiotemporal variables include cadence, stride length, step length and velocity. When able-bodied individuals walk at their preferred speed, *cadence* varies from a mean of 101 to 122 steps per minute and is reported to be slightly higher in women than in men (Winter 1991). *Stride length* is approximately 1.4 m with a *step length* of 0.7 m in able-bodied young subjects walking at their preferred speed. Walking *velocity* for adult pedestrians aged between 20 and 60 years, who were unaware they were being observed, was on average 1.4 m/s for males and 1.2 m/s for females (Finley and Cody 1970).

Kinematics

Kinematic variables provide information about angular displacements, paths of body parts and centre of body mass (CBM), with angular and linear velocities and accelerations. These variables do not give information about the forces that cause the movement. As Winter (1987) points out, the number of kinematic variables required to describe one gait stride is very high and some serious compromise is necessary to make any gait description manageable.

In level walking, the *path of the CBM* describes a sinusoidal curve along the plane of progression. The peak of the oscillations of this path occur at about the middle of the stance phase. The path of the CBM also moves laterally and describes a sinusoidal curve alternating from right to left in relation to support of the weightbearing limb (Saunders et al. 1953). These motions are related to each other in a systematic fashion, a smooth passage of the CBM being essential for efficient walking.

Major *angular displacements* of lower limb joints during gait take place in the sagittal plane as the body moves forward and can be seen by a careful observer.

Sagittal plane angular displacements at hip, knee and ankle in able-bodied subjects walking at a natural cadence are shown in Figure 3.2. These average values provide a set of reference norms that can be used to guide clinical observation of gait. Normally individual variations in the magnitude of angular displacements are relatively small, with the greatest variations occurring in the less obvious movements of ankle and foot (Sutherland et al. 1994).

The mass of the upper body, including the pelvis and trunk, responds to the needs of the individual to advance the lower limb and to transfer body weight from one supporting limb to the other. For example, the pelvis (moving at hip joints and joints of lumbar spine) rotates, tilts, lists and shifts laterally, governed by such factors as muscle length and length of stride. Shoulders rotate and arms swing out of phase with displacement of pelvis and legs.

In level walking, the pelvis rotates around a vertical axis with the magnitude of this rotation approximately 4° on either side of the central axis. Since the pelvis is itself a rigid structure, this rotation occurs alternately at each hip joint which passes from relative internal rotation to external rotation in the stance phase (Saunders et al. 1953). Rotation also occurs in the spinal joints. The amount of rotation is related to stride length, with older individuals showing less rotation than younger individuals (Murray 1967).

| **FIGURE 3.2** | *Intersubject ensemble averages of hip, knee and ankle angles in the sagittal plane during a single gait cycle. Flexion is positive, extension is negative. CV, coefficient of variation; 0–60%, stance phase; 60–100%, swing phase. (Reproduced from Winter 1987, University of Waterloo Press, with permission.)* |

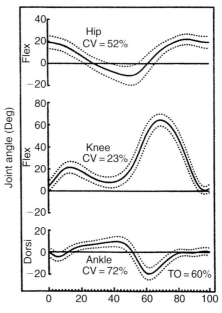

The pelvis also tilts forward and backward, movement occurring at hip joints and joints of lumbar spine. Maximum forward tilting through a mean excursion of 3° occurs in mid to late stance and terminal swing. The movement is controlled by gravity, inertia and hip flexor and extensor muscle action (Sutherland et al. 1994), as well as soft tissue length.

Lateral horizontal pelvic shift occurs as the CBM is displaced laterally in preparation for single support. This displacement involves adduction at the stance hip. The tibiofemoral angle acts as a mechanical constraint, allowing the tibia to remain vertical while the hip adducts slightly. The extent of lateral shift (4–5 cm) is governed in part by activation of hip abductors and muscles extending the knee by mid-stance.

In association with this shift, the pelvis lists downward relative to the horizontal plane toward the side opposite to the stance limb. The displacement occurs at the hip joints, with adduction of the stance hip and abduction of the swing hip, and at joints of the lumbar spine. To overcome the effect of this 'leg-lengthening' on the swing leg, the knee joint of that leg flexes to 'shorten the limb' and allow it to swing through (Saunders et al. 1953).

Trunk movement, in terms of specific movements of spinal joints during gait, has not been studied extensively; however, current research utilizing three-dimensional measurement systems is enabling more discrete examination of the complex spinal movements. The extent of trunk rotation about the longitudinal axis may be greater than previously reported (Krebs et al. 1992) and may be an optimal means of increasing step length when conditions demand. A study in which the movement patterns of lower thoracic, lumbar and pelvic segments were examined found consistent patterns within and between different segments. When walking speed increased, range of motion in each segment increased. The results suggest that spinal movements are linked to motion of the pelvis and lower limbs (Crosbie et al. 1997a,b). This study also found a significant decrease in spinal range of motion in elderly individuals during walking.

Kinetics

These variables are calculated from force plate and kinematic data. They include vertical and horizontal ground reaction forces (GRF) (Newtons per kilogram), moments of force at the joints (Newton-metres per kilogram), power transferred between body segments (watts), and mechanical energy of body segments (joules). Moments of force are the net result of muscular, ligamentous and friction forces acting to change the angular rotation at a joint. Net moments can be interpreted as resulting principally from muscle forces (Winter 1991).

GRFs are the simplest kinetic variables to record. Although internally generated forces are required to move body segments, the forces responsible for displacement of the body mass are external to the system. In an action such as walking in which the feet are on the ground, these forces are called ground or supportive forces. They occur in response to muscle activity and segmental movements when body weight is transmitted through the feet (Fig. 3.3).

FIGURE 3.3   *Averaged horizontal and vertical ground reaction forces. Horizontal force has a negative phase during the first half of stance, indicating a slowing down of the body, and a positive phase, indicating forward acceleration of the body, during the latter half of stance. Vertical force has the characteristic double hump, the first related to weight-acceptance and the second to push-off. CV, coefficient of variation. (Reproduced from Winter 1987, University of Waterloo Press, with permission.)*

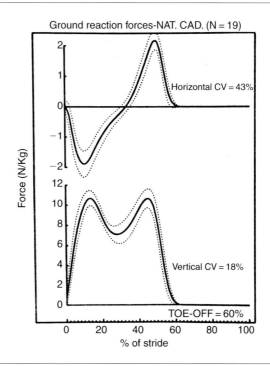

There are many combinations of muscle forces occurring across hip, knee and ankle joints that can result in similar patterns of movement. There are also many combinations of muscle activity that can produce the same *moments of force* at a specific joint. However, in the stance phase, muscles across the three joints act cooperatively and ensure support of the body mass through the lower limb and prevent collapse of the limb. Winter (1980) has shown that collapse is prevented by an overall extensor moment of force called a *support moment of force* (SM). SM, an algebraic summation of forces at hip, knee and ankle, is consistently extensor despite the variability that may occur at the individual joints. While ankle moment of force remains relatively consistent at different speeds, hip and knee moments covary, a decrease in extensor moment at the knee, for example, being countered by an increase in extensor moment at the hip.

Mechanical power is the rate at which energy is generated and absorbed and is the product of the net moment and angular velocity at the joint. An analysis of power provides information about which muscles are generating mechanical energy and which are absorbing it (Winter 1987). Power is generated when muscle contraction is concentric (positive power) and is absorbed when muscle contraction is eccentric (negative power). Power profiles of the three lower

FIGURE 3.4	*Power profiles of hip, knee and ankle during a single gait cycle indicating the most important power phases. Power generation is positive, absorption is negative. CV, coefficient of variation. (Reproduced from Winter 1987, University of Waterloo Press, with permission.)*

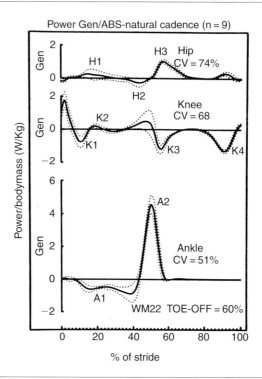

limb joints in able-bodied subjects are shown in Figure 3.4. These profiles describe the magnitude and direction of the flow of energy in and out of muscle and reveal that the major power generation occurring in gait occurs at the ankle for push-off (about 80%), with the second most important source being the generation of a flexion force at the hip for pull-off during late stance and early swing (Winter 1983). These two major bursts of power are said to provide the propulsive force necessary for forward level progression. The actual energy to swing the leg through comes from pendulum action (the conversion of potential energy to kinetic). Magnitudes of power profiles vary according to speed but tend to remain constant in shape.

Muscle activity

Evidence suggests that, when subjects walk at their preferred speed, muscles produce only a small amount of the total force required to propel the body mass forward, with other contributions coming from ground reaction and inertial forces. Muscles contract and relax in a precise, orchestrated manner (Rab 1994). Their major role is to provide bursts of muscle activity at the appropriate time to initiate, accelerate, decelerate and control movement throughout the gait cycle. As the cycle progresses, muscle action becomes primarily isometric or eccentric, both of which are energy efficient forms of contraction to maintain

FIGURE 3.5 *Changes in EMG pattern of six major muscle groups associated with three different gait cadences (n = 11). Note the change in EMG pattern is primarily in amplitude, the shape remaining similar. The degree of amplitude change was muscle specific. (Reproduced from Yang JF, Winter DA (1985) Surface EMG profiles during different walking cadences in humans.* Electroencephalography and Clinical Neurophysiology, 60, 485–491, with permission.)*

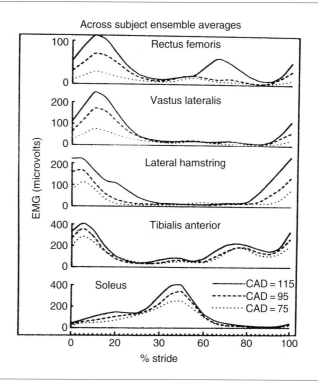

Across subject ensemble averages

upright posture against gravity and to transfer energy between segments. Shortening (concentric) contractions are used to provide brief bursts of power for forward motion when required (Winter 1987).

Surface electromyography (EMG) enables the determination, using a threshold signal, of when in the gait cycle a given muscle or muscle group is active. Since many factors affect the magnitude of EMG, including sensitivity to gait speed, electrode size, shape, placement and amount of fatty tissue, there are numerous problems in recording and reporting the electrical signals.

Winter (1991) reports EMG values for 25 lower limb muscles during gait. There is considerable variability across subjects, some of which can be explained by biological differences. Ankle muscle activity appears the most consistent, which may reflect the joint's position closest to the base of support. Knee and hip muscles, however, have multiple roles, particularly during stance, and tend to show more variability. Signals from monoarticular muscles are less variable than those from biarticular muscles, which may reflect different roles in producing power bursts (monoarticular muscles) and transferring power between segments (biarticular muscles) (Ingen Schenau et al. 1987). However, the patterns of EMG for five major muscles at three different cadences (Fig. 3.5) indicate that the shape of the signal remains similar despite changes in amplitude due to variations in speed.

Walking in different environments

Slopes

Slopes are frequently encountered in everyday life. Although muscle weakness and many joint pathologies are known to interfere with slope walking, few studies have investigated the effects of slopes on gait. Ramps are increasingly being provided for access to buildings, one of the intentions being to reduce the number of falls occurring on steps. Ramps, however, provide their own hazards. This is particularly the case when walking down the slope due to the potential for slippage and loss of balance. Slippage is a problem when walking down because of the generation of high shear forces which increase as ramp angle increases.

The most significant finding in a study of urban pedestrians walking up and down slopes of up to 9° was that step length decreased with increasing slope in descent (Sun et al. 1996). This may reflect the need to accommodate the increased friction demand with increasing slope. Another study comparing able-bodied subjects' level walking with downhill walking at a gradient of −19% indicated that kinematic adjustments for downhill walking occurred primarily at the knee joint (increased flexion) during stance and at the ankle and hip joints during swing to compensate for the slope. Peak moments and powers were much higher at the knee joints in downhill walking compared with level walking (Kuster et al. 1995, Redfern and Di Pasquale 1997). Ankle dorsiflexion moments also increase with slope angle during the first 20% of stance (Redfern and Di Pasquale 1997). In walking uphill, subjects demonstrated a reduction in walking speed, cadence and step length with increasing slope. In walking up a slope with a 20% gradient, increases in hip and knee flexion were reported during late swing and the initial part of support phase (Wall et al. 1981).

Obstacles and kerbs

A common obstacle encountered in everyday life is a kerb or a single step indoors. Negotiating obstacles has been investigated in the laboratory (Patla et al. 1991, Grabiner et al. 1993). Obstacle crossing requires many adaptations that depend on such factors as height, width and nature of obstacle, gait speed, degree of lighting and position of object within step or stride. Modification to gait may include changes in foot clearance, in step length and step time, and in gait speed. Obstacle crossing requires clearance of an obstacle by both the lead limb (clears the object first) and the trail limb.

A recent study observed a group of young able-bodied subjects negotiating a standard kerb on the edge of a footpath in a natural setting outdoors (Crosbie and Ko 2000). All subjects were able to make accurate and appropriate adjustments to their step pattern to negotiate the obstacle without any loss of fluency, regardless of gait speed or cadence. Planning for obstacle negotiation appears to be made some distance from the obstacle. Several critical requirements emerged from analysis of the data. During kerb ascent, enough of the foot is placed on top of the kerb to enable balance and stability during the swing phase of the contralateral limb, and to enable propulsion from the stance foot once the kerb had been negotiated. Another imperative appears to be that the toe of the swing limb does not catch on the kerb as the foot is swung upward and forward. Kerb descent appeared to require a more conservative step adjustment in which the foot of the swing limb was either well short of, or well over, the kerb.

Stair walking

Stair walking is mechanically different from level walking in terms of joint range, muscle activity and joint forces. Lowering and raising the body mass while progressing forward to another step level requires increased angular displacements at the lower limb joints, increased duration and intensity of muscle activity and increased magnitude of joint forces (Andriacchi et al. 1980). Considerable demands are also placed on balance, particularly during the period of single stance when the body mass is moving forward.

An essential feature of stair ascent is the forward translation of the body mass over the foot by ankle dorsiflexion. The body remains in the same relative alignment while forces produced by the back limb push the body mass diagonally in a forward and upward direction over the forward foot. Extension at the hip, knee and ankle of this leg raises the body mass as the back foot is lifted forward on to the next step. Thus a smooth ascent results from the coordination of forces produced by both legs. In contrast, during stair descent, the body mass is kept back over the supporting leg which flexes at hip, knee and ankle to lower the body for foot placement on to the next step. Stair descent has a shorter double support phase than stair ascent, probably reflecting different mechanical demands.

Extensor muscle strength is particularly critical to stair walking since the body mass must be raised or lowered essentially supported on one limb. In contrast to level walking, it is the knee which generates most of the energy (Bradford et al. 1988). During ascent, concentric contraction of lower limb extensor muscles raises the body mass vertically; stair descent is achieved through control of gravitational forces by eccentric muscle contraction. Stair ascent, descent and level walking all exhibit a support moment of similar shape. However, the magnitude of support moment for stair walking is greater. During ascent it is twice the magnitude produced during level walking (Bradford et al. 1988).

AGE-RELATED CHANGES

The ability to maintain effective gait function with increasing age is important for the health and well-being of older people. Although it is a common observation that the walking pattern changes with increasing age, how many of the changes observed in the older individual are due to an ageing process and how many to reduced physical activity and the pathology that may accompany ageing is not clearly understood. Due to fear of falling and the possible consequences of a fall, apprehension may also influence performance. The changes observed in walking pattern may also reflect slower walking speeds commonly reported in the elderly. Cross-sectional studies have repeatedly shown decreases in walking speed and stride length, and increases in duration of double support phase in older subjects.

Investigators have also described age-related decreases in vision, cardiovascular capacity, muscle strength, joint flexibility and bone mass, all of which could impact on walking performance. Many of the above decrements are similar to those associated with extended periods of bed rest and relative inactivity (Bortz 1982). Gabell and Nayak (1984), using stringent subject selection criteria, failed to find significant age effects on spatiotemporal gait variables in a group of healthy elderly subjects aged between 66 and 84, suggesting that pathology rather than age may be the major contributor to variability in gait. Stride width and duration of double support phase, however, showed less consistency than step length and stride time.

Falls are a frequent hazard for elderly individuals. The reduction in frequency of falls among the elderly is a public health issue and a major goal of researchers and health workers. Epidemiological data have implicated initiation of walking, turning, walking on uneven surfaces and stopping in almost all incidences of falls (Prudham and Evans 1981, Gabell et al. 1986). Increased stride width, erratic floor clearance and increased stride time variability (Hausdorff et al. 2001) are three parameters that distinguish between fallers and non-fallers.

Recovery from an obstacle-induced anteriorly directed stumble appears to depend upon lower extremity muscle power and ability to restore control of hip/trunk flexion (Grabiner et al. 1993). Individuals with limited ankle joint mobility may be particularly at risk of stumbling, tripping and falling. Range of motion and joint stiffness studies suggest that decreased mobility at the ankle joint may be a characteristic of ageing associated with an increasingly sedentary life style, and acute and chronic pathology (Vandervoort et al. 1990). Muscle weakness, especially in the ankle musculature, seems to be another factor contributing to falls and variability in gait. Reduced push-off power in subjects aged between 62 and 78 years compared with younger subjects has been reported (Winter et al. 1990), and significantly smaller peak torque and power values were found in ankle and knee muscles in a group of fallers compared with a group of non-fallers (Whipple et al. 1987).

Several studies of older individuals show beneficial effects of muscle strengthening exercises and aerobic exercises in preventing falls, increasing gait speed, and aerobic capacity (Fiataroni et al. 1990, Krebs et al. 1998). Vandervoort (1999) reported positive effects of strengthening and stretching exercises even in very old residents in long-term care. Interestingly, in a longitudinal study of aerobic capacity of master athletes aged between 50 and 82 years, those who continued competitive levels of training maintained their aerobic capacity. Those who decreased training showed significant decreases in aerobic capacity (Pollock et al. 1987).

ANALYSIS OF MOTOR PERFORMANCE

Certain gait abnormalities are evident following stroke. In part they arise as a result of different patterns and degrees of muscle weakness/paralysis and lack of coordination, and in part as a result of adaptations as the person attempts to walk despite muscle weakness, balance deficits, changes in muscle length and stiffness.

Over the past decade or so the increasing use of movement analysis systems that enable measurement of kinematic and kinetic variables, together with EMG analysis, have provided data that not only have greatly increased our understanding of gait adaptations associated with neurological dysfunction but have also enabled clinical gait analysis to be more objective. Descriptive variables for measurement include gait speed, stride length, cadence and joint angles, whereas moments of force and power profiles along with EMG signals help to explain why a given movement pattern might occur.

Research findings

In an attempt to investigate whether or not there is a typical pattern of muscle weakness in the lower limbs, Adams et al. (1990), using myometry, examined the voluntary strength of eight muscles of the lower limb (flexors and extensors of hip, knee, ankle and hallux) in able-bodied subjects and in both the weak and clinically unaffected lower limbs of stroke subjects. No consistent pattern of muscle weakness was found in the hemiplegic limb. Sometimes the flexors were more affected than the extensors at one joint with the converse at another joint. The strength of muscles tested on the clinically unaffected side was also reduced compared with controls. On average, one of the most affected groups was the ankle plantarflexors.

Given the high energy cost of walking in the presence of muscle weakness, decreased motor control and adaptive soft tissue changes it is not surprising that the most consistent research finding is that individuals following stroke walk more slowly than able-bodied age-matched subjects (e.g. von Schroeder et al. 1995). Slow walking disrupts the dynamics of the action and many of these spatiotemporal characteristics are also found in able-bodied subjects walking at these very slow speeds. Consistent with a decrease in speed are decreases in stride length and changes in cadence, and increased duration of double support phase (Olney and Richards 1996). Several differences in proportion of time spent in stance and swing phases have been reported. A typical finding is that the stance phase of the non-paretic limb is both longer and occupies a greater proportion of the gait cycle than that of the paretic limb.

Studies of joint angle displacements following stroke, focused in general on sagittal plane movements, have shown variability in magnitude of angular displacements at a particular point in the gait cycle compared with able-bodied subjects. The major differences are (Burdett et al. 1988, Lehman et al. 1987):

- decreased hip extension at the end of stance
- decreased hip flexion in mid-swing
- decreased knee flexion at toe-off and mid-swing
- decreased ankle dorsiflexion at foot contact, and during stance associated with a hyperextended knee
- decreased ankle plantarflexion at toe-off
- increased knee flexion at foot contact.

Note that some of these changes in angular displacement can be attributed to differences in walking speed. The data from one group of stroke subjects were divided into three groups according to speed. In the fastest group, the hip extended an average of 10° beyond neutral in late stance, but only about 2° beyond neutral in the medium speed group. Extension was a few degrees short of neutral in the slowest group (Olney and Richards 1996). The clinically unaffected limb showed similar trends although the average hip extension always exceeded neutral.

While spatiotemporal and kinematic variables have descriptive value in clinical practice, kinetic variables have particular explanatory value for our understanding of the underlying reasons for a particular movement pattern. Kinetic variables are of value in determining, for an individual patient, where in the support phase to focus intervention. They can also be used to evaluate the effect of intervention.

Several vertical GRF variations in stroke patients have been reported compared with able-bodied subjects (Carlsoo et al. 1974). These variations included decreased magnitude of vertical GRFs, particularly associated with push-off. Rather than the characteristic two peaks and intermediate trough there was a relatively constant magnitude of force throughout the support phase. As an example of how such information is of clinical value, the absence of vertical GRF peak representing push-off suggests the need to strengthen the calf muscles, increase their length, and emphasize push-off in walking training.

The propulsive force for forward progression comes mainly from generation of power at the ankle for push-off and at the hip for pull-off (Winter 1987). A consistent finding in able-bodied individuals is a relationship between gait speed and power bursts at pull-off and toe-off. A recent study provides profiles of moments of force and powers at hip, knee and ankle for two hemiplegic subjects compared with values obtained in slow walking in able-bodied subjects (Richards et al. 1999). One patient who walked very slowly (0.15 m/s), maintained hip, knee and ankle flexion throughout most of the gait cycle. This was associated with high extensor moments at hip and knee and low or absent plantarflexor moments. Power generation was very low at push-off and pull-off. In contrast, profiles of a second hemiplegic subject walking a little faster (0.57 m/s) showed mechanical power values that were much closer to slow normal values but less sustained than normal. It is noteworthy for clinical practice that significant increases in push-off and pull-off power generation and in walking speed have been reported after 4 weeks of intensive task-specific exercise and training which included muscle strength training and treadmill walking (Dean et al. 2000).

Olney and Richards (1996) also report exaggerated extensor moments at hip and knee throughout stance. It is often observable in the clinic that the hemiplegic leg is held stiffly during stance. This stiffness may be misinterpreted as reflecting 'spasticity'. However, the exaggerated extensor moments may reflect increasing muscle co-contraction to prevent collapse of the limb. This would indicate the need for weightbearing exercises to strengthen lower limb muscles and improve control of the limb during both concentric and eccentric activity (i.e. flexion and extension) in addition to walking practice.

There is a great deal of variability in the reporting of EMG activity in stroke patients, reflecting differences in speed, motor control deficits and adaptations (Peat et al. 1976, Knutsson and Richards 1979). Low levels of muscle activity have been reported in some muscles (e.g. gastrocnemius). In other muscles, levels of activity were increased in some phases of the gait cycle and decreased in others. As would be expected, abnormal patterns of EMG activity during walking have also been reported for the clinically unaffected limb (e.g. Shiavi 1985).

Observational analysis

A clear distinction should be made between measurement, i.e. the collection of objective data, and observational analysis. Visual observation, which therapists must rely on for ongoing gait analysis and as a guide to intervention, is dependent on the clinician's skill and knowledge of normative biomechanical values. There are some major drawbacks to observational assessment. Critical biomechanical characteristics such as angular velocities, ground reaction and muscle forces cannot be observed but they can be inferred. Several clinical studies have indicated the problems, showing lack of reliability in observational assessment (Wall 1999), erroneous and incorrect conclusions (Malouin 1995), and lack of familiarity with normative values (Eastlake et al. 1991).

It is not possible or practical for every individual with stroke to have a full biomechanical gait assessment. However, researchers are continuing to investigate the nature of gait deficits and attempting to explain the reasons for functional limitations observed by clinicians. This ongoing research continues to direct clinical practice.

In the clinic, the only directly observable movement characteristics are kinematic, particularly angular displacements and paths of body parts, and such spatiotemporal characteristics as speed, step length and stride width. Spatiotemporal and kinematic variables can also give clues to the underlying dynamics. For example, collapse of the lower limb at the knee suggests muscle weakness and insufficient control of extensor forces. In order to increase observational accuracy, both sagittal and frontal views are necessary for the clinician to analyse the relationships between multiple segments. Videotaping is recommended to enable multiple viewing opportunities and avoid the patient becoming frustrated and fatigued.

Biomechanical studies indicate that there are several key kinematic characteristics that are necessary for effective and efficient gait. These characteristics or components are based on data provided by able-bodied subjects walking at their preferred speed. Although there are variations between individuals or within the one individual as a result of such factors as change in speed or alteration in footwear, there are certain observable events shared by all (Fig. 3.6). Individual variations, for example in the magnitude of angular displacements are relatively small.

The essential components listed below provide a basic structure or model upon which observational analysis is carried out. The patient's attempts at walking (the performance) are observed and compared to this 'normal' model.

FIGURE 3.6   *Gait cycle in an able-bodied subject illustrating major kinematic components in the sagittal plane.*

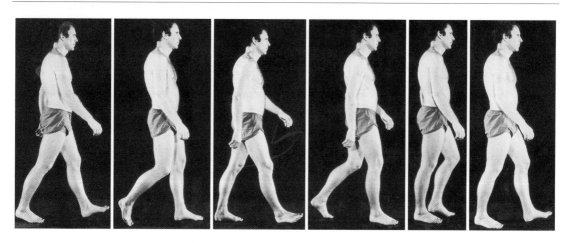

Although components are listed separately, they are of course integrated during the gait cycle.

Stance phase

- Ankle dorsiflexion for heel contact, plantarflexion to foot flat, dorsiflexion as body mass progresses forward over the foot, pre-swing ankle plantarflexion for push-off
- Knee flexion at heel contact (approximately 15°) to absorb body weight and momentum, extension by mid-stance, flexion (35–40° pre-swing)
- Hip extension to advance body mass forward over the foot (approximately 10–15° beyond neutral) together with ankle dorsiflexion
- Lateral horizontal pelvic shift (approximately 4 cm from side to side) involving adduction at stance hip

Transition from stance to swing

Several events in late stance appear to set up the conditions for swing. Hip extension in late stance is associated with moving the body mass forward over the stance foot, which provides the hip flexors with a mechanical advantage to generate power for pull-off at the start of swing (Teixeira-Salmela et al. 2001). Step length and walking velocity depend principally on plantarflexor activity at push-off and hip flexor activity at pull-off (Winter 1987).

Swing phase

- Hip flexion (pull-off) to swing lower limb forward
- Knee flexion to shorten lower limb (35–40° pre-swing, increasing to 60°)
- Lateral pelvic list downward (approximately 5°) toward swing side at toe-off
- Rotation of pelvis about the vertical axis (approximately 4° to either side)
- Knee extension plus ankle dorsiflexion for heel contact

| FIGURE 3.7 | *Normally the knee flexes at the start of stance and provides shock absorption. Note the hyperextension of the knee. (Reproduced from Perry J (1992) Gait Analysis. Normal and Pathological Function. Slack, Thorofare, NJ, with permission.)* |

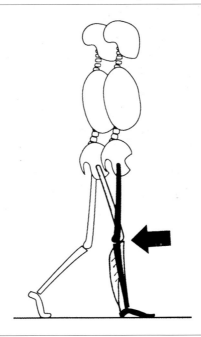

The challenges to stability during locomotion are complex. They present major difficulties for the patient and can instill fear of walking. The base of support during both single and double support phases is small, and the CBM is a considerable distance above it. Balance control is concentrated in muscles linking thigh to pelvis and shank to foot.

The individual's ability to walk varies with the severity of impairments, the ability to utilize adaptive movements and the extent of secondary soft tissue contracture. Although the mechanisms underlying gait limitations are complex and multifactorial, it is possible to identify some causes of observed functional limitations to guide intervention (see also Adams and Perry 1994, Olney and Richards 1996).

Typical kinematic deviations and adaptations

Initial stance (heel/foot contact and loading)

- Limited ankle dorsiflexion
  - decreased activation of anterior tibial muscles
  - contracture and/or stiffness of calf muscles with premature activation.
- Lack of knee flexion (knee hyperextension) (Fig. 3.7)
  - contracture of soleus
  - limited control of quadriceps 0–15°.

FIGURE 3.8   *(a) The knee remains flexed throughout stance. Soleus weakness fails to stabilize the tibia. As a result, without a stable base the quadriceps cannot extend the flexed knee. (b) The mechanism is made clear by the stick figure. (Reproduced from Perry J (1992) Gait Analysis. Normal and Pathological Function. Slack, Thorofare, NJ, with permission.)*

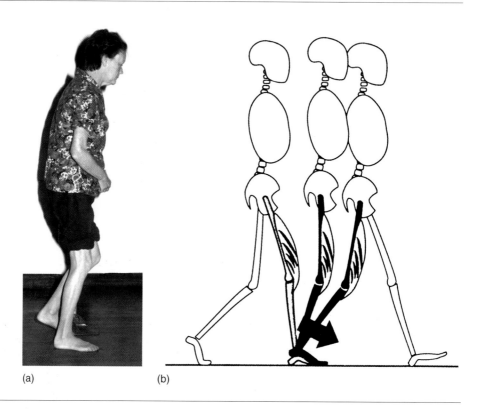

(a)   (b)

Mid-stance

- Lack of knee extension (knee remains flexed 10–15° with excessive ankle dorsiflexion) (Fig. 3.8)
    — decreased activation of calf muscles to control movement of shank forward at ankle (ankle dorsiflexion)
    — limited synergic activation of lower limb extensor muscles.
- Stiffening of knee (hyperextension). This interferes with preparation for push-off
    — contracture of soleus (Fig. 3.9)
    — an adaptation to fear of limb collapse due to weakness of muscles controlling the knee.
- Limited hip extension and ankle dorsiflexion with failure to progress body mass forward over the foot
    — contracture of soleus (Figs 3.9, 3.10).
- Excessive lateral pelvic shift (Fig. 3.11)
    — decreased ability to activate stance hip abductors and control hip and knee extensors.

FIGURE 3.9   *Lack of forward movement of the shank on the foot (ankle dorsiflexion) and knee hyperextension are compensated for by forward movement of the trunk at the hip (hip flexion). Note the short contralateral step. (Reproduced from Perry J (1992)* **Gait Analysis. Normal and Pathological Function.** *Slack, Thorofare, NJ, with permission.)*

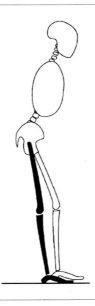

FIGURE 3.10   *Left mid-stance. Failure to transport body mass over the foot due to a short soleus which prevents ankle dorsiflexion and hip extension and hyperextends the knee.*

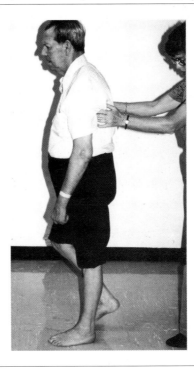

FIGURE 3.11   *Increased lateral pelvic shift to the R and downward list of the pelvis on the L.*

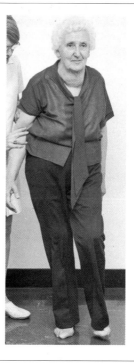

FIGURE 3.12   *Bold limb shows inadequate knee flexion, and ankle plantarflexion with prolonged foot contact in pre-swing. (Reproduced from Perry J (1992)* **Gait Analysis. Normal and Pathological Function. Slack, Thorofare, NJ, with permission.)**

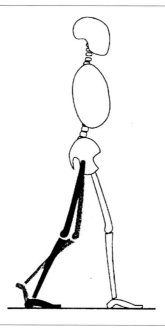

FIGURE 3.13   *(a,b) Inadequate hip and knee flexion at the beginning of swing with toe drag (bold limb). (Stick figure from Perry J (1992)* **Gait Analysis. Normal and Pathological Function.** *Slack, Thorofare, NJ, with permission.)*

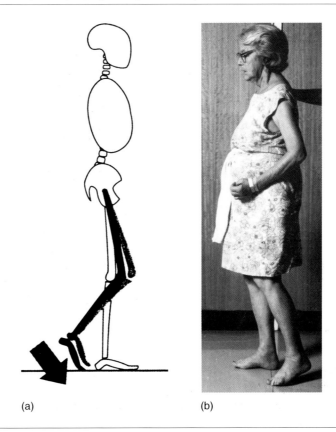

(a)   (b)

Late stance (pre-swing)

- Lack of knee flexion and ankle plantarflexion, prerequisites for push-off and preparation for swing (Fig. 3.12)
  — weakness of calf muscles.

Early and mid-swing

- Limited knee flexion (Fig. 3.13). Normally 35–40° increasing to 60° for swing and toe clearance
  — increased stiffness in or unopposed activity of two-joint rectus femoris
  — decreased activation of hamstrings.

Note

The mechanisms that prevent knee flexion in pre-swing reduce the potential for normal limb advancement. Insufficient knee flexion requires adaptive action of

FIGURE 3.14 *Backward trunk movement with posterior pelvic tilt to advance the leg forward when hip flexion is reduced. (Reproduced from Perry J (1992)* **Gait Analysis. Normal and Pathological Function.** *Slack, Thorofare, NJ, with permission.)*

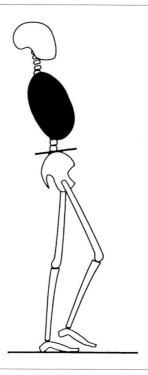

adjacent segments to achieve limb advancement and foot clearance (Adams and Perry 1994). Typical adaptations to limited knee and hip flexion are hip hiking and increased posterior pelvic tilt, or limb circumduction.

- Limited hip flexion at toe-off and mid-swing (Fig. 3.14)
  — decreased activation of hip flexors.
- Limited ankle dorsiflexion*
  — may be slowness in flexing knee rather than decreased dorsiflexor activity
  — stiffness and contracture of calf.

Late swing (preparation for heel contact and loading)

- Limited knee extension and ankle dorsiflexion jeopardizing heel contact and weight-acceptance (Fig. 3.15)
  — contracted or stiff calf muscles
  — decreased dorsiflexor activity.

*Strength requirements of dorsiflexors vary throughout the gait cycle. Functional demands during loading far exceed requirements during swing (Adams and Perry 1994).

FIGURE 3.15 *(a) Normally the hip flexes, the knee extends and foot dorsiflexes as the leg reaches out to make heel contact. Note the lack of ankle dorsiflexion and the very short step. (b) The seven figures to the R illustrate one gait cycle.*

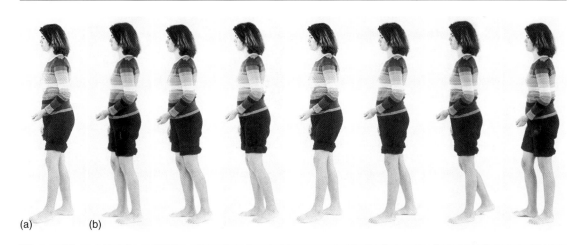

(a)   (b)

FIGURE 3.16 *A frontal plane view showing increased stride width. Note she is not moving her body weight forward and diagonally to the L but keeping her weight back on her non-paretic leg as she steps forward.*

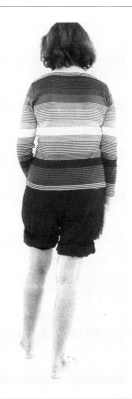

Spatiotemporal adaptations

These include:

- decreased walking speed
- short and/or uneven step and stride lengths
- increased stride width (Fig. 3.16)
- increased double support phase
- dependence on support through the hands.

Note

Although symmetry is frequently an unquestioned goal of gait rehabilitation, an investigation of 34 gait variables failed to provide evidence that symmetry promotes an increase in walking speed (Griffin et al. 1995). It was pointed out that there are several reasons for expecting to see asymmetric rather than symmetric variables in individuals whose limbs have unequal capabilities. Knowing gait is asymmetrical is, therefore, not helpful in planning intervention. The goals should be directed toward impairments causing the asymmetry – weakness and lack of control of segmental movement in the context of walking. Promoting the rhythmic nature of walking (e.g. on a treadmill) should be more of a focus than symmetry which will improve when lower limb muscles are stronger and gait speed is increased.

GUIDELINES FOR TRAINING

Intervention aims to optimize walking performance by:

- preventing adaptive changes in lower limb soft tissues
- eliciting voluntary activation in key muscle groups in lower limbs
- increasing muscle strength and coordination
- increasing walking velocity and endurance
- maximizing skill, i.e. increasing flexibility
- increasing cardiovascular fitness.

These aims are addressed by a combination of treadmill and overground walking practice, strength training and soft tissue stretching. In general, it is the tendency for the stance limb to collapse, lack of forward propulsion and poor balance that interfere most with gait. Although in the acute phase walking capacity may be limited, it is only by integrating strength gains into meaningful function (i.e. walking) that performance will improve.

Given the mechanics of the action, the major emphasis in walking training is on:

- support of the body mass over the lower limbs
- propulsion of the body mass
- balance of the body mass as it progresses over one or both lower limbs
- controlling knee and toe paths for toe clearance and foot placement
- optimizing rhythm and coordination.

Since support (loading the limb) is a prerequisite for upright stance, and push-off sets up the conditions for propulsion and swing, training focuses initially on these. Note that support, balance and stepping are trained only when the individual practises walking itself. A treadmill with harness provides some body weight support and safety, enabling early walking for those who would otherwise not be able to practise. The use of hands for balance and support is discouraged to enable the regaining of dynamic balance and the ability to support the body mass through the lower limbs.

The following guidelines provide what can be considered a critical pathway for optimizing gait for individuals following stroke. The guidelines are individualized according to each patient's impairments, level of functional ability and needs. The guidelines are set down with no intention of a prescribed sequence. They address the essential requirements for effective gait, synthesized from research. Many of the exercises can be practised as part of circuit training or in a group with minimal supervision.

Walking training

When to commence walking practice and what criteria to use have been critical clinical questions in stroke rehabilitation. Conventional gait training has focused on part-practice of components of gait in preparation for walking. Gait training on a treadmill with a harness and partial body weight support, however, enables walking training to commence far earlier than has been possible. It is also a method of enabling repetitive leg exercise. Patients as early as 1 month after stroke have commenced training on a treadmill (Malouin et al. 1992). Reservations have been expressed about the studies so far, for example, the variations in methodology and small sample sizes which may bias the size of the treatment effect (Dobkin 1999). Without a doubt randomized controlled studies are necessary. However, all of the studies show effective results, some showing substantially better results than the usual methods of therapy provided in rehabilitation (see Table 3.1).

Walking on a treadmill with harness and partial body weight support (Fig. 3.17)

- Adjust treadmill speed to achieve an optimal step length (Moseley and Dean 2000). Treadmill speeds as low as 0.5 km/h or 0.1 m/s may be required for some patients. However, if speed is too slow, a rhythmical, cyclic gait pattern is not stimulated.
- Use the minimum amount of body weight support and arm support to maintain hip and knee extension of stance limb. A maximum of <30% body weight support appears to result in the most normal gait pattern. Any more than 50% body weight support results in the patient walking on their toes (Hesse et al. 1997).
- Decrease body weight support when patient is able to swing leg through.

TABLE 3.1	*Gait: clinical outcome studies*			
Reference	Subjects	Methods	Duration	Results
Hesse et al. 1995	7 Ss > 3 months post-stroke Mean age 60.3 Age range 52–72 yrs	A-B-A design **A**: PWS treadmill training **B**: Bobath	3 weeks each treatment **A** – 30 min/day **B** – 45 min/day	Gait velocity increased significantly during treatment **A** only
Sharp and Brouwer 1997	15 Ss > 9 months post-stroke Mean age 67 ± 10 yrs	Pre-test, post-test design Warm up, stretches, isokinetic strengthening exercises for paretic leg, cool down	6 weeks 3 days/week, 40 mins	Significant increases in muscle strength (p < 0.05), gait velocity (p < 0.05), overall physical activity scores (HAP) (p < 0.003) Improvements in stair climbing and Timed 'Up and Go' test were not significant No increase in spasticity Follow-up at 4 weeks – gait velocity and HAP scores continued to increase
Visintin et al. 1998	79 Ss (**E**: 43, **C**: 36) < 6 months post-stroke Mean age 65.2 ± 11.1 yrs	Randomized controlled trial Treadmill training: **E**: PWS up to 40% **C**: no PWS	6 weeks On average 15 min/day	79% of **E** Ss were training without PWS at end of study **E** scored significantly higher than **C** on Berg Balance Scale (p = 0.001), overground gait velocity (p = 0.02), overground walking endurance (p = 0.01) Follow-up at 3 months: **E** group continued to have significantly higher scores for overground gait velocity (p = 0.006)
Duncan et al. 1998	20 Ss 30–90 days post-stroke Mean age **C**: 67.8 ± 7.2 yrs **E**: 67.5 ± 9.6 yrs	Randomized controlled trial **E**: Exercise programme (warm-up, stretches, assisted/resisted exercises, balance, progressive walking or bicycle ergometer, functional activities with upper limb) **C**: Usual care (highly variable in intensity, frequency and duration. No subject received endurance training)	12 weeks (8 of which were therapist supervised) 3 days/week, 1.5 hours	Significant differences in gait speed*, Fugl-Meyer scores for lower extremity* between **E** and **C**. Changes in Berg score, 6 min walk test favoured **E** but were not significant. No between-group differences in Barthel Index, Jebsen Test of Hand Function, Lawton ADL Scale, MOS-36, apart from Physical Function Scale

(Continued)

TABLE 3.1 *(Continued)*

Reference	Subjects	Methods	Duration	Results
Teixeira-Salmela et al. 1999	13 Ss 9 months post-stroke Mean age 69.42 ± 8.85 yrs	Randomized controlled pre-test, post-test design Warm up, aerobic exercises, lower limb strengthening, cool down	10 weeks 3 days/week	28.3% improvement in gait speed (p = 0.00); 37.4% improvement in stair climbing (stairs/min) (p = 0.00); 42.3% improvement in mean peak torque generated by all muscle groups of affected leg (p = 0.00); 39.2% improvement in functional activities on adjusted activity score (HAP) (p < 0.001) No increase in spasticity
Mercier et al. 1999	1 S 19 months post-stroke 39 yrs	Single case design Training on static dynamometer (S produced submaximal static forces in 16 sagittal plane directions with computer-generated feedback on direction and intensity of applied force)	6 weeks 3 days/week, 1 hour	Improvements in Timed 'Up-and-Go' test (26.9%), comfortable gait speed (72.0%), 2 min walk test (121.4%) Follow-up at 6 weeks – some loss of function which was still considerably improved compared with baseline values
Dean et al. 2000	9 Ss > 6 months post-stroke Mean age **E**: 68.8 ± 4.7 yrs **C**: 64.8 ± 3.3 yrs	Randomized pre-test, post-test group design **E**: Circuit training (reaching in sitting and standing, sit-to-stand, step-ups, heel lifts, isokinetic strengthening, treadmill walking, walking over obstacles, up and down slopes) **C**: Training of affected upper limb	4 weeks 3 days/week, 1 hour	**E** scored significantly higher than **C** on gait velocity and endurance, VGRF produced through affected leg in STS and number of repetitions in step test (p ≤ 0.05) Follow up at 2 months – improvements retained
Teixeira-Salmela et al. 2001	13 Ss > 9 months post-stroke Mean age 67.7 ± 9.2 yrs	Pre-test, post-test design Warm-up, aerobic exercises, lower extremity muscle strengthening, cool down	10 weeks 3 days/week	Gait speed increased 37.2%, associated with increases in cadence and stride length (p < 0.001) Post-training profiles showed that subjects generated higher power levels, with increases in positive work by ankle plantarflexors, hip flexor/extensor muscles

ADL, activities of daily living; C, control group; COG, centre of gravity; E, experimental group; HAP, Human Activity Profile; MOS-36, Medical Outcome Study-36 Health Status Measurement; PWS, partial body-weight support; Ss, subjects; STS, sit-to-stand; VGRF, vertical ground reaction force.

FIGURE 3.17   *(a,b) Treadmill training with supportive harness. (b) The physiotherapist assists with toe clearance and step length during swing phase of the paretic leg.*

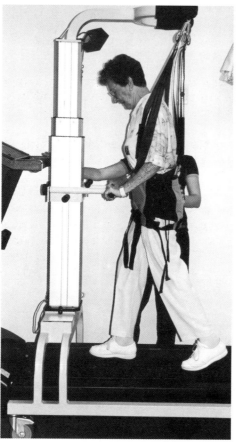 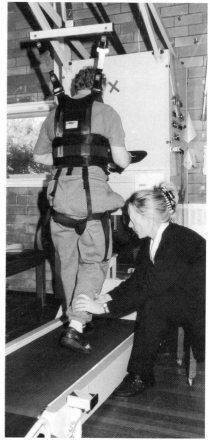

(a)   (b)

- Encourage patient to decrease arm support.
- Increase treadmill speed as soon as possible, using clinical judgement, ensuring that step length is not compromised, i.e. avoid an increase in cadence with a decrease in step length.

Check
Therapist may need to swing affected lower limb forward (Fig. 3.17b) and to stabilize the knee in stance to avoid hyperextension.

Walking on a treadmill with harness and no body weight support

- Increase speed, slope and duration (with warm-up and cool-down periods).
- Encourage decrease in arm support.

- Encourage increase in step length.
- Progress to treadmill walking without harness.

Note
This training, if done intensively, can increase endurance and aerobic fitness.

A recent study demonstrated that increasing treadmill speed in a structured manner (using an interval paradigm) led to significantly greater overground walking speed than training with limited progression (Pohl et al. 2002).

A useful description of the advantages and disadvantages of training walking on two commercially available machines (TR Spacetrainer* and Lite Gait†) has recently been published by clinicians experienced in their use (Crompton et al. 2001). Both the TR Spacetrainer and Lite-Gait can pull the patient up from sitting to standing. This is a useful feature for heavy, dependent patients and enables walking practice while complying with a no-lift policy. The Lite-Gait has the additional capacity of use without a treadmill for walking overground. The authors suggest that the harnesses provided need to be more adjustable and available in different sizes.

Overground walking

A Lite-Gait may help the individual make the transition from treadmill walking to walking overground. In particular, such an aid enables the individual to focus on walking without fear of falling. The Lite-Gait frame needs to be pushed by the therapist or aide since it is quite large and difficult to manoeuvre.

Walking forward   Starting with body erect, i.e. hips extended, patient steps forward with non-affected limb then affected limb.

- Initiating gait with affected limb in stance may set up the best conditions for the subsequent swing phase.
- The goal of the first few steps is for the patient to get the idea of producing a basic locomotor rhythm, while supporting, propelling and balancing the body mass.
- Steady patient at upper arm or at safety belt. Do not interfere with progression forward.
- Stand to the side of patient or if necessary behind, so as not to impede vision.
- Encourage patient to step out and take even steps. Foot prints on the floor may give the idea of an optimal step length and stride width and provide a stimulus to increasing step length and decreasing stride width.

*TR Equipment, S-57322 Trenas, Sweden.
†Mobility Research, Tempe, Arizona, USA.

Check
- Do not hold patient too firmly as this may offer resistance to translation of body mass forward or interfere with dynamic balance of the linked segments over the feet.
- Do not confuse patient – give only brief instructions during walking; for example, 'Take a longer step', 'Step out' or 'Just do it' may be enough to stimulate an attempt at a person's 'normal' walking.

Note
- Encourage patient to walk faster and take longer steps. This may be counter-intuitive to therapists who have worked with patients at relatively slow speeds with the intention of improving the quality of movement. It is difficult to develop an effective locomotor rhythm when walking very slowly. Slow walking disrupts the dynamics of the action in both able-bodied and disabled subjects and it has been demonstrated that when stroke patients walk at their maximum speed they show more symmetry (Wagenaar 1990). A significant relationship has been found between speed and gait parameters (Wagenaar and Beek 1992).
- An early goal for the patient can be to walk to the next appointment as an alternative to being transported in a wheelchair, or at least part of the way, with the explicit aim of increasing the distance walked each day.
- Patient selects a distance to walk independently and safely. It may only be the length of the bed initially. The goal is to walk this distance five times a day, increasing it as soon as possible. The number of sessions per day can be decreased as walking improves and distance increases. At home, the patient continues with a regime of increasing both distance walked and duration of walk.

As soon as the patient achieves a degree of independence, practice of negotiating ramps, stairs, kerbs and obstacles needs to be introduced. The evidence from follow-up studies is that few patients when discharged are able or confident enough to walk ouside the house (Hill et al. 1997). Patients are discharged from a flat, protected environment one day and expected to deal with the complexities of the built and natural environments the next day, often with little practice in such environments.

Soft tissue stretching

Preservation of the extensibility of soft tissue, in particular calf muscles and rectus femoris, is critical to the patient's ability to stand up, walk and stair walk. Preserving functional muscle length involves both passive and active stretching.

Brief sustained passive stretches are carried out immediately before exercise to decrease muscle stiffness. Active stretching occurs during the strengthening exercises given below.

Calf muscles: passive stretch in standing (Fig. 3.18a)
Rectus femoris: passive stretch in prone (Fig. 3.18b) or side lying

FIGURE 3.18   *(a) Stretching calf muscles in standing. Ensure the knee is straight with hips extended. (b) Stretching rectus femoris in prone. (c) Prolonged stretch to calf muscles on a tilt table. Note: positioning the R leg on a stool ensures paretic limb is loaded. (d) *Another way to stretch the calf muscles in standing that ensures the paretic limb is loaded. He also practises heel raise and lower in this position. (*Courtesy of K Schurr and S Dorsch, Physiotherapy Department, Bankstown-Lidcombe Hospital, Sydney.)*

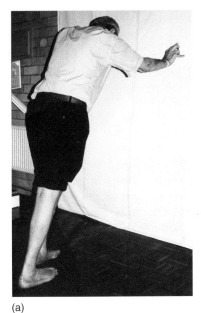

(a)

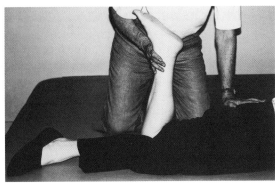

(b)

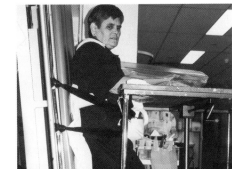

(c)

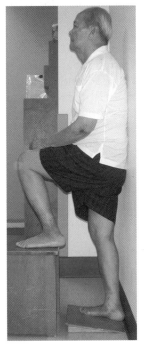

(d)

Note
- Hold stretch for approximately 20 s, relax, repeat 4–5 times.

Patients with severe muscle weakness who are physically inactive require periods of prolonged passive stretching during the day.

Soleus: in sitting (see Fig. 4.14)
Gastrocnemius–soleus: in standing on a tilt table (Fig. 3.18c)

Note
- Hold prolonged stretch for 30 min.
- Ensure that the tilt table is as erect as possible. Backward leaning should be avoided as it may interfere with regaining a perception of the vertical.

Eliciting muscle activity

Patients who are unable to produce sufficient muscle force to support the body mass in standing may require intervention to elicit muscle activity in lower limb extensor muscles. *Simple exercises*, such as the examples below, may stimulate muscle activity in a simplified context. Equipment such as an electrical stimulator, EMG biofeedback monitor and dynamometer may be required.

Electrical stimulation has a role in preserving muscle fibre contractility and, since it can be done with minimal supervision, increases the time during which muscles are being exercised. *Augmented sensory feedback* using an EMG signal in either visual or auditory form may assist the patient to activate weak muscles.

During *isokinetic dynamometry*, muscle activity may be elicited more easily in the eccentric mode. Isokinetic eccentric training has been shown to be superior to concentric training for the knee extensors (Engardt et al. 1995). However, weightbearing through the limbs and practice of walking itself are critical for promoting functional muscle activity in the lower limbs.

Simple active exercise

Simple exercises may give the patient the idea of activating muscles of the lower limb (e.g. hip extensors and quadriceps). Below are some examples (Fig. 3.19).

Hip extension. Supine, affected leg over side of bed, practise small-range hip extension by pushing down through heel (Fig. 3.19a).

Check
- Knee at less than 90° flexion.
- Discourage movement of the other leg and plantarflexion of affected leg.
- If the foot slides forward, stabilize foot on the floor by pushing down along the line of the shank.

FIGURE 3.19   *Simple exercises to elicit muscle activity. (a) Therapist may need to stabilize foot to prevent it from sliding forward. (b) Therapist flexes the knee to 90° and patient tries to activate the hamstrings to lower the leg slowly (eccentric mode). It may be possible to elicit an eccentric contraction before a concentric contraction.*

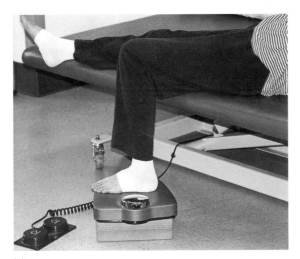

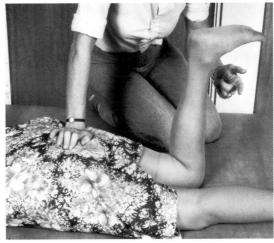

(a)

(b)

Note
- This exercise involves extensors of both hip (gluteus maximus and hamstrings) and knee (quadriceps). Hamstrings contraction, by its action at the knee, also stabilizes the foot on the ground, preventing it from sliding forward. Encourage patient to sustain muscle activity by counting.
- Incorporate muscle activity into loading the limb in standing.
- This exercise is particularly useful for assisting the patient to achieve alignment of the lower limb and pelvis in standing.

Patient sitting. Therapist extends the knee. Patient attempts to activate the quadriceps to lower the leg slowly and repeat several times.

Note
- It may be possible to elicit an eccentric contraction before a concentric contraction.

Walking sideways

This exercise involves practice of a simple locomotor action in which the number and extent of joint displacements to be controlled are reduced compared to forward walking.

Starting with feet together, patient steps laterally while supporting and balancing the body mass on one leg then the other. Swing and stance: hips should remain in neutral extension while stepping.

- Major angular displacements in the frontal plane are abduction and adduction at the hips.

Check

- Foot placement should progress in a straight line laterally.
- Placing toes along a line may give the patient the idea of this; however, continually looking down at the feet should be discouraged.

Note

- A patient can practise walking sideways unsupervised or with minimal supervision while resting hands on a raised bed rail (Fig. 3.20a).

Walking backward

Walking backward exercises the hip extensors particularly hamstrings.

| **FIGURE 3.20** | *(a) Walking sideways. Once she got the idea, she was able to practise semi-supervised. (b) Walking backward.* |

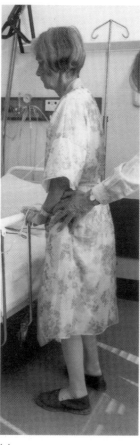 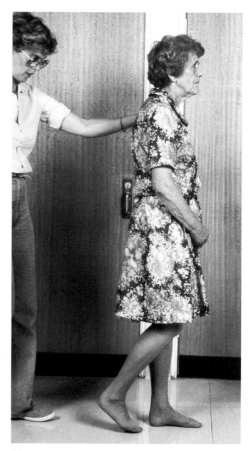

(a)   (b)

Note
- This exercise is only useful if the patient has some ability to flex the knee while extending the hip (Fig. 3.20b).
- The hamstrings act over two joints and must be critical to gait. For at least two reasons little is understood about their actual function: (1) paucity of investigation involving all three muscles in the group; (2) difficulty in interpreting the electrical activity of two joint muscles in functional actions.

Strength training

There is evidence that muscle weakness is modifiable in individuals following stroke (Bohannon and Andrews 1990, Sharp and Brouwer 1997, Teixeira-Salmela et al. 1999) and in the elderly (e.g. Fiatarone et al. 1993, Wolfson et al. 1993, Sherrington and Lord 1997). Increases in lower limb strength are associated with improved walking speed, with the greatest impact from strength increases in the weakest patients (Buchner et al. 1996). There is increasing evidence that quadriceps muscle strength is critical for dynamic stability in stance (Scarborough et al. 1999).

Emphasis in strength training is on lower limb muscles, in particular extensors such as gluteus maximus, gluteus medius, hamstrings, quadriceps and calf muscles, since these muscles provide the basic support, balance and propulsive functions during stance. Abductors and adductors are major muscles controlling lateral movement of the body mass. An increase in strength, however, may not be sufficient to bring about improved walking performance without practice of the action itself which is necessary for neural adaptation to task and context to be regained (Rutherford 1988).

Note
- Amount and intensity of strength training (i.e. resistance, repetitions) are graded to individual patient's ability.
- Patient is encouraged to work as hard as possible.
- As a general rule, a maximum number of repetitions should be performed, up to 10 without a rest and repeated three times. No increase in spasticity with strength training has been reported (Sharp and Brouwer 1997, Teixeira-Salmela et al. 1999).

Functional weightbearing exercises

These exercises are designed to improve force generation, speed of muscle contraction and synergistic muscle activity in the context of stance.

Simple loading of the affected limb

Generation of sufficient extensor force in the weightbearing limb is critical to support of the body mass while the contralateral leg is raised and lifted forward. The action in this exercise is similar to gait initiation (Brunt et al. 1999).

FIGURE 3.21 *Stepping with the non-paretic limb to load the paretic limb. (a) She has not moved far enough forward (inadequate hip extension and ankle dorsiflexion). (b) A better performance.*

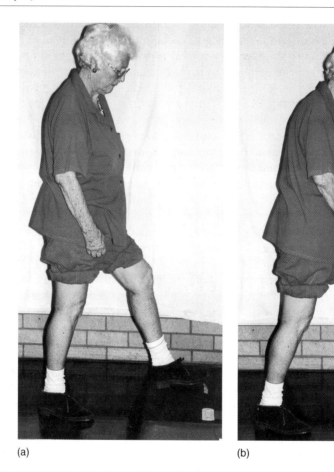

(a)   (b)

Standing, stepping forward and backward with the contralateral limb (Fig. 3.21). The body mass is moved diagonally and forward over the stance limb to place the contralateral foot on a step.

Check

- Ensure that stance hip extends (approximately 15°) and ankle dorsiflexes (shank rotates forward over foot).
- Step needs to be approximately 15 cm away from the toe of the stance limb (depending on height of individual) to encourage hip extension and forward movement of body mass. A footprint can be used to indicate how far to step.
- When stepping back, upper body should not flex forward over hip.
- If body mass cannot be supported over foot without the leg collapsing or the knee hyperextending, apply strapping or a splint to give some support to the knee while exercising (see Fig. 1.6b).

Note

- In standing, movement of the body mass laterally to the stance limb is preceded by movement of centre of pressure initially to the opposite side before it moves to the stance side (Rogers and Pai 1990). Since this exercise requires the coordination of forces produced by both legs, it is practised to both sides.
- Rapid stepping forward to place the non-paretic foot up on to a 15 cm step placed 15 cm in front of the stance limb, without transferring all the body weight, provides a particular challenge to mediolateral stability and to gluteus medius (Sims and Brauer 2000). This is, therefore, an important exercise for increasing strength of the gluteus medius and hip stability, a problem following stroke and a known source of falls. Previous studies have demonstrated that the hip adductors (Rogers and Pai 1993) and superior portion of the gluteus maximus of the stepping limb can also assist in control of the frontal plane movement.

Step-up/step-down exercises

These exercises train hip, knee and ankle extensors to work together, both concentrically and eccentrically, to raise and lower the body mass. Step-up exercises also train ankle dorsiflexors.

Forward step-ups (Fig.3.22a)
Foot of affected leg on a step (approximately 8 cm high). Forward and upward translation of the body mass over the foot with upper body remaining erect.

- Forces produced by the back limb move the body mass in a forward and upward direction over the forward foot (ankle dorsiflexion). Extension of hip, knee and ankle of the affected limb raises the body mass as the back foot is lifted on to the step.
- When stepping back down, flexion of hip, knee and ankle of support leg lowers the body mass until the foot touches the ground.

Check

- Therapist places the foot on to the step if necessary.
- Ensure that the shank rotates forward at the ankle (dorsiflexion). This brings the body mass forward over the foot.
- Shank and foot may need to be stabilized to provide a stable shank over which the knee can extend and prevents knee hyperextension.

Note

- Major extensor force generation of support limb is relatively evenly distributed over the three lower limb joints in forward step-ups (Agahari et al. 1996).

Lateral step-ups (Fig. 3.22b)
Foot of affected leg on a step. Step up with unaffected limb with body mass remaining erect.

- Extension of hip, knee and ankle of affected limb raises the body mass, and adduction of hip moves the body mass laterally as the contralateral foot is lifted on to the step.

FIGURE 3.22   *Step-ups: (a) forward; (b) lateral; (c) step-downs. (d) The therapist holds her foot to stop external rotation as she steps down. Note (a) and (b) can be practised in a harness.*

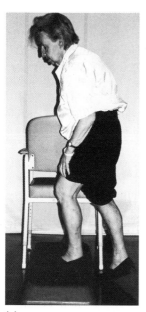

(a)

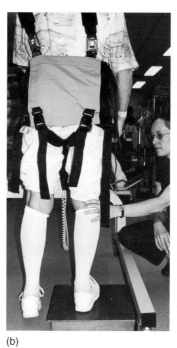

(b)

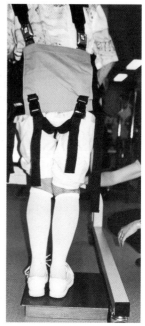

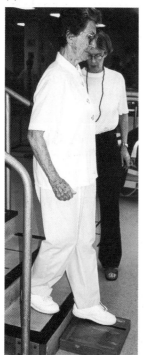

(c)

(d)

- When stepping down, flexion at hip, knee and ankle lowers the body mass until the foot touches the ground.

Check
- Therapist places the foot on the step if necessary.

Note
- Major extensor force generation of the support limb in lateral step-ups is concentrated at the knee with some involvement at the ankle, and strong adductor/abductor forces at hip (Agahari et al. 1996).
- Forward and lateral step-ups can be practised in a harness.

Forward step-downs (Fig. 3.22c)
Both feet on step, step down with the unaffected leg.

- Body mass remains supported and balanced on the affected limb which flexes at hip, knee and ankles to lower body mass for foot placement on to the floor.
- When stepping up backward, hip, knee and ankle of the support limb extend to raise body mass while foot is lifted back on to step.
- Force is also produced by the front limb to move body mass backward and add propulsive force to the upward movement.

Note
- Do not allow the support (paretic) limb to externally rotate during step-downs (Fig. 3.22d). This happens if soleus is stiff or contracted.

Progress step-up and step-down exercises by increasing the height of the step, number of repetitions and speed, by stepping without stopping (i.e. no foot placement) (Fig. 3.23), and by practising reciprocal stair walking (average riser height 17 cm).

Heels raise and lower

Since the major power generator during the gait cycle is ankle plantarflexion during push-off (Winter 1987) every effort is made to strengthen and train plantarflexor activity. This pre-swing muscle activity accelerates the lower limb into swing phase. During stance phase, ankle plantarflexors also contribute to ankle and knee stability and to the control of forward translation of the body mass over the foot.

Forefeet on step, heels free (Fig. 3.24). Heels are lowered as far as possible then raised to plantigrade.

Check
- Hips and knees remain extended throughout. Knee flexion may indicate that patient is having difficulty coordinating synergistic activity of knee extensors which contract to counter flexion of the knee by two-joint gastrocnemius.
- Ensure weight is over affected leg.
- Running shoes should be worn.

FIGURE 3.23   *Repetitive semi-supervised continuous lateral step-ups. Note the paretic limb is on the edge of the block to prevent foot placement. (Courtesy of K Schurr and S Dorsch, Physiotherapy Department, Bankstown-Lidcombe Hospital, Sydney.)*

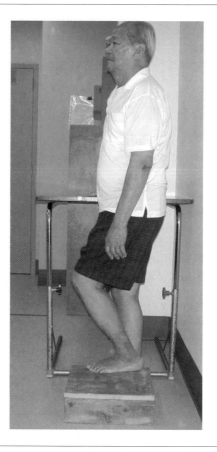

Note

- Increased stiffness in ankle plantarflexors may be largely due to mechanical changes in muscle fibres (e.g. Dietz et al. 1981).
- As strength increases the exercise is done on one leg (Fig. 3.24b).
- Increased stiffness and contracture of calf muscles commonly have a negative effect on function. Maintaining length and flexibility of these muscles is a priority.
- This exercise places an active stretch on the plantarflexors as the heels are lowered (eccentric contraction). It also gives the idea of activating the plantarflexors (concentric contraction) from a lengthened position similar to that of push-off at end of stance.
- It is clinically evident that this exercise decreases stiffness in the calf muscles. There is no evidence that the exercise increases spasticity.
- Walking up a ramp is another exercise for stretching and strengthening calf muscles (Fig. 3.25).

FIGURE 3.24   *(a) Heels raise to plantigrade and lower to strengthen and stretch plantarflexors. This exercise trains the calf muscles specifically at the length required for push-off at end of stance. Patient is holding on to a stable object. (b) With improvement in strength and skill, the exercise is performed on one leg.*

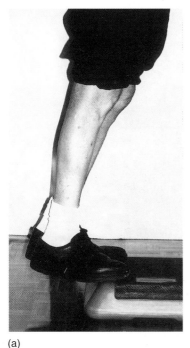
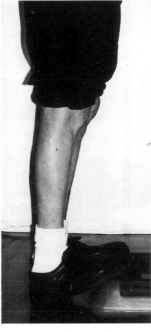
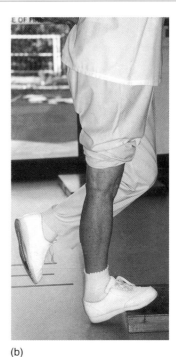

(a)

(b)

Non-weightbearing strength training

These progressive resistance exercises are designed to improve force generation, speed and sustainability of muscle contraction (Fig. 3.26). However, as Scarborough and colleagues (1999) comment, integrating strength changes into meaningful function needs practice of the action itself.

Isokinetic dynamometer
Elastic band resistance exercises

Note
- These exercises can be done as part of circuit training.
- Encourage patient to do a maximum number of repetitions, up to 10, without stopping. Repeat three times. Aim to train at 80% maximum isometric voluntary contraction (Ch. 7).
- Muscles apart from the target group are also active as synergists (e.g. as stabilizers). Some increase in strength in these muscles also can be expected (Fiatarone et al. 1990).
- Increase resistance on the dynamometer by upgrading to the next rubber band. Bands are coloured, each colour representing a certain tension, yellow has the least tension, black the most (Ch. 7).

FIGURE 3.25   *Walking up a ramp. She needs to be encouraged to use her calf muscles to push off.*

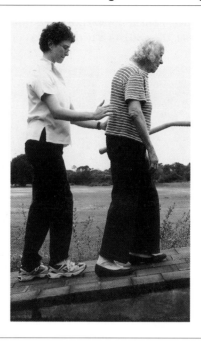

FIGURE 3.26   *Some examples of semi-supervised exercising. (a) The MOTOmed provides resistance or assistance in response to the patient's performance (Reck, Reckstrasse 1-1, D-88422 Betzenweiller, Germany). (b) Exercising on the Orthotron to strengthen knee extensor muscles concentrically and eccentrically or isometrically (Cybex Human Performance Rehabilitation, 2100 Smithtown Ave, Ronkon Koma, NY 11779, USA).*

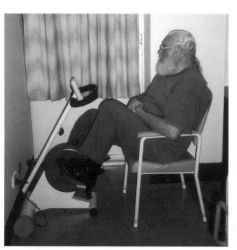

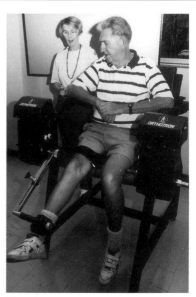

(a)   (b)

FIGURE 3.26   *(c) The elastic band should be under tension at all parts of the range.*

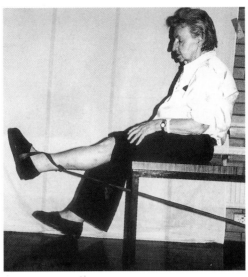

(c)

Maximizing skill

Walking involves a basic locomotor pattern which is normally adapted in the presence of obstacles such as kerbs and steps, speed demands and other environmental factors. The opportunity for challenging and variable practice is critical to optimize performance in everyday terrains and contexts. Variable practice (Fig. 3.27) involves walking in a busy corridor, walking at speeds required to cross a street safely, practice of stepping on and off moving walkways and escalators, walking through automatic doors, under and over obstacles, up and down ramps and kerbs, under different lighting conditions. The patient needs practice in identifying potential threats to balance and making the appropriate avoidance strategies. The ability to increase walking speed to avoid a moving obstacle is an important safety issue. A recent study has demonstrated the difficulty patients have in stepping over obstacles of different heights and widths (Said et al. 1999). Patients need to practise coping with this common everyday hazard (Fig. 3.28). Turning while walking, stopping, and reciprocal stair walking all need to be practised.

Increasing aerobic capacity has been found not only to improve cardiorespiratory function in stroke patients but also to increase functional ability (Ch. 7). Treadmill walking, bicycle ergometry and adapted cycle ergometry are used to increase fitness.

FIGURE 3.27   *Training flexibility by practising on an obstacle course.*

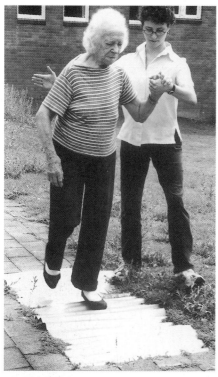

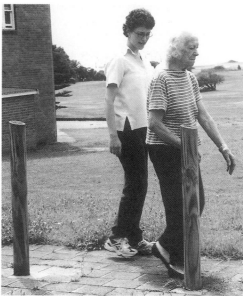

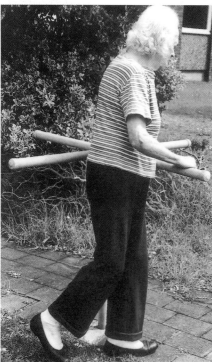

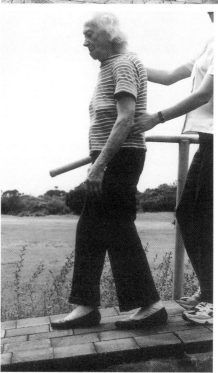

FIGURE 3.28 *Walking over obstacles can be started once the person can walk independently. This figure illustrates some common difficulties. (a) She steadies herself with the rail, and has positioned her L foot so only a small step is needed. Note the path of the R limb – R hip abducts excessively, hip flexion and ankle dorsiflexion are reduced. (b) She has increased step length and can clear the obstacle without needing support. (c) She catches her heel on the flexible obstacle. Poor placement of supporting (trail) foot may contribute to this. Practice should include walking over wider obstacles requiring both limbs to step over. Obstacle crossing provides practice of balancing on one leg, controlling the body mass as it moves forward and controlling step length and foot.*

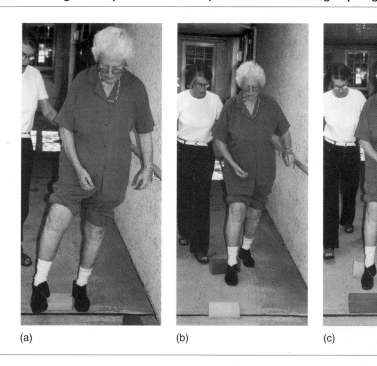

(a)   (b)   (c)

MEASUREMENT

An important concern for a therapist is to determine which aspects of performance should be measured to make a valid assessment of progress. Observational analysis gives uncertain results. Valid and reliable tests enable the documentation of the patient's progress and the effects of intervention. Standardized protocols should be followed in administering all walking tests. Even the level of encouragement provided by a test supervisor to subjects undergoing walking tests can have a large effect on their performance (Guyatt et al. 1984). The tests listed below have been shown to be reliable if performed under standardized conditions.

Walking velocity may be the most important objective clinical measure of functional ability. It is simple to administer and is easily understood and accepted by patients. Almost all other gait measures are speed dependent (Andriacci et al. 1977); for example, as speed increases so does the extent of hip extension and amount of push-off. Another critical measure involves the testing of walking ability outside the house, within the community.

Functional tests

These include:

- *10 m walk test*
- *6- or 12-minute walk test* (McGavin et al. 1976, Guyatt et al. 1985)
- *Motor Assessment Scale:* Walking item (Carr et al. 1985)
- *Timed 'Up and Go' Test* (TUG) (Podsialo and Richardson 1991)
- *Step Test* (Hill et al. 1996)
- *Obstacle Course Test* (Means et al. 1996)

10 m walk.   The subject is timed while walking between two marks on the floor, using a stopwatch. Velocity is calculated, as distance/time, in m/s. To avoid the effects of acceleration and deceleration, the subject is timed only over the middle 10 m of a 14 m walkway. The 10 m walk test is useful in the early stages as a guide to progress. It should not be taken to reflect functional walking as it involves a very short distance. This has been confirmed recently (Dean et al. 2001).

Other clinically feasible spatiotemporal measures that yield valid quantitive data include include step and stride length, stride width and cadence. Stride and step lengths are measured using foot switches, an instrumented walkway or a Stride Analyser*. Attaching felt pens to the heels can provide a simple and inexpensive method of collecting these data.

The 6- or 12-minute walk test   measures the distance walked in 6 or 12 minutes. These tests are used extensively in individuals with cardiorespiratory conditions. The 6-minute test is particularly useful since there are some normative data available for comparison (Enright and Sherrill 1998). This test may provide a more realistic appraisal of function and enable an accelerated programme of training to prepare the patient for independent life after discharge.

TUG.   Patient stands up from a chair, walks 3 m, turns around, returns to chair and sits down. Time taken to complete the test is measured with a stopwatch. Able-bodied subjects are able to perform this test in less than 30 s.

Step test   is used to evaluate the ability to support and balance the body mass on the affected lower limb while stepping with the unaffected limb. Starting with feet parallel and 5 cm in front of a 7.5 cm high block, patient steps forward and backward repeatedly as fast as possible for 15 s. The number of steps is counted.

Where a biomechanical laboratory is attached to the rehabilitation centre, comparative *biomechanical tests* can be used to evaluate progress.

*B & L Engineering, 3002 Dow Ave, Suite 416, Tustin CA 92780, USA.

Biomechanical tests

Variables to be tested include:

- angular displacements
- ground reaction forces
- moments of force, power, energy.

Matching observations with biomechanical test results enables physiotherapists to get feedback on and improve their observational skills.

Calf muscle length test

A reliable method of measuring passive ankle dorsiflexion in a clinical setting is described by Moseley and Adams (1991). It involves the use of skin surface markers (head of 5th metatarsal, lateral malleolus and head of fibula), polaroid photography and the application of a known torque, using a specially designed template. The knee is held at a constant angle in extension with a velcro strap over the shank (see Fig. 7.4).

Physiological tests

Physiological tests have shown that speed and energy costs during gait are valid parameters in assessment of walking capacity. Fitness is typically tested using a treadmill, bicycle ergometer or MOTOmed Pico Leg Trainer. Fitness tests are described in Chapter 7. The fitness test most specific to gait uses the treadmill. Monitoring heart rate is a simple method of ensuring that exercise is sufficiently vigorous.

NOTES

Treadmill training

The rationale for considering treadmill training in rehabilitation of gait follow-ing stroke arose from animal research investigating motor control mechanisms in lesioned animals (Grillner and Shik 1973). There have been several recent clinical studies showing the positive effects of treadmill training on individuals with stroke, although such training has yet to be widely used in clinical set-tings. Several studies have demonstrated effects superior to those obtained by neurodevelopmental therapy (Bobath) intervention (Fig. 3.29) (Richards et al. 1993, Hesse et al. 1995, Pohl et al. 2002). There is no evidence that treadmill training causes 'mass synergies' or increases spasticity (Hesse et al. 1995, Hesse 1999), a concern which may be expressed by clinicians.

Many of the gait deviations seen in stroke patients result from their inability to adequately bear weight through the affected lower limb during the loading phase of the gait cycle (Carr and Shepherd 1998). Treadmill training using a

FIGURE 3.29 *Means and standard deviations of walking velocity over time. Walking velocity increased during treadmill training (A1, A2) but did not increase during conventional therapy. B, Bobath. (Reproduced from Hesse et al. 1995, with permission.)*

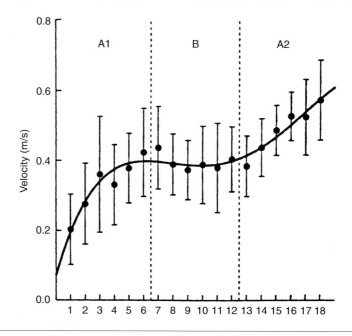

harness for partial body weight support (PWS) seems to address this problem and can allow a patient with severe weakness of lower limb extensor muscles to go through the gait cycle with some assistance from the therapist. The harness also provides a sense of security for the patient who need not fear falling.

Hesse and colleagues (1997) investigated the influence of various amounts of PWS compared with full weightbearing. Their data suggest that 30% PWS results in the most normal gait. A recent randomized clinical trial involving stroke subjects reported better outcomes for the experimental group who trained with PWS (decreased as subjects' gait improved) compared with subjects who trained on the treadmill bearing full weight on the lower limbs (Visintin et al. 1998). At the end of 6 weeks, 79% of PWS subjects were training with full weight. This group scored significantly higher than the non-PWS group on overground walking speed and endurance and on balance using the Berg Scale (Table 3.1).

The major benefits from training on a treadmill with PWS include the following.

- Task-specific gait training can be started early after a stroke even before the patient is able to support 100% of the body mass on the affected lower limb.
- The patient can practise the complete gait cycle, i.e. support, balance and stepping.

- Inter- and intralimb timing parameters are practised before the patient has sufficient muscle strength to fully support body weight.
- Loading the affected limb can be varied according to ability to support weight.
- The harness eliminates the need to use adaptive movements that favour an asymmetrical gait.
- Speed of the treadmill can be increased, thereby stimulating the patient to walk faster.
- If performed intensively (progressively increasing speed, slope and duration), without PWS, treadmill walking can increase muscular endurance and cardiovascular fitness (Ch. 7).

Treadmill walking represents a biomechanical stimulus that may lead to improved motor control. There are many similarities between treadmill and overground walking (Strathy et al. 1983, Murray et al. 1985, Arsenault et al. 1986). A biomechanical study investigating the equivalence of treadmill walking with PWS and overground walking in healthy subjects at different speeds and different percentages of support reported only minor differences (Finch et al. 1991). The major differences between treadmill walking and overground walking are in the visual and kinesthetic information perceived by the walker. Therefore, once a patient is able to walk unaided, training incorporates walking in more natural environments and for different goals.

Certain characteristics of treadmill walking are probably beneficial to the training of gait by externally forcing a rhythmical and dynamic gait pattern. The moving belt 'forces' hip extension and ankle plantarflexion in support phase. With the treadmill moving at a reasonable speed, the relatively strong stretch applied to the hip flexor and calf muscles at the end of stance may enhance muscle activity for swing.

As Hesse (1999) points out, further comparative studies are needed to meet the criteria for evidence-based practice (e.g. large randomized controlled multicentre trials). Meanwhile treadmill training in neurorehabilitation has a sound scientific rationale, and many clinical studies have compared its efficacy with the lack of efficacy of conventional intervention in the training of gait. We suggest that treadmill walking is likely to be maximally effective when combined with functional lower limb strength training and practice of walking overground.

Electrical stimulation

Electrical stimulation (ES) has had a long and varied history in rehabilitation post-stroke. There is evidence that ES has the potential for positive effects on muscle. These include stimulating muscle fibre contractility, increasing strength (Glanz et al. 1996), decreasing contracture (Hazlewood et al. 1994) and preventing a build up of connective tissue (Williams et al. 1988).

Early in stroke, while the patient is relatively inactive, ES can be used as an adjunct to exercise to maintain the integrity of muscles. It should be given in particular to those muscles likely to adapt negatively to physical inactivity (e.g. calf muscles, quadriceps, tibialis anterior) as a means of stimulating muscle fibre contractility. ES units are relatively inexpensive, extremely durable and reliable and can be used by the patient or a family member after instruction.

A meta-analysis (Glanz et al. 1996) of four randomized controlled trials testing the effect of functional electrical stimulation (FES) on muscle force post-stroke, supports its efficacy in improving muscle strength. Studies of FES-assisted gait, involving the use of multichannel stimulators (e.g. Malezic et al. 1987, Bogataj et al. 1989), have also reported to improved aspects of gait performance. Whether or not either of these effects is lasting or transfers into clinically significant improvement is so far unclear.

Aids and orthoses

An *orthosis* is defined by the International Society for Prosthetics and Orthotics as an externally applied device used to modify structural and functional characteristics of the neuromuscular system. The most commonly prescribed orthosis with a view to improving gait is an *ankle–foot orthosis (AFO)*.

A major consideration in determining the use of an orthotic device is that the device, by constraining motion at one joint, alters body mechanics which necessitates adaptations at other joints. These adaptations may increase energy cost during gait. One study compared a group of able-bodied subjects who wore either a narrow or wide semi-rigid plastic AFO set in neutral position (Balmaseda et al. 1988). When walking with either AFO there was a decrease in the duration of stance phase of the ipsilateral leg, centre of pressure was shifted to a more lateral position throughout stance, and the point of impact at heel contact was more posterior. In these subjects the magnitude of vertical force at toe-off was increased, indicating that more muscle force was required to overcome the resistance of the AFO and propel the body mass forward. An AFO has, therefore, the potential to impact negatively on aspects of gait performance.

Research into the potential of AFOs to control foot/ankle mechanics during gait, and thereby improve gait performance following stroke, has equivocal results and the issue of whether or not to prescribe some form of AFO remains controversial. There are several descriptive studies comparing the effects of different types of AFO on aspects of gait after stroke (Lehmann et al. 1987, Burdett et al. 1988, Beckerman et al. 1996). However, for methodological and theoretical reasons it is difficult to draw specific conclusions from these studies. One of the problems in evaluating this literature is the theoretical assumption that it is calf muscle spasticity that is impeding gait, and that the AFO will affect foot position. Where the term spasticity is used in a generic sense, it is not clear whether the problem is soft tissue contracture, increased muscle stiffness or hyperreflexia.

Rigid or semi-rigid AFOs are often prescribed for patients with 'foot drop'. Both anterior tibial muscle weakness and contracture of calf muscles can interfere with ankle dorsiflexion during swing phase, impeding toe clearance and heel contact. Although a rigid AFO holds the foot in some dorsiflexion during swing, it imposes a mechanical resistance to plantarflexion for push-off. Use of a muscle stimulator to produce anterior tibial muscle activation, strengthening exercises and stretching for calf muscles are likely to be more effective for such a problem and enable a more energy-efficient gait.

From the evidence so far, hinged AFOs that allow dorsiflexion and/or plantarflexion are preferable to fixed orthoses. Ankle orthoses that provide mediolateral stability at the subtalar joint without resistance to dorsiflexion or plantarflexion, such as an Air Stirrup Brace*, may be useful for patients whose gait is impeded by such instability (Burdett et al. 1988).

Until there is more research that addresses these issues, we suggest that the essential prerequisites in prescribing an AFO, should it be considered necessary, are that:

- biomechanical gait mechanisms underlying gait dysfunction have been identified
- relative contribution of active and passive soft tissue components has been determined
- orthotic device fits, neither allowing unwanted movement nor restricting desired motion, and can be shown to improve the effectiveness and efficiency of gait for that individual.

Where plantarflexor muscles are very stiff, hyperreflexic and/or there is soft tissue contracture, low-dose botulinum toxin or serial casting combined with walking training may be necessary. An AFO is unlikely to produce a measurably more effective gait under these conditions. Reiter and colleagues (1998), using a combination of low-dose botulinum toxin and ankle–foot taping, reported a decrease in Ashworth scores and increases in gait velocity and step length.

Walking aids

Walking aids – parallel bars, walking frame, three/four point stick (tripod, quadrupod), stick, an assistant's arm – have a number of predictable drawbacks. They unload the weightbearing structures of the lower limb and can increase muscle activity and support in the upper limb (Winter et al. 1993). They may compromise an already reduced gait velocity.

Walking sticks or *canes* have been prescribed following stroke for many years although their efficacy in increasing stability and improving gait has not been documented. It is only recently that the effects of different types of sticks have been compared. A quadrupod stick offers no advantage over a standard stick in terms of standing balance (Milczarek et al. 1993) or in spatiotemporal variables in walking (Joyce and Kirby 1991). In a comparative study of stroke patients walking with and without a stick there was no increase in speed with the stick compared with no stick (Kuan et al. 1999). However, step and stride length with the affected leg were increased and cadence and stride width decreased when the stick was used, suggesting that a stick may have a greater effect on spatial variables (stride length and stride width) than on temporal variables (speed and gait phases). A recent study found that individuals post-stroke

*Aircast Inc., PO Box T, Summit, NJ 07901, USA.

walking with stick assistance relied mostly on the unaffected limb for propulsion, while using the affected limb and stick for braking (Chen et al. 2001).

Walking with a *pick up walking frame* is constrained by the structure of the frame. There are periods of motion and of stasis with the result that gait velocity is markedly decreased and hips remain flexed (Crosbie 1993). Roller walkers, if they are high enough to prevent hip flexion, may be a better option for the very frail individual, who should be encouraged to take longer steps and to increase the distance walked each day.

Parallel bars are designed for arm support with partial weightbearing through the lower limb(s). They are, therefore, useful for training patients with spinal cord injuries who have to rely on upper limbs for support and balance. Although sometimes used in stroke rehabilitation, walking in parallel bars has major disadvantages, encouraging use of non-paretic limbs and preventing the regaining of appropriate balance mechanisms.

Propelling a *one-arm drive wheelchair* with the intact arm and leg may promote early independence in getting from one place to another. However, it focuses attention on the intact side and is likely to contribute to learned non-use.

In summary, although all walking aids impose some mechanical constraint, a simple walking stick interferes least with balance and walking yet provides some stability (Kuan et al. 1999). Further research on the effects on gait of different types of orthoses and walking aids would assist clinicians to prescribe an aid, or not, with some understanding of the potential mechanical and physiological effects.

4 *Standing up and sitting down*

CHAPTER CONTENTS

- **Introduction**
- **Biomechanical description**
  Standing up
  Sitting down
- **Age-related changes**
- **Analysis of motor performance**
  Research findings
  Observational analysis
- **Guidelines for training**
  Standing up and sitting down practice

Soft tissue stretching
Eliciting muscle activity
Strength training
Maximizing skill

- **Measurement**
  Functional tests
  Biomechanical tests
- **Notes**
  Augmented feedback

INTRODUCTION

The ability to stand up (STS) and sit down (SIT) is essential to an independent lifestyle. Standing up is a prerequisite for other actions such as overground and stair walking which require the ability to get into the standing position. Its incidence in daily life is high, an early study reporting that able-bodied individuals stand up on average four times an hour (McLeod et al. 1975).

Standing up is one of the most mechanically demanding daily activities, requiring greater range of motion at the knee and higher moments of force at both hip and knee than gait or stair climbing (Andriacchi et al. 1980, Berger et al. 1988). Lower limb muscle strength, balance and control of the total body segmental linkage are therefore critical for effective performance.

Inability to stand up is common early on following stroke and difficulty performing the action may continue beyond discharge, limiting independence and participation in everyday life. Inability to stand up independently predisposes the individual to further decreases in muscle strength and physical fitness, and to adaptive soft tissue changes, particularly in soleus muscle, associated with disuse and physical inactivity.

Difficulty standing up is reported to be a common source of falls (e.g. Sorock and Pomerantz 1980, Yoshida et al. 1983, Tinetti et al. 1988), with a report that 20% of falls occurred while getting out of a wheelchair and 22% while getting out of bed (Sorock and Pomerantz 1980). The tendency to fall during attempts at standing up is not surprising given the deficits in muscle strength and postural stability following stroke, and lack of independence in standing up has been found to be one of the most likely factors associated with an increased risk of institutionalization (Branch and Meyers 1987).

Despite the significance of this action to daily life, until recently there has been little focus in clinical practice on the specific training of STS and even less on SIT. We have argued for some time (Carr and Shepherd 1987, 1998) the importance of intensive practice designed to improve the performance of STS/SIT, together with methods of increasing lower limb muscle strength and weightbearing through the paretic limb. Over the last decade there has been more clinical focus due in large part to an increasing number of biomechanical studies reporting the principal dynamic features of the action and some clinical studies showing that training can be effective in improving motor performance (see Table 4.1).

BIOMECHANICAL DESCRIPTION

Standing up

The majority of biomechanical studies have focused on movement in the sagittal plane, using two-dimensional video analysis systems with subjects standing up with feet on one or two force plates. Results of investigations performed in the laboratory provide biomechanical data which are used to guide the development and testing of training protocols. These data also enable a rational analysis of a patient's performance. Without such information about the dynamic characteristics of the action and the effects of different task and environmental conditions, the therapist can only guess at what constitutes 'normal' movement.

STS requires translation of the body mass in a horizontal and vertical direction from a relatively stable sitting position with thighs and feet as base of support, to a period of relative instability when the thighs leave the seat and the feet become the base of support (Fig. 4.1). Generating the angular and linear momentum to perform the horizontal to vertical translatory movements of the body mass is potentially destabilizing. Postural stability is most threatened around the time the thighs lift off the seat. At this point, angular displacement of the relatively large upper body (head, arms and trunk) pivoting at the hips changes from flexion to extension, and linear momentum of the body mass changes from horizontal to vertical. Braking forces are required to control horizontal momentum, ensuring a stable transition from horizontal to vertical movement. Translation of the body mass forward depends on strength and control of muscles crossing hip, knee and ankle. These muscles generate the necessary forces to support and balance the body mass while at the same time propelling it vertically. In everyday life, such factors as foot position and weight distribution between the two feet vary, adapting to task and environmental demands.

For ease of description, STS can be divided into a pre-extension and an extension phase (Carr and Gentile 1994, Shepherd and Gentile 1994), the transition occurring at thighs-off (TO). Although other methods of identifying phases of the action have been reported, this may be the simplest division for clinical purposes. In reality, the pre-extension and extension phases form one continuous

FIGURE 4.1   *Standing up. Horizontal movement of the body mass: forward rotation of the trunk at the hips and of the shank at the ankles. Vertical movement: extension of hips, knees and ankles.*

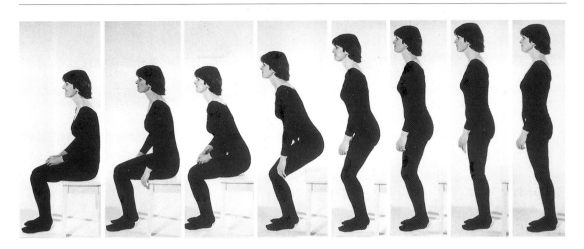

translatory movement of the body mass horizontally, changing to movement vertically without a pause (Fig. 4.2).

Kinematics and kinetics

In the *pre-extension phase* the feet are placed well back so that when the upper body is rotated forward at the hips, lower limb muscle activity and segmental movement generate the posteriorly directed component of ground reaction forces, thus propelling the body mass forward. Biomechanical investigations of STS typically model the pelvis and spine as one segment called 'trunk' in order to capture the action of the upper body as it rotates forward. These segments act together functionally as a 'virtual' segment with minimal motion occurring within the spine itself and between the spine and pelvis. Rotation forward of this virtual segment by flexion at the hips, together with rotation of the shank at the ankle by dorsiflexion, move the body mass forward over the feet. That is, the trunk and shank segments act as a functional unit for bringing the body mass forward (Pai and Rogers 1991). In the *extension phase*, vertical movement is brought about by extension at hips, knees and ankles in a typical sequence of onsets, the knees starting to extend (at TO) before the hips and ankles (Shepherd and Gentile 1994).

Since the feet are on the supporting surface, horizontal and vertical *ground reaction forces* (GRFs) play an important part in the movement. Prior to TO, horizontal GRFs generated in a posterior direction (approximately 10% body weight) serve to propel the body mass forward. These are followed by anteriorly directed forces to brake the forward momentum. At TO, there is a rapid rise in amplitude of vertical GRFs to a peak of approximately 150% of body weight depending on factors such as speed (Fig. 4.3). These forces decrease

FIGURE 4.2 *Superimposed stick figures graphed from x/y coordinates. Shoulder and knee paths can be seen. Note knee moves forward early in movement (ankle dorsiflexion and knee flexion) and then backward as hips, knees and ankles extend. Final standing alignment: hip marker is in front of ankle marker (lateral malleolus).*

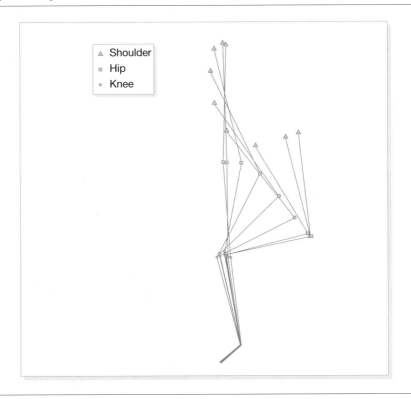

FIGURE 4.3 *Typical vertical (z) ground reaction force profile of an able-bodied subject standing up at a preferred speed of approximately 1.5 s. Vertical line indicates thighs-off. Arrows indicate movement start and end.*

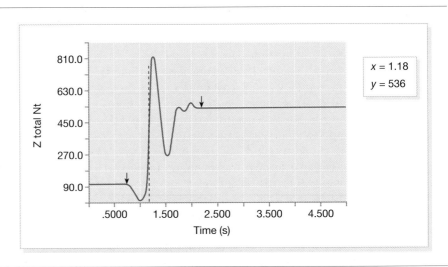

after TO and stabilize at body weight when standing is reached. This pattern reflects the requirement to generate force greater than body weight to accelerate the body vertically.

The major extensor muscle forces occur therefore at TO. As in the stance phase of gait, peak extensor *moments of force* at individual joints can vary cooperatively. However, for each limb overall, support moment (an algebraic summation of hip, knee and ankle moments of force) of approximately four times the body mass peaking at TO, propels the body mass vertically (Shepherd and Gentile 1994).

STS under different conditions

Identifying the fundamental biomechanical determinants of STS enables the clinician to organize training with a greater understanding of the major dynamic interactions occurring within the segmental linkage. Certain biomechanical variables under constrained conditions across different age groups have been found to be remarkably consistent and repeatable within and between subjects, for example, angular displacements, sequence of joint onsets, linear paths of body parts and support moments of force.

However, for daily life, flexibility of performance is essential. Normally we adapt the action to the prevailing internal (pregnancy, joint pain) and external (seat type, task) constraints. For example, the extent of angular rotation varies depending on height of stool in relation to leg length, extent of thigh support and type of chair. Investigations of several external conditions of relevance to clinical practice (foot placement, initial trunk position, speed of movement, seat height) have been found to affect the dynamics of the action in ways that could impact negatively for a patient with motor system impairments including muscle weakness. Understanding these effects makes it possible to set up optimal practice conditions for patients who are having difficulty performing the action effectively.

Foot placement.   Several studies have investigated the mechanical effects of different foot placements (Fleckenstein et al. 1988, Shepherd and Koh 1996), i.e. the angles at ankle and knee prior to the start of the action. Prior to standing the feet are normally drawn back so that they are placed posterior to the knees. The position of the feet affects the distance the body mass has to be moved forward. Laboratory studies have shown that the further forward the feet, the greater the magnitude of hip flexion and the greater the velocity required to overcome the potential braking force created by the anterior foot position (Vander Linden et al. 1994) and to move the body mass the additional distance forward (Shepherd and Koh 1996). Anterior foot placement was shown to be associated with an increase in peak hip moments of force and an increase in the duration of the extension phase, with muscle force therefore being sustained for a longer period than when the feet were back (Vander Linden et al. 1994, Shepherd and Koh 1996).

The clinical implication from these studies is that for ease of standing up the most biomechanically effective foot position is with the ankles at approximately

FIGURE 4.4   *Preferred foot placement is, on average, 10 cm from a vertical line drawn from the middle of the knee joint (approximately 75° dorsiflexion). Distance was calculated from Shepherd and Koh 1996.*

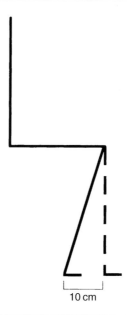

10 cm

75° dorsiflexion (Fig. 4.4). For this to be possible after stroke it is necessary to preserve the extensibility of soleus muscles by both passive and active stretching. Repetitive practice of STS with the feet placed back is itself a method of providing active stretch to soleus.

Timing and speed of trunk rotation.   Several studies have described the *contribution of trunk flexion* to STS (Pai and Rogers 1990, Schenkman et al. 1990, Shepherd and Gentile 1994). It is evident that a timing relationship between flexion of the trunk at the hips and onset of lower limb extension may be a critical feature in the movement's organization. The extension phase of STS starts at the knee while the trunk is still flexing at the hip. Peak hip angular acceleration has been found to occur simultaneously with the onset of knee extension. This means that the body mass starts moving upward while it is still moving forward. There is a smooth continuous transition from pre-extension to extension phase that occurs as a result of intersegmental coordination. This mechanism of momentum transfer is probably a major factor in conserving energy. It is possible to stand up from a position with the upper body already forward at the hips, but as one of the following studies shows there is a cost in terms of additional extensor muscle force.

Angular momentum produced by the trunk as it rotates forward at the hips is the major contributor to horizontal momentum of the body mass (Pai and Rogers 1991) and appears to facilitate the lower limb extension that raises the body mass to the standing position. A study in which the initial trunk angle at the start of STS was varied from erect (0°) to flexed (60°) provides evidence in support of this mechanism. The results indicated that a high level (more than three times body mass) of support moment of force over the three lower limb joints was produced for longer when subjects stood up from the 60° position, i.e. without the facilitatory effects of active hip flexion, than when the movement started with the trunk erect (Shepherd and Gentile 1994).

Speed of movement   also impacts on the extension phase. In a study in which subjects stood up at three different speeds (slow, preferred, fast), it was evident that increased hip flexion velocity when subjects moved fast had a potentiating effect on the production of lower limb extensor force. When subjects moved slowly, however, a significantly longer period of time was spent producing a high level of support force, illustrating the effect of reduced velocity of trunk movement, and therefore momentum, on the production of lower limb muscle forces (Carr et al. 2002).

The findings from these studies show that if patients do not rotate the upper body segment through a range of 30–40°, at a reasonable speed, and do not move the body mass forward and upward without a pause between the two, they will have to work harder to stand up. The clinical implications are that active rotation of the upper body should start with the upper body erect, and there should be no pause between the pre-extension and extension phase. These conditions may optimize the transfer of momentum from horizontal to vertical and potentiate lower limb extension.

Seat height*.   Studies designed to investigate the effect of different seat heights on moments of force at lower limb joints have found that seat height can have significant effects on performance (Burdett et al. 1985, Rodosky et al. 1989). Rodosky and colleagues reported a greater than 50% decrease in the moment of force at the knees from the lowest to the highest seat height. There was a relatively small change in peak moments at the hips, while peak moments at ankles were unaffected by chair height (Fig. 4.5). As chair height was increased peak angular displacements at hip, knee and ankle were also decreased.

The clinical implications from this work are related to training methods and selection of chair type for individuals with difficulty getting into standing. Raising seat height enables an individual with weak muscles to practise STS and SIT. As strength increases, seat height is lowered, providing progressive strength training for lower limb extensors.

Important factors in *chair type* to assist STS are, therefore, the height of the seat and the absence of any structural block to posterior foot placement at

---

*During STS the hips are flexed when the largest hip moments are being produced (Andriacci et al. 1980). In individuals with joint disease or endoprostheses, the stresses created may accelerate hip damage or loosen a prosthesis (Fleckenstein et al. 1988). STS from a relatively high chair with feet placed back decreases the magnitude of hip flexion required to get the body mass forward. Such individuals may also need to use arm rests for assisting STS in order to decrease the hip moments.

FIGURE 4.5 *An illustration of the change in peak moments of force occurring with different chair heights at hips, knees and ankles. (Reproduced from Rodosky et al. 1989, with permission.)*

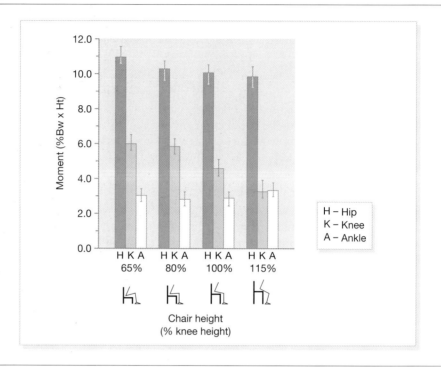

approximately 75° dorsiflexion. Seats need to be high enough to enable the individual to stand up without gross adaptation (e.g. most of the weight through the non-paretic limb). A survey in which elderly people were asked to rank the five factors they considered important in terms of chair design found that 'Easy to get out of' was the most important factor when choosing a chair. 'High seat' was ranked third, before comfort (Munton et al. 1981). It is notable that a chair specially designed for comfort in sitting with a deep, posteriorly slanted seat was found to involve greater quadriceps activity and greater hip and knee flexion, and therefore appeared more difficult to stand up from, than a standard armchair (Wheeler et al. 1985). Recommendations for chair type must therefore take into account both ease of standing up and comfort (Fig. 4.6).

Muscle activity

The principal muscles in the pre-extension phase are hip flexors and ankle dorsiflexors to move the body mass forward. There is some isometric contraction of spinal and abdominal muscles to stabilize the extended trunk. Rectus abdominus activity has been found to be minimal and sporadic (Millington et al. 1992, Vander Linden et al. 1994). Hip, knee and ankle extensor muscles propel the body mass vertically in the extension phase.

Electromyographic (EMG) studies (Fig. 4.7) have shown that tibialis anterior is activated early in the action, reflecting its contribution to foot placement

FIGURE 4.6   *An 'easy to get out of' chair with adjustable seat height.*

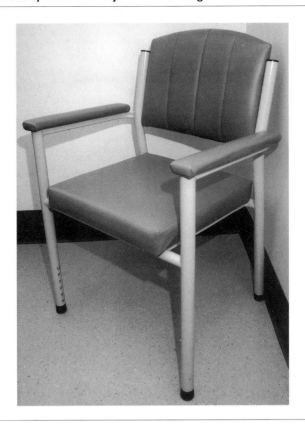

FIGURE 4.7   *Illustration of mean muscle onsets and duration of activity from able-bodied subjects standing up at their preferred speed. Left and right error bars indicate standard error of onset and duration time respectively. TA, tibialis anterior; RF, rectus femoris; BF, biceps femoris; VL, vastus lateralis; GAST, gastrocnemius; SOL, soleus; 0%, movement onset; 31%, thighs-off; 100%, movement end. (Reproduced from Khemlani et al. 1998, with permission.)*

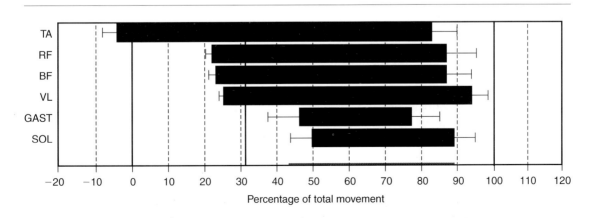

backward, stabilizing the shank and foot, and moving the body mass forward (Khemlani et al. 1998). Onsets of hip and knee extensor muscles (gluteus maximus, biceps femoris, rectus femoris, vastus lateralis and medialis) tend to occur almost simultaneously (Kelley et al. 1976, Millington et al. 1992, Khemlani et al. 1998), demonstrating peak activity around TO which diminishes as standing is reached. Variable patterns of EMG activity have been found in gastrocnemius and soleus muscles, probably reflecting their additional role in balancing the body mass throughout the action (e.g. Khemlani et al. 1998).

Rectus femoris is not activated early enough to be associated with initial hip flexion (Kelley et al. 1976, Millington et al. 1992, Khemlani et al. 1998) and iliopsoas, by its action on the pelvis and thigh, would be the major initiator. The simultaneous onsets of biarticular rectus femoris and biceps femoris (Khemlani et al. 1998) may reflect their contributions to controlling hip flexion and therefore body movement forward, with rectus femoris contributing to flexion and biceps femoris exerting a braking moment at the hip that serves to decelerate upper body movement prior to the onset of extension. Both biceps femoris and rectus femoris continue to contract after thighs-off. The co-contraction of two theoretically antagonistic muscles such as these is efficient, each muscle reinforcing the other as they combine to extend hip and knee (Roebroeck et al. 1994).

Sitting down

On observation, STS and SIT appear fundamentally the same action only in reverse. Certainly, angular displacements at hip, knee and ankle joints are similar (Kralj et al. 1990). Mechanically, however, the two actions are different and independent. SIT involves flexion at hips, knees and ankles controlled by extensor moments of force at these joints, i.e. the lower limb extensor muscles spanning the three joints are generating and sustaining lengthening (eccentric) contractions throughout the movement. The body mass moves back as well as down, the upper body flexing forward. SIT lacks the propulsive component that is so critical in STS. Movement duration tends to be longer, a precaution due to lack of visual information and uncertainty about seat location (Kralj et al. 1990). Since balance mechanisms differ in this action compared to STS, it is critical that it is trained specifically.

AGE-RELATED CHANGES

Difficulty standing up from a seated position is common in elderly people. Undoubtedly factors such as joint pain, muscle stiffness, muscle weakness and decreased range of motion arising from pathology and physical inactivity can affect the performance of both STS and SIT in this age group. However, healthy elderly subjects standing up under constrained laboratory conditions without arm use have demonstrated motor performance similar to young adults in terms of angular displacements, timing of joint onsets and moments of force normalized to subject's body mass (Ikeda et al. 1991, Saravanamuthu and Shepherd 1994). Although increased movement duration has been reported in older individuals, elderly subjects are able to increase speed of rising when asked to stand up as fast as possible (Vander Linden et al. 1994).

A study of STS examined a group of able-bodied elderly people, a group of elderly who could not stand up without using their arms and a group of young able-bodied adults (Schultz et al. 1992). Medical histories and physical findings were essentially normal in the young group but were important in differentiating the elderly groups. Every subject in the group who had to use their arms had some degree of lower limb muscle weakness and joint deformity (primarily due to osteoarthritis), and problems such as dizziness and decreased vision. Movement time was similar in the young and able-bodied elderly groups but significantly longer in the group who used their arms. Both older groups had significantly increased angular displacements at hip and knee joints compared to the young, but only moderate differences in joint moments of force at thighsoff. The larger joint displacements resulted in a more anterior position of the centre of body mass at thighs-off. This strategy may provide greater stability, since the centre of body mass at thighs-off would be within the foot support area. The results suggest that hands may be used to gain more postural stability, particularly at TO, rather than to reduce joint moments. However, using the hands at TO may also be a strategy to decrease force requirements at the knee in individuals with substantial joint pain.

ANALYSIS OF MOTOR PERFORMANCE

Research findings

Despite the importance of STS as a precursor to getting out of bed and walking there has been little investigation of this fundamental action following stroke. In general, movement time and vertical ground reaction forces (GRF) under each foot are the variables that have been tested. Although different methodologies and protocols have been used, there are two consistent findings:

- Stroke patients take significantly longer to stand up than age-matched able-bodied subjects (Yoshida et al. 1983, Engardt and Olsson 1992, Hesse et al. 1994). Sitting down is also slower (Yoshida et al. 1983, Engardt and Olsson 1992).
- Amplitude of vertical GRF under the paretic lower limb is markedly decreased compared with the non-paretic lower limb (Engardt and Olsson 1992, Hesse et al. 1994, Fowler and Carr 1996).

Able-bodied subjects of different ages stand up at their preferred speed in approximately 1.6 s, with the pre-extension phase occupying approximately 30% and the extension phase 70% of the total movement time. Differences in defining movement onset and movement end make it difficult to generalize. However, in one study, stroke subjects tended to stand up very slowly, taking on average 2.3 s to complete the extension phase (Ada and Westwood 1992).

Associated with this latter finding were angular displacements at hip and knee that occurred at low velocities with no discernible peak. After specific training

---

Typical vertical ground reaction force (GRF) profile during STS performed by a stroke patient. Lower trace shows the hemiparetic limb.

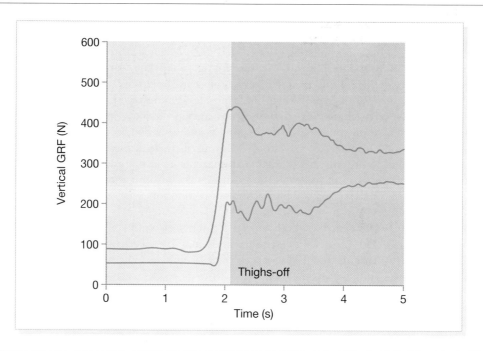

of STS, however, duration of the extension phase decreased to 1.5 s. Knee and hip velocities showed a definite peak, the plots assuming a clear bell shape typical of well-coordinated movement, i.e. as performance improved, coordination between hips and knees was regained. The change from independent action at each joint to a more normal coupling of the joints demonstrates the development of the basic synergy required for unaided standing up. The coordination changes shown in this study are similar to those of able-bodied people developing skill (Ada et al. 1993). Another study also reported an increase in speed after training of the action (Engardt et al. 1993). Although both studies involved small samples, these results illustrate the potential of stroke patients to improve with appropriate and intensive training (Table 4.1).

Vertical ground reaction force graphs typically show either no discernible peak at thighs-off for the paretic leg or peak force occurring later in the action (Fig. 4.8). Fluctuations in vertical force both during the action and in quiet standing (Yoshida et al. 1983, Fowler and Carr 1996) can indicate difficulty in balancing the body mass over both feet.

Observational analysis

The therapist observes the performance of STS and SIT or the patient's attempts at these actions, comparing performance with a list of key components derived from biomechanical data reported consistently in able-bodied subjects across

TABLE 4.1   *Sit-to-stand: clinical outcome studies*

Reference	Subjects	Methods	Duration	Results
Ada and Westwood 1992	8 Ss Early post-stroke Mean age 65 ± 8.9 yrs	Pre-test, post-test design Task-specific training of STS	4 weeks 5 days/week, 10–20 mins	Significant decrease in movement duration (p < 0.005), increased amplitude of peak angular velocities (p < 0.01). All subjects reached 6 on Motor Assessment Scale (Item 3) Coordination of hip and knee angular velocity more discernible
Engardt et al. 1993	40 Ss <3 months post-stroke Mean age E: 64.6 ± 6.7 yrs C: 65.1 ± 9.0 yrs	Pre-test, post-test design Randomly assigned to two groups: C: Task-specific training of STS/SIT E: Task-specific training of STS/SIT with auditory feedback about force produced by paretic leg	6 weeks 5 days/week, 15 mins 3/daily	STS – significant increase in force through paretic leg in both groups (p < 0.01) SIT – significant increase in force produced through paretic leg in **E** group only (p < 0.001).
Fowler and Carr 1996	12 Ss <3 months post-stroke Mean age 63.5 (43–79) yrs	Pre-test, post-test design Randomly assigned to two groups: 1: Task-specific training of STS 2: Task-specific training + auditory feedback about force produced by paretic leg	3 weeks 25 repetitions twice daily	All subjects but one produced peak force ≥ 50% body weight through paretic leg at end of study

(Continued)

TABLE 4.1	(Continued)			
Reference	Subjects	Methods	Duration	Results
Hesse et al. 1998	35 Ss 3–23 weeks post-stroke Mean age 64.8 (59–79) yrs Note: all subjects could stand up independently with minimum help	Pre-test, post-test design Bobath techniques (tone inhibiting, trunk control in lying and sitting, pelvic tilting, weight shift in standing, facilitated walking)	4 weeks 4 days/week, 45 mins	STS – no change in movement duration, horizontal and vertical GRFs Gait – no change in speed, cadence, stride length. Rivermead Motor Score, Ashworth score, Motricity Index showed little or no relevant change
Cheng et al. 2001	54 Ss <4 months post-stroke Mean age 62.7	Randomly assigned to 2 groups: **C:** (neuromuscular facilitation, FES, mat exercises, therapeutic exercises) **E:** (symmetrical standing and repetitive STS training with visual and auditory feedback)	**C:** not specified **E:** 3 weeks 5 days/week, 50 mins	Follow-up at 6 months – **C:** no significant differences between initial and follow-up tests of STS and SIT **E:** significant differences between initial and follow-up tests – decrease in duration of STS ($p < 0.001$) and SIT ($p < 0.01$); decrease in L/R vertical GRF – STS ($p < 0.005$), SIT ($p < 0.001$); decrease in COP sway STS (x: $p < 0.01$, y: $p < 0.05$), SIT (x: $p < 0.005$); increase in rate of rise in force in STS ($p < 0.001$) Significantly fewer falls in **E** ($p < 0.05$)

C, control group; COP, centre of pressure; E, experimental group; FES, functional electrical stimulation; GRF, ground reaction force; SIT, sitting down; Ss, subjects; STS, sit-to-stand.

different age groups. The following components appear to be critical to effective performance:

- initial foot placement backward (approximately 10 cm from a vertical line dropped from the knee joint, approximately 75° ankle dorsiflexion)
- flexion of the extended trunk at the hips* to move the body mass forward, together with dorsiflexion at the ankles
- knee, hip and ankle extension.

The above list comprises sagittal plane angular displacements at hip, knee and ankle which are easily observable by the clinician. Also observable are paths of the shoulder and knee as the individual performs the action. The shoulder moves along a smooth, continuous curvilinear path forward and upward. As the hips flex, the knees move forward along a linear path for a few centimetres, movement occurring at the ankles.

These components provide a structure or a model of the action with which to compare the patient's performance and determine major adaptations and possible causes. Although it is not possible to observe the underlying momentum and force characteristics of the action it is possible to make inferences from observational analysis about these characteristics. Knowledge of three mechanical requirements for effective standing up is necessary as a reference:

- generation of sufficient speed and therefore horizontal and vertical momentum to propel the body forward and upward over the feet
- generation and sustaining of lower limb joint forces to support and raise the body mass into standing
- postural stability at thighs-off, controlling the centre of body mass in relation to foot support area.

Some *common motor problems* evident on observational analysis and possible explanations are described below. They include the following.

- Inability to stand up independently
  — lower limb muscle weakness and lack of coordination.
- Absent/insufficient foot placement backward (flex knee and dorsiflex ankle) (Fig. 4.9a)
  — weakness of hamstrings and ankle dorsiflexors
  — decreased extensibility of soleus.
- Decreased projection of body mass forward in pre-extension phase (flex hips and dorsiflex ankles) (Fig. 4.9b)
  — inadequate foot placement backward
  — inability to stabilize the paretic lower limb, in particular the shank and foot. Normally the lower limbs are used actively for balance and propulsion in the pre-extension phase
  — flexion of spine instead of at hips (Fig. 4.9c)
  — moving very slowly

*Although the pelvis is the segment linking the lower limbs to the spine, during STS the pelvis and spine act together as a virtual segment as the upper body pivots forward at the hips. Minimal movement in the spine and between the spine and the pelvis has been reported. Although sometimes referred to in the clinic as forward pelvic tilt, the movement is actually a rotation of the pelvis–spine unit by flexion at the hips.

FIGURE 4.9   *(a) Failure to place paretic leg back. Adaptations: weight concentrated on non-paretic R leg; increased distance between feet. (b) Failure to move body mass forward over feet (insufficient hip flexion and ankle dorsiflexion). Note adaptive use of arms. (c) Failure to move body mass forward (flexing lumbar spine instead of hips). Note adaptive use of arms. (d) In sitting down, body mass has not stayed forward over the feet as hips, knees and ankles flex. As a result she has lost balance backward and falls to the seat. (e) Feet have not been moved backward and arms are swung forward to aid propulsion forward and up.*

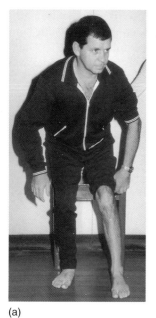

(a)

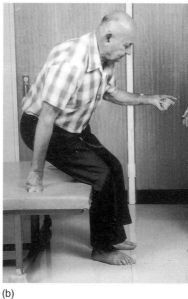

(b)

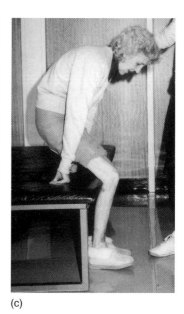

(c)

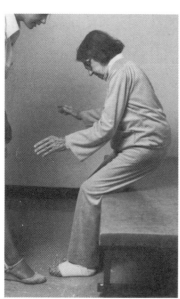

(d)

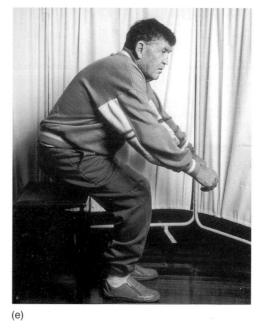

(e)

    — fear of falling forward

    — lack of vigour.

- Decreased control of body mass sitting down (Fig. 4.9d)
  - weakness of eccentric control of lower limb extensor muscles.
- Decreased stability, particularly at TO when horizontal momentum of the body mass must be controlled and flexion of upper body at hips changes to extension
  - weakness of lower limb muscles and slowed reaction times (muscles that link the shank and foot are particularly critical to balancing the body mass as it pivots over the feet)
  - lack of intersegmental coordination and poor timing.

There are several predictable *adaptations* to muscle weakness, lack of segmental coordination and decreased stability. They include:

- weight borne principally on stronger and more easily controlled leg
- body mass can be observed to shift laterally toward non-paretic leg at TO (Fig. 4.9a)
- positioning of foot of stronger leg behind foot of weaker leg (the most posterior foot bears most weight)
- use of hands for balance or support
- arms swung forward to aid horizontal and vertical propulsion of the body mass (Fig. 4.9e)
- distance between feet increased (Fig. 4.9a)
- action is performed slowly with a pause between pre-extension and extension phases.

GUIDELINES FOR TRAINING

Training of STS and SIT following stroke is critical for the regaining of independence and mobility. Inability to perform these actions effectively and efficiently predisposes the individual to dependence on others for mobility and to an increasingly sedentary lifestyle. It has also been reported that being assisted to stand up by another person can be a common cause of damage to the soft tissues around the shoulder complex and the development of pain (Wanklyn et al. 1996).

Immediately following stroke, patients naturally adapt their performance as they attempt to become independent and learn to manage daily activities. The principal adaptation is to bear weight mainly through the stronger leg and use the non-paretic upper limb. If these adaptations persist, the patient may learn not to use (i.e. neglect) the affected limbs. It appears from stroke rehabilitation texts that therapy methods may reinforce this adaptation. The emphasis in clinical practice may not be on training standing up and sitting down and on strengthening lower limb muscles, but on teaching what is to the patient the novel task of 'transferring' from one seat to another. There are several variations of the transfer (low transfers, pivot transfers, STS transfers). All involve the patient being taught to bear weight on the stronger leg and arm, with minimum support from the affected leg, in order to move from one sitting surface to another. Although it may be a practical necessity for patients to be able to move from, say, wheelchair to toilet, this manoeuvre can be practised by the patient in the appropriate environment rather than taught as a general strategy.

Every effort should be made to train STS and SIT intensively, since real world independence requires not the ability to transfer from one surface to another by pivoting on the non-paretic limb but the ability to stand up and sit down. There is some evidence that repetitive training of STS and SIT has some generalizability. The more the paretic limb is loaded during STS and SIT the better the individual performs in other activities of daily living as measured on the Barthel Index and the Fugl-Meyer Scale (Engardt et al. 1993).

Physiotherapy intervention has the potential to train most patients to gain independence in these actions. Although muscle weakness is a limiting factor immediately after stroke, there are several key mechanical factors arising from biomechanical research which can be utilized to make it possible for even a frail patient to practise the action:

- initial foot position at approximately 75° ankle dorsiflexion as this requires less effort
- vary seat height depending on strength of lower limb extensors
- active hip flexion initiated with the trunk vertical (90° to horizontal) to optimize horizontal momentum of the body mass
- no pause between pre-extension and extension phases
- speeding up the action.

For training to be effective, given the impairments following stroke, it is also necessary to:

- prevent adaptive soft tissue shortening
- increase lower limb muscle activation, strength and coordination.

The following guidelines provide what can be considered a critical pathway for optimizing STS/SIT for most individuals following stroke. The guidelines are individualized according to each patient's impairments, level of functional ability and needs, and are set down with no intention of a prescribed sequence. They address the essential requirements for effective performance, synthesized from research.

Standing up and sitting down practice

Standing up

Start with upper body vertical and feet placed back. Patient swings upper body forward at the hips and stands up (Fig. 4.10).

- *Patient sits on a firm flat surface.*
- *No arm rests.*

FIGURE 4.10 *Practice of standing up and sitting down. (a) Therapist stabilizes paretic foot on the floor by pushing down along the line of the shank. (b) As she stands up therapist moves her body mass laterally to increase loading of the L leg. (c) Lateral view illustrates how the therapist can give guidance for relative intersegmental alignment. It is important that the patient does not extend her upper body at the hips before the body mass is far enough forward.*

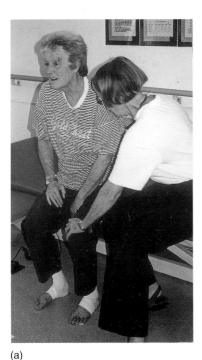 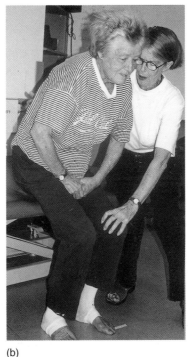 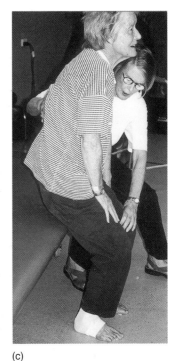

(a)   (b)   (c)

- *Feet flat on floor (vary thigh support so ankles are dorsiflexed to 75°).*
- *No flexion within upper body throughout action, eyes on target.*
- *Choose a seat height to encourage weightbearing through the affected lower limb and discourage adaptive loading of the non-paretic limb (Fig. 4.11).*

Note
- Directing vision and attention toward a target during STS/SIT assists appropriate body alignment by affecting head position and sense of verticality. Target is placed 2–3 m in front at eye level.
- If necessary, therapist assists foot placement so the action is practised from an optimal starting position. Voluntary activation of hamstrings and ankle dorsiflexors for foot placement are trained specifically in sitting.
- For patients with severe muscle weakness, therapist stabilizes the foot on the floor and encourages weightbearing through the affected leg by pushing down and back along the line of the shank. This ensures that quadriceps activity moves the thigh on the shank to extend the knee

FIGURE 4.11   *(a) Although she can stand up independently, she loads the L leg more than the R. Note that she has moved the foot of her non-paretic L leg further back just before thighs-off. (b) It is better for her to practise repetitively from a higher seat. Left: on her early attempts she moved the L foot behind the paretic foot. Right: the physiotherapist suggests the R foot is placed further back to force more loading of the paretic R leg.*

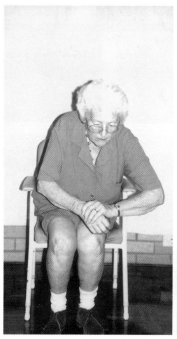
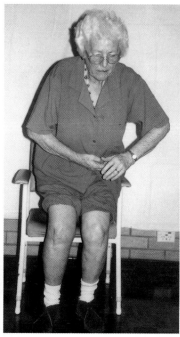

(a)

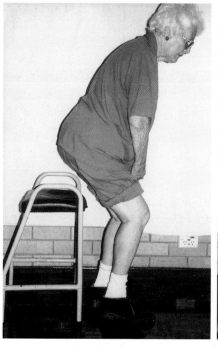
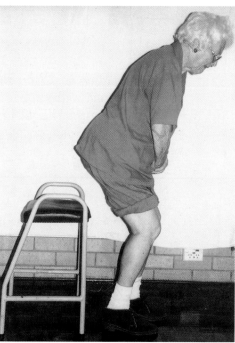

(b)

FIGURE 4.12   *(a) Vertical ground reaction forces during unconstrained standing up. (b) The effect of the therapist stabilizing the affected foot on the floor with some external pressure down and back along the line of the shank. Note the redistribution of the vertical ground reaction forces through the two legs.*

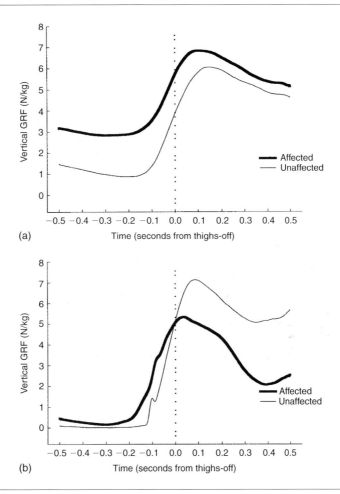

(a)

(b)

rather than the foot sliding forward. Guiding the knee forward along a horizontal path may help the patient move the body mass forward over the feet.

Check

- Do not block forward movement of the body mass by standing too close to the patient, i.e. blocking shoulders or knees from moving forward.
- Give instructions that identify body part to be moved, e.g. 'Swing your shoulders forward and stand up'. The instruction 'Lean forward' is not an appropriate cue as it does not identify what body part is to be moved or take account of the generation of horizontal momentum.
- Discourage use of hands.
- Discourage holding paretic hand in other hand. This does not increase weightbearing on paretic lower limb or symmetry (Seelen et al. 1995).

- If patient is flexing within the spine and not at the hips, direct attention (vision) toward the target.
- Final standing alignment is with hips and knees extended, angles at approximately 0°. Avoid assisted extension of the knee while the hips are still extending or patient will overbalance backward.

Seating.   Chairs provided for stroke patients frequently enforce passivity. In choosing a seat, a compromise should be achieved between comfort and ease of standing up. Patients early after stroke and those who are weak are not able to stand up unaided without the provision of such a chair. If there is no supportive muscle activity around the shoulder, the arm should be supported when the patient is sitting (see Fig. 5.23).

Sitting down

Patient flexes hips, knees and ankles to lower body mass toward the seat.

- *Upper body flexes forward at the hips as body mass is lowered.*
- *Weight remains supported over the feet. Nearing the seat, body mass is moved back to enable seat contact.*

Note
- Assist initiation of knee flexion by moving the knee forward.
- Stabilize shank and foot to assist weightbearing on affected leg.
- Specific training of SIT with weight through the affected leg appears necessary to improve performance (Engardt et al. 1993).

Soft tissue stretching

Extensibility of soleus muscle is critical to foot placement backward and to weightbearing through the affected leg. Preserving functional muscle length involves both passive and active stretching.

A brief passive stretch is given immediately before exercises to decrease muscle stiffness. Active stretching occurs during practice of STS and SIT and the weightbearing exercises below if the paretic limb is loaded and ankles are initially dorsiflexed.

Soleus: stretch in sitting (Fig. 4.13).

Note
- Hold stretch for approximately 20 s, relax, repeat 4–5 times. Patients can learn to do this themselves.

Patients with severe muscle weakness who are physically inactive require periods of prolonged passive stretching during the day.

Soleus: stretch in sitting (Fig. 4.14).
Gastrocnemius–soleus: prolonged stretch in standing (see Fig. 3.18c).

FIGURE 4.13   *Patient stretches her L soleus for 20 s prior to practice of STS and SIT.*

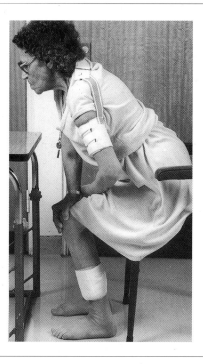

FIGURE 4.14   *Sustained passive stretch to soleus. (Conceived and developed by K Schurr and J Nugent, Physiotherapy Department, Bankstown-Lidcombe Hospital, Sydney.)*

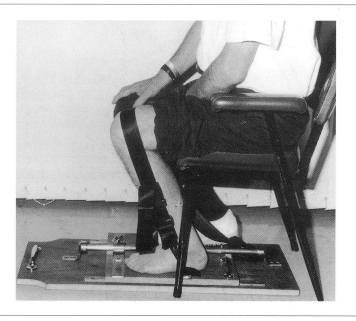

FIGURE 4.15   *A roller skate reduces the friction between the shoe and floor while she practises activating hamstrings and muscles crossing the ankle to move her foot back. She aims to move her toes behind a line on the floor (concealed under rear wheel).*

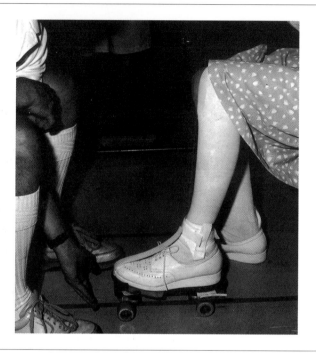

Note
- Hold prolonged stretch for 30 min.

Eliciting muscle activity

Initial foot placement backward is critical to the ease of STS since it minimizes the distance the body mass is moved forward over the feet. Specific training to activate hamstring and anterior tibial muscles may be necessary. The therapist can palpate hamstrings to ensure they are active or use an EMG monitor. Activity of tibialis anterior is easily observable.

Foot placement backward

Patient sits with feet flat on floor and slides foot backward and forward. Decreasing resistance using a slippery surface or roller skate may encourage this action (Fig. 4.15).

Note
- Encourage patient to lift thigh slightly to reduce friction under the foot.
- Once patient voluntarily activates these muscles and gets the idea of the movement, encourage an increase in speed.

FIGURE 4.16	*Getting the idea of moving the body mass forward and backward over the feet by flexing at the hips and dorsiflexing at the ankles. This is useful when the patient is fearful of moving forward. Paretic foot may need to be stabilized.*

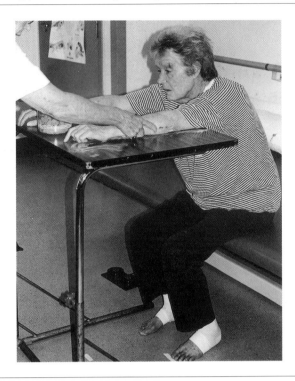

- Incorporate into STS practice, i.e. expect the patient to move the foot back without assistance.

Electrical stimulation to ankle dorsiflexors in sitting may assist the movement.

Moving the upper body forward and backward at the hips

Fear of falling may be a major barrier to moving the body mass forward in some patients early after stroke. This action may require some practice briefly at the start of rehabilitation to increase the patient's confidence.

Patient sits with arms on a table at approximately shoulder height, trunk and head erect. She flexes the upper body forward at the hips by sliding her hands to the edge of the table and back to the erect position (Fig. 4.16). Maintenance of erect trunk and head is encouraged by having the patient look ahead at target. The far edge of the table needs to be a distance of at least 1.5 times arm length to enable body mass to move forward over the feet.

Check
- Assist movement of paretic arm if necessary.
- Stabilize the foot on the floor to encourage generation of ground reaction forces and activity in anterior tibial muscles as the person moves forward.
- Encourage patient to take weight through the feet and to speed up the movement.
- Incorporate into STS practice.

Strength training

Lack of strength, particularly in the lower limb extensor muscles, is a major limiting factor in the ability to stand up and sit down, together with lack of intersegmental coordination and postural instability. Functional strength training includes repetitive practice of the action itself.

STS and SIT with progressive body weight resistance

Practice of STS/SIT with maximum repetitions and against an increasing load (body weight) can increase and maintain strength in the lower limb extensor muscles (Kotake et al. 1993, Carr and Shepherd 1998). Progressive strength training involves lowering seat height and increasing number of repetitions. Patient is encouraged to do a maximum number of cycles of STS/SIT for a selected seat height, up to 10, repeated three times. When this can be achieved, the seat is lowered. Seat height selection is determined by observation of the ability to bear weight relatively evenly through both lower limbs.

Note
- Many repetitions without pause are necessary to improve strength and control, so a target number should be set and repetitions counted (Fig. 4.17a).
- Placing foot of weaker limb behind other foot forces weightbearing through the weaker leg (vertical GRF are greater under the backward placed foot, particularly at TO)
- Lower limb muscle strength enhances the generation and control of momentum and dynamic stability, ultimately influencing the ability to stand up and sit down (Scarborough et al. 1999).
- As strength increases, encourage an increase in speed. Reduce upper limb assistance by folding arms (Fig. 4.17b).
- This is a suitable home exercise to be carried out long-term, particularly by elderly individuals, to preserve lower limb muscle strength and functional ability.

The patient may also benefit from strengthening exercises that have similar dynamics to STS/SIT, i.e. flexion and extension of the lower limb joints to raise and lower the body mass over the feet:

- *step-ups (see Fig. 3.22)*
- *heels raise and lower (see Fig. 3.24).*

| FIGURE 4.17 | (a) Partially supervised repetitive practice of STS and SIT. She is getting feedback about loading the limb from a limb load monitor and is recording the number of repetitions on a counter. (b) Repetitive practice with arms folded increases lower limb extensor force requirements.* (*Courtesy of K Schurr and S Dorsch, Physiotherapy Department, Bankstown-Lidcombe Hospital, Sydney.) |

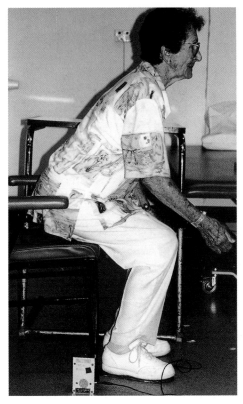

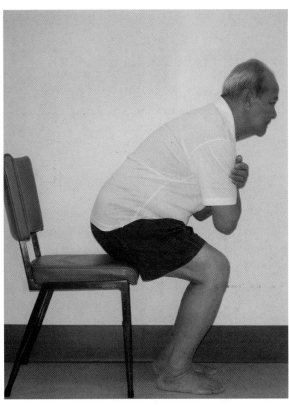

(a)   (b)

Note
The above exercises can be practised in group circuit training with minimal supervision.

Maximizing skill

In the initial stages of rehabilitation the patient and therapist focus on developing the basic movement coordination, i.e. the essential spatial and temporal components of STS/SIT, using many repetitions. Although repetitive practice plays an important role in tuning motor activity to become effective and more reliable (Gallistel 1980), variable practice – what Bernstein (1967) has described as 'repetition without repetition' – is necessary to develop skill. There is a great improvement in morale and lifestyle when a person can stand up from a chair unaided. However, for

FIGURE 4.18   *Training to increase stability and skill: balancing the mugs on the tray changes the focus of attention.*

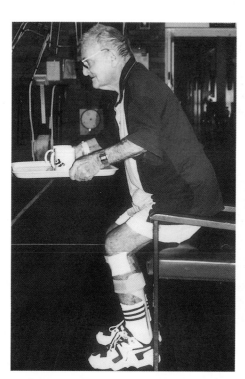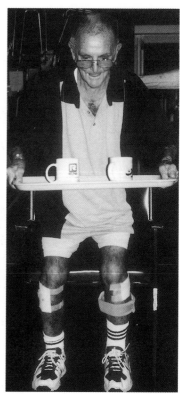

flexibility of performance, practice has to provide the opportunity for the individual to learn how to adapt performance to different contexts.

Training for skill therefore includes practice of STS/SIT under different regulatory conditions:

- Holding a glass of water, tray with utensils (Fig. 4.18), objects of different sizes and weights; carrying on a conversation (to decrease conscious attention to performance); varying speed.
- Performing action sequences: STS → walk to the right or to the left, to another chair → SIT → STS → walk back → SIT.
- Stopping on request (immediately after thighs-off or before thighs-on) without losing balance.
- STS/SIT from different types of seat.

MEASUREMENT

The most commonly reported motor problems in STS and SIT are moving slowly compared with age-matched able-bodied subjects, decreased weightbearing on the affected lower limb and poor balance. Since observational analysis gives uncertain results, valid and reliable tests are necessary to document progress and the effect of intervention. The following tests have been found to be reliable if performed under standardized conditions.

Functional tests

These include:

- *Motor Assessment Scale:* Standing up item (Carr et al. 1985)
- *Timed 'Up and Go' Test* (Podsialo and Richardson 1991)
- *Quadriceps strength* using a hand-held dynamometer.

Note
Timed STS tests may also provide an indirect measure of knee extensor muscle strength (Fiatarone et al. 1990, Bohannon et al. 1995). Bohannon and colleagues reported a curvilinear relationship between isometric knee extension strength measured with a dynamometer and the number of STS/SIT performed in 10 s. The number of repetitions also correlated with maximum gait speed.

Movement duration can be tested simply, using a visual estimate of the start and end of STS and SIT. Starting and finishing positions for both must be standardized. Movement is said to begin when the subject's head starts to move anteriorly and ends when no further displacement of the pelvis occurs. SIT begins when the head starts to move and ends when the pelvis rests on the seat. The technique on which this is based was found to be reliable when observed time values were compared with data from a motion analysis system (Engardt and Olsson 1992). The tester stands at the side of the subject with a stopwatch.

Biomechanical tests

Variables that can be tested include:

- movement duration
- magnitude and timing of vertical ground reaction force
- coordination of angular displacement and velocity – phase–plane plots (Cahill et al. 1999).

NOTES

Augmented feedback

Results of research on the efficacy of providing auditory feedback, whether using a specially designed vertical ground reaction force feedback device (Engardt et al. 1993) or a Limb Load Monitor* (Fowler and Carr 1996), are

*Electronic Quantification, Model 101-1.

equivocal. It may be that focusing on making the auditory signal can become the goal of the action rather than loading the limb and developing an internal representation of the action. In addition, an auditory signal about force already produced may come too late to allow modification of the action (Fowler and Carr 1996). A visual template of the specific force–time curve required may, therefore, be a more beneficial form of feedback than information about peak force itself. However, as with the use of any external feedback, the patient must be able to move on to use naturally occurring feedback about weight distribution.

5 Reaching and manipulation

CHAPTER CONTENTS

- **Introduction**
- **Biomechanical description**
  Reaching to grasp
  Manipulation
- **Recovery of upper limb function after stroke**
- **Analysis of motor performance**
  Research findings
  Observational analysis
  Critical components of reach, grasp, manipulation
- **Guidelines for training**
  Soft tissue stretching

Eliciting muscle activity
Reaching and balancing practice
Manipulation and dexterity practice
Bimanual practice
Strength training
Shoulder pain prevention
- **Notes on specific methods**
  Forced use: 'constraint-induced movement therapy'
  Computerized training
  Electrical stimulation
- **Measurement**

INTRODUCTION

Much of what we do with our arms is related to carrying out complex tasks involving one or both hands. We move our arms in order to place our hands at the appropriate place for manipulation in the working environment and to transport objects from one place to another. The distance we can reach is a function of arm length. If the object to be reached is beyond arm's length, protraction of the shoulder girdle and movement of the body mass forward at the hips and ankles extends the reachable distance. If the object is out of reach in standing a step is taken. The muscle forces produced and the timing and sequencing of joint movements involved in a specific action are a function of the task being performed, the object, the individual's position relative to the object, and the constraints of the environment. The way we move is controlled by the context; for example, both the shape of an object and what is to be done with it determine the type of grasp. The location of glass relative to mouth determines how the hand moves through space, and the amount of rotation of shoulder and forearm. Bernstein observed that dexterity is never present in the motor act itself but only in the interaction of the act with the changing environment (cited in Latash and Latash 1994).

The large variety of motor actions performed by the arm and hand illustrate two fundamental problems in motor control raised originally by Bernstein (1967): the many degrees of freedom available in the neuromusculoskeletal system and the need for context-specific or context-conditioned variability. Here also is a dilemma for stroke rehabilitation. As a result of the lesion there are a very large number of actions, ranging from simple to complex, which the patient must relearn in the contexts of independent daily life. Most important therefore is functional training in which the person learns to optimize motor control. Training is designed to help the patient regain the ability to harness the degrees of freedom available so the limb functions as a coordinated unit in functional actions with many different goals.

Skilled motor actions are characterized by patterns of segmental movement which best address the spatiotemporal demands of the action. Although theoretically there are many movement options due to the flexibility of the neuromusculoskeletal system (the degrees of freedom), the most parsimonious (cost-efficient) options are used (Kelso et al. 1994). Normally, the control system utilizes 'simplifying' strategies made possible by anatomical configurations, neuronal connections and biomechanical characteristics of linked segments. For example, the arm and hand appear to function as a single coordinated unit in reaching and manipulation as do the fingers in grasping; in bimanual actions the two limbs may initiate and end motion simultaneously despite differing constraints for each arm. The concept of simplification also enables the development of exercises, the effects of which are likely to transfer to improved performance of a number of different tasks.

Although there are a large number of actions that we carry out every day, they fall into different categories. Some have high externally imposed temporal demands, such as catching a ball; others have high precision demands, such as picking up a pin or keyboard typing. Many tasks involve both hands if they are to be carried out easily and effectively. In bimanual actions such as opening a can of drink the two limbs are constrained to function as a coordinated unit. This means it is unlikely that individuals with predominantly unilateral impairments will function effectively if they are not specifically trained in bimanual actions. This creates another dilemma in planning intervention. Exercises are necessary to activate and train weak muscles of the affected limb, yet emphasis must also be on bimanual practice. For many patients the optimal intervention for avoiding learned non-use and for training functional use of the affected limb involves intensive exercise and training of the affected limb, in some cases forcing use by constraint of the non-paretic limb. Daily training sessions have to be planned, however, to incorporate intensive training of bimanual tasks.

Most actions specifically involving the upper limbs also involve the whole body due to the dynamics of the segmental linkage. The arms also play a part in balancing mechanisms (Gentile 1987). When the centre of body mass moves too close to the limits of stability they may play a stabilizing and supportive function. If balance is lost and the person falls, the arms can play a supportive role or, at the very least, serve to break the fall.

The function of the hands is sensory as well as motor (Hogan and Winters 1990). Tactile receptors in the palm convey critical information for the identification of objects and their properties. Tactile information is obtained from the feel of the object in the hand, the recognition of its nature (size, shape, form in three dimensions, composition and texture) and its position in the hand. Proprioceptive information involves awareness of the relationship of parts of the hand to each other, and their position in space. A significant aspect of sensory discrimination for manipulation is the appreciation of the compressibility of an object – a combination of dynamaesthesia (the awareness of force applied in a motor act), kinaesthesia (appreciation of change in position of fingers) and counter-pressure of fingertips (Roland 1973).

Vision plays a critical role in reaching and interacting with objects. The dynamic linkage between eye, head and upper limb movements enables skilled hand use. Information of importance to understanding motor control comes from the work of Gibson (1977), who used the term 'affordances' to refer to the properties of the environment to which we are attuned. When we ask a person to look at what he or she is doing, we expect the person to pick up information about the object and the environment (the affordances or possibilities offered for interaction) that will assist in task performance.

Major prerequisites for hand use are therefore the ability:

- to move the hand to the scene of the action
- to look at and pay attention to both object and environment
- to make the postural adjustments which occur with arm movement
- to utilize somatosensory information.

BIOMECHANICAL DESCRIPTION

Many early scientific investigations of upper limb function examined arm and hand movements in simple reaching actions or manipulation under relatively constrained conditions. More recently, researchers have studied the interactions between reaching and manipulation in real-life functional tasks.

Reaching to grasp

Reaching to grasp an object can be divided into two components: transportation and manipulation (Jeannerod 1981). The transport component is performed relatively ballistically. The manipulation component, however, requires visual feedback to ensure an accurate approach with appropriately sized grasp aperture. Studies of the relationship between these two phases (Marteniuk et al. 1990, Hoff and Arbib 1993, Rosenbaum et al. 1999) show that the arm and hand function as one unit during the reach, with the hand starting to open around the time the reaching action begins. Final adjustment to the grasp aperture occurs at the end of the reach just prior to grasp (Fig. 5.1). The magnitude of grasp aperture reflects the size of the object, with an extra few centimetres as a margin for error. Grasp aperture is also related to the speed of the movement, wider apertures being observed with faster movements (Wing et al. 1986). Stabilization of the thumb in abduction may provide a focus for monitoring the relationship between grasp aperture and object size (Fig. 5.2). Just before the object is grasped the aperture decreases and aperture adjustment

FIGURE 5.1

A cinematographic study by Jeannerod of reaching toward an object. Dots represent successive positions of the hand every 20 ms. Note the hand slows on approach to the object. Lines represent the size of the grasp aperture every 40 ms. Note that aperture formation starts soon after movement onset, reaches a maximum of 3 cm, then decreases until it is appropriate for the size of the object. (We thank the International Association for the Study of Attention and Performance for permission to reprint from Long and Baddeley 1981, as cited in Jeannerod 1981.)

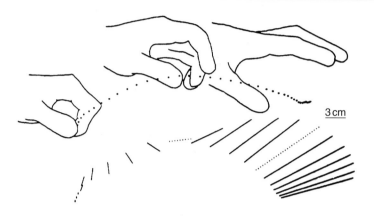

3 cm

FIGURE 5.2

The aperture opens and closes by movement of the fingers to and from the abducted thumb. Figure shows the marker positions used in the kinematic investigation. (Reproduced from Wing and Fraser 1983, with permission.)

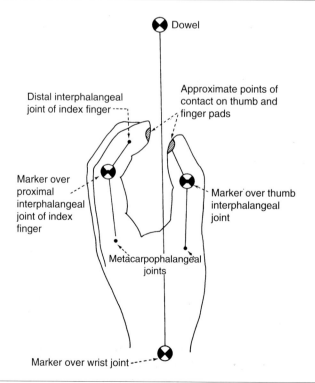

appears to be a function of finger movement to the already abducted thumb (Wing and Fraser 1983).

The spatiotemporal organization of these transportation and manipulation components varies according to whether one or both hands are used (Castiello et al. 1992). It takes into account the shape and other physical characteristics of the object, including its fragility, and what is to be done with it (Iberall et al. 1986, Rosenbaum et al. 1992, van Vliet 1993, Smeets and Brenner 1999).

The organization of transport and manipulation components differs according to whether subjects reach to grasp with the whole hand or with a precision grasp. In opening a can, for example, one hand reaches to hold the can and stabilize it, the other reaches to grasp and pull the ring with thumb and index finger. A study of this action in able-bodied subjects (Castiello et al. 1993) showed that both hands started and finished the movement together, although the kinematic details varied for each hand (Fig. 5.3). In particular it was noted that the precision hand reached a smaller value of peak velocity earlier and started to decelerate earlier than the other hand. The longer deceleration time illustrates the relative complexity of the ring pulling task compared to the holding task. A similar relationship between the two limbs was found in another task that involved opening a drawer with one hand and taking out a small rod from the drawer with the other (Wiesendanger et al. 1996).

Cooperation between the two hands and the predictive nature of some tasks are also shown by an experiment in which the subject dropped a ball into a cup held in the other hand (Johansson and Westling 1988). The grip force of the cup hand was found to increase in anticipation of the ball's impact, i.e. before the ball hit the cup. Findings from such studies confirm the view that a patient with a unilateral lesion is unlikely to regain the ability to perform bimanual actions unless such actions are practised. It is only by practising tasks with both hands that interlimb timing parameters can be regained. In addition, bimanual exercise addresses the issue of poor dexterity (clumsiness) in non-paretic hand use, which may be present due to the effects of the brain lesion on ipsilateral pathways.

The upper limbs are also involved in throwing and striking actions. Most of these actions are characterized by sequential movement of the segments within the upper limb linkage, proximal segments moving first. This sequencing imparts maximum speed effects on the distal segment and therefore the ball (Putnam 1993).

Any movement of the body mass toward the limits of stability, such as reaching beyond arm's length, has the potential to destabilize the individual. In both sitting and standing, movement of the body over the base of support is normally countered both before and during the reach by postural leg muscle activity which is linked to the arm movement (Ch. 2).

There are a number of degrees of freedom to be harnessed in actions involving the arm in sitting and standing. Studies of the relative contributions of trunk and arm movement in reaching beyond arm's length in sitting have shown

FIGURE 5.3   *A single trial of a bilateral task, reaching to grasp a can with one hand and pull the tab with the other hand, showing linear wrist velocity (top) and acceleration (middle), and grip size (lower). Both hands reach the can together, with peak velocity, acceleration and deceleration occurring earlier and with less amplitude of peak velocity for the precision hand than for the whole-grasp hand. (Reprinted from* **Behavioral Brain Research,** *Vol. 56, U Castiello, KMB Bennett and GE Stelmark, The bilateral reach to grasp movement, p. 48, copyright 1993, with permission from Elsevier Science.)*

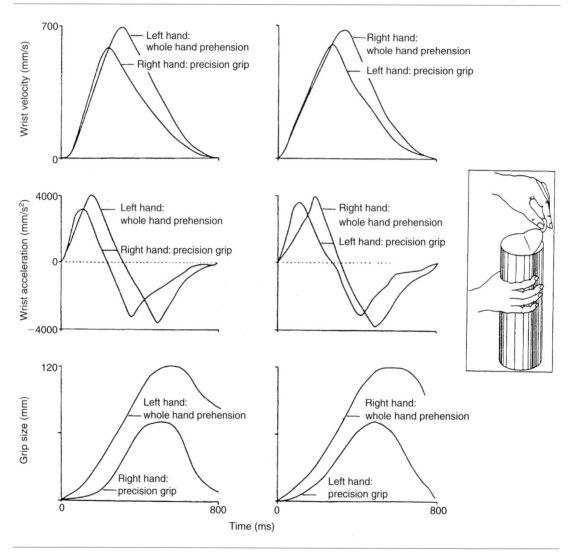

variability in performance according to task and context, but consistency in performance between subjects (Kaminski et al. 1995, Dean et al. 1999a,b, Seidler and Stelmach 2000). The task itself affects temporal aspects of coordination, with simple tasks (pressing a switch) being carried out faster than more complex ones (reaching to pick up a full glass of water) (Dean et al. 1999a). On the other hand, distance to be reached affects spatial and temporal coordination between trunk and arm (Saling et al. 1996, Dean et al. 1999a), with magnitude of trunk and arm motion increasing and elbow motion decreasing as reaching distance is increased. The lower limbs play an important role in balancing and supporting the body mass during long reaches (Dean et al. 1999a). Overall, it seems that the trunk plays a general transport role with the arm playing a corrective role, countering any variability in the movement as the hand approaches the target (Seidler and Stelmach 2000).

Manipulation

The hand is the principal means of interacting with people and objects in the environment. Grasp has been categorized as either precision or power (Napier 1956), the former involving pads of digits, the latter the whole hand. Although this general distinction remains, modern biomechanical research is casting light on the dependence of grasp configuration on the object and the task to be performed.

Grasping is a complex action involving movement at several joints. The hand takes on many different configurations in the performance of complex and skilled manipulations. It is becoming evident, however, that control is simplified to some extent by certain anatomical configurations and patterns of force production (Fig. 5.4); for example, many tasks involve interactions between object, thumb and index finger. The thumb abducts and rotates and the index finger flexes while force is exerted on the object through the pads of the digits, primarily by long flexors of thumb and finger. Each digit is stabilized by a combination

| FIGURE 5.4 | *Task-related grasps showing the different patterns of force production. (Reproduced from Iberall et al. 1986, with permission.)* |

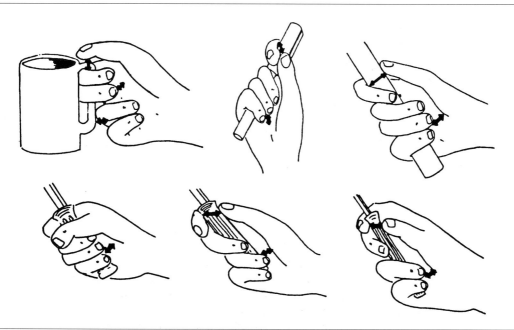

of joint geometry and intrinsic muscle action. The force produced on the index finger by the thumb is countered by the first dorsal interosseus muscle and the force produced on the carpometacarpal joint of the thumb is constrained by activity of all the thenar muscles. The resulting axial rotary moments of force are balanced by contraction of other muscles crossing the hand and wrist (Lemon et al. 1991). The relative contributions of muscles differ and are task related.

For some tasks, 'locking' (holding cutlery or a tool) and 'supporting' (holding a loaded plate or tray) grasps involving the 4th and 5th fingers and thumb are required. These grasps are described in detail by Bendz (1993), but a brief description taken from Bendz's work is given here.

In the locking grasp (Fig. 5.5a), the implement is locked into the palm of the hand by the 4th and 5th fingers flexed at all joints and rotated at the metacarpophalangeal (MCP) joints. The 5th metacarpal is flexed (at the carpometacarpal joint) by hypothenar muscles, with opponens digiti minimi acting directly on the metacarpal. Abductor digiti minimi and flexor brevis flex the metacarpal indirectly through their common attachment to the proximal phalanges of the little finger. The major function of abductor digiti minimi is therefore the application of the flexing and rotational force to the proximal phalanx of the 5th finger. The force produced by this muscle is augmented by the action of flexor carpi ulnaris via their common attachment to the pisiform bone. In the supporting grasp (Fig. 5.5b), flexion of the 5th metacarpal enables the little finger to prop up the plate and keep it horizontal. The work of Bendz is interesting as it examines closely the contribution of the ulnar side of the hand, in particular the 5th finger, to the

---

FIGURE 5.5   *(a) The locking grasp is used in holding cutlery. The 4th and 5th fingers hold the implement firmly in the palm. (b) In the supporting grasp, the 4th and 5th fingers are instrumental in keeping the plate level.*

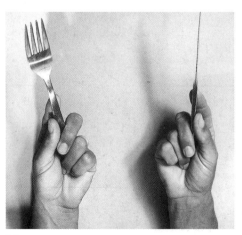

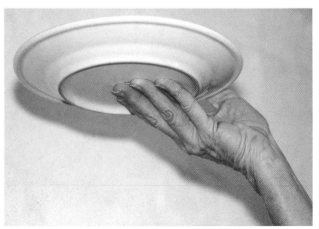

(a)   (b)

shaping of the hand. His work also makes clear the importance of specifically training these two grasps in the contexts of the tasks in which they occur.

Shaping the hand appropriately for any object or task involves the carpal and metacarpal bones giving the hand a concave shape by the combined action of intrinsic muscles. Lemon et al. (1991) call this a 'postural set' for the promotion of precision movement. A similar concept is that a group of fingers acts as a single functional unit, a 'virtual finger' (Arbib et al. 1985, Li et al. 1998a,b). When an object is gripped strongly between thumb and four fingers, forces are shared between the four fingers in the functional unit, the fingers acting cooperatively (Li et al. 1998a). Figure 5.4 shows how, in holding a mug, three functional units, each producing force in different directions, cooperate to ensure a stable grasp.

The anatomical structure and the corticomotoneuronal connections to hand muscles allow a great variety of joint configurations and functional possibilities. Monosynaptic corticomotor axons diverge intraspinally and make functional contact with a small number of different target muscles making up the 'muscle field' of the corticomotoneuronal cell. In playing a musical instrument, the dominant pattern may be one of fractionation, or the fingers can move together in a pattern of co-contraction when force is required as in gripping (Lemon et al. 1991). During strong gripping actions, the contribution of each finger to the force produced varies according to the finger's position relative to the thumb (Zatsiorsky et al. 1998). Contributions both to force sharing and to co-activation of muscles that are not primarily involved in a strong grasp may be mechanical coupling effects (Kilbreath and Gandevia 1994), with neural factors such as a widespread neural interaction controlling different muscles (Zatsiorsky et al. 2000). These investigations illustrate how a large number of muscles (a synergy) can cooperate to produce a required common output (Li et al. 1998b). Since the object and task are themselves driving the control of the hand, the importance of patients practising real tasks with real objects is quite evident.

Since shaping the hand for manipulation is partly a function of the anatomy of the hand, it is critical to preserve the integrity of bony relationships of the hand (i.e. joint flexibility and muscle length) in the early stages after stroke to allow recovering muscle activity to be channelled into the ability to hold and manipulate objects.

While reaching for an object appears to be largely under visual control, once the hand comes in contact with the object, the major sensory inputs contributing to movement control come from cutaneous tactile and pressure sensors in the hand. These help us identify objects and classify them according to properties such as texture, shape, weight and potential for slippage, enabling the motor output (muscle force) to be adjusted accordingly. The two forces produced to respond to weight of the object and its frictional properties are called, respectively, the 'vertical lifting force' and the 'slip-triggered grip force' (Johansson and Westling 1984, 1990, Johansson et al. 1992a,b,c). The extent of sensory control may, however, depend on the predictability of the task, being used more intermittently when the object's properties are predictable (Johansson and Westling 1990).

Another factor of interest is that changes in grip force occur while an object is being moved in response to the inertial forces produced by movement. Many patients having difficulty maintaining their grasp on an object while moving the arm may be demonstrating deficits in adaptive force control, lacking the ability to adjust force sufficiently rapidly.

RECOVERY OF UPPER LIMB FUNCTION AFTER STROKE

There is increasing evidence that recovery is minimal in some individuals, particularly those with an initially severely paretic limb (Nakayama et al. 1994, Coote and Stokes 2001). Reports of recovery of functional use irrespective of severity of initial impairment vary from 5% (Gowland 1982) to 52% (Dean and Mackey 1992). Such studies do not give any indication of the differences in recovery between those whose initial paresis is severe and those with moderate or mild impairment. It is only recently that studies have begun reporting measures of actual arm use as a real indicator of functional ability (Liepert et al. 1998, Kunkel et al. 1999). In addition, for results to be meaningful, a study of recovery needs to provide details of type and intensity of interventions since the process of rehabilitation itself affects brain reorganization (Liepert et al. 2001) and therefore recovery.

An early report indicated that only 20% of patients with a flaccid upper limb 2 weeks after stroke regained any functional use of the hand (Wade et al. 1983). There have also been previous reports that absence of a measurable grip by 1 month after stroke indicates poor functional recovery (Sunderland et al. 1989). According to another recent study (Pennisi et al. 1999), individuals with paralysis of the hand muscles in the first 48 hours of their stroke, who have an absence of motor-evoked potentials in response to transcortical magnetic stimulation (TMS), are likely to have a very poor prognosis. This severely affected group of patients is the group that typically receives the most intervention, and this may be at the expense of those with the potential for regaining usable function. Clinical research reporting the details referred to here is critical in order to be able to specify interventions appropriately to different groups of patients.

What is not so clear is the potential for recovery of those patients with a mild to moderate degree of disability. This group may be particularly susceptible to the methods of intervention used. Several studies have reported positive effects of interventions involving repetitive exercise and practice of task-oriented and functionally relevant actions (Sunderland et al. 1992, Butefisch et al. 1995, Duncan 1997, Kwakkel et al. 1999, Parry et al. 1999b, Nelles et al. 2001), and evidence comes from a growing number of studies reporting positive effects of intensive task-oriented exercise of the affected limb during constraint of the non-paretic limb in individuals with some ability to activate hand muscles (e.g. Taub et al. 1993, Liepert et al. 2001). However, as Butefisch et al. (1995) point out, many interventions still in common use do not emphasize voluntary activation of the distal arm and hand musculature, but utilize more passive cutaneous and proprioceptive facilitation techniques and aim for more proximal control of the limb before the hand.

Encouraging results of the effects of interventions such as task-specific exercise and training and forced use are slowly transferring to clinical practice, a necessary step for the ongoing testing of such interventions. Much therapy, however, still focuses on slings and splints which constrain the affected limb, one-arm wheelchairs propelled by the non-paretic limb, and passive manipulations of the paretic limb. In addition, only a small percentage of a day may be spent on upper limb function – 10 minutes per day according to one audit (Goldie et al. 1992).

Although it has typically been assumed that most recovery after stroke takes place within the first 3 months, clinical studies of motor training have shown improvements in functional upper limb performance more than 1 year post-stroke in patients who have some active finger and wrist movement (Taub et al. 1993, Liepert et al. 1998). Therefore, it is probably more accurate to say that although the most rapid recovery typically takes place very early (Duncan et al. 1994) as a result of spontaneous processes involving post-lesion reparative mechanisms in the brain, such as resolution of oedema, functional recovery may go on for much longer in those with some active use of the limb. This later recovery reflects the ongoing nature of reorganizational processes in the nervous system in response to use and activity. It is becoming increasingly likely that these processes are use dependent.

Reorganizational processes in the brain have been demonstrated both early and late after stroke, associated with intensive use of the the affected limb. A recent randomized and controlled study (Nelles et al. 2001) reported brain changes evident on positron emission tomography in a small group of patients after intensive 3-week training of task-oriented functional arm exercises based on a programme published in an early version of this book (Carr and Shepherd 1987). The authors concluded that the training induced functional brain reorganization in bilateral motor and sensory systems (Fig. 5.6).

A second study examined the changes occurring in the brain at 4–8 weeks after stroke when use of the affected hand was made mandatory by constraint of the non-paretic limb in nine individuals who had moderate ability to use the hand (Liepert et al. 2001). After 1 week of constraint of the non-paretic limb and physiotherapy (unspecified), the motor output map in the affected hemisphere was significantly enlarged. Associated with this increase in motor cortex excitability was significant improvement in dexterity. The authors suggested that the major contributing factor was the more frequent use of the affected hand. A study of individuals several years after stroke reported significant enlargement of the hand muscle output area in the affected hemisphere, suggesting recruitment of adjacent brain areas (Liepert et al. 1998). These changes remained 6 months later (2000). These findings are of interest as they provide a link between imposed use of the affected limb, brain reorganization and improvements in functional performance.

The real picture of recovery may, therefore, reflect not only the level of initial impairment, but also the amount and type of training and practice available and whether or not the patient is compelled to use the hand.

FIGURE 5.6   *Functional reorganization in bilateral motor and sensory systems illustrated by increases in regional blood flow when the subjects' paretic arms are moved passively. Areas of activation: (top) before training, (middle) after task-oriented training in the experimental group, (lower) in the control group. (Reproduced from Nelles et al. 2001, with permission.)*

TRAINING INDUCED PLASTICITY AFTER STROKE

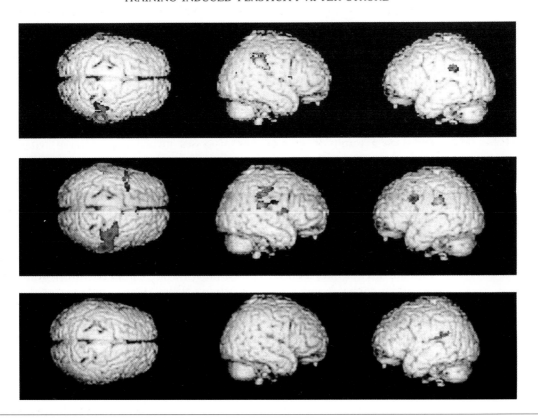

Preventing the non-paretic limb from reorganizing itself into the 'only available limb' and forcing activity of the impaired limb may be critical to stimulate the brain recovery processes that lead to the recovery of effective upper limb function in patients with some active use of the hand. The complexity of hand use and the imperative to be independent in such functions as eating, drinking and dressing are factors that need to be taken into account in planning intervention.

As an interesting aside, there is no empirical support for the view espoused by Brunnstrom (1970) that there is a 'natural' four-stage recovery pattern for the upper limb in individuals following stroke. Recent studies have shown that the kinematic patterns of movement used by patients as they reached forward to a target were due to impaired interjoint coordination and unrelated to the Brunnstrom stages (Trombly 1992, Levin 1996). Several other studies report recovery patterns that vary considerably from those observed by Brunnstrom (Wing et al. 1990, Trombly 1993). Recent research makes it clear that use and context have an effect on the motor pattern, and the pattern of muscle activity reflects the biomechanical demands of the task and the distribution of muscle weakness rather than a stereotyped neurological linkage (Trombly 1993). Nevertheless, these stages form the basis of a measurement tool (the Brunnstrom–Fugl-Meyer scale) still used in clinical practice and in research despite its questionable validity (Malouin et al. 1994).

In conclusion, it appears likely that many patients with paralysed hand muscles early after stroke recover little if any functional limb use. Those with some hand muscle activity, however, appear to do well if intervention begins early and emphasizes repetitive exercise, meaningful task-oriented training, intensive, forced use of the paretic limb, and bimanual exercise. It is these patients on whom intensive upper limb training and exercise should be focused.

ANALYSIS OF MOTOR PERFORMANCE

Impairments such as depressed motor output, decreased rate of neural activation, poor timing and coordination of segmental movements and sensory deficits impact severely on upper limb functional performance. Muscle weakness and loss of manual dexterity may be compounded by the development of soft tissue changes and shoulder pain, and by the natural tendency for patients to focus on their non-paretic limb for their daily activities (Carr and Shepherd 2000). Muscle weakness and impaired motor control affect motor performance according to the distribution of muscles involved. Abnormalities of movement also reflect the adaptations made as the individual attempts to move.

Research findings

There are relatively few biomechanical and physiological studies of arm function after stroke. Findings from such studies are gradually increasing our understanding of upper limb function and are helping to explain clinical observations. There is no typical pattern of weakness in the upper limb after stroke (Colebatch and Gandevia 1989, Duncan et al. 1994). Weakness is no greater distally than proximally or in extensors more than flexors. There is also no evidence that recovery takes place from proximal to distal.

There is relative sparing of some proximal muscles which have bilateral innervation, such as shoulder adductors (pectoralis major) (Colebatch and Gandevia 1989). A study of corticospinal influences on two antagonistic muscles – deltoid and pectoralis major – showed that inputs from both hemispheres appeared to be particularly marked for the adductor muscle, and provided evidence of direct corticospinal projections to the deltoid muscle (Colebatch et al. 1990). These results provide some evidence of the possible mechanisms underlying the clinical observation that some active shoulder adduction is often present while the converse is true for the deltoid muscle.

Rapidly conducting corticospinal neurons may be preferentially damaged in stroke (Hauptmann and Hummelsheim 1996). Slower recruitment times of upper limb muscles (flexor and extensor carpi radialis longus, biceps and triceps brachii) and difficulty sustaining a contraction have been reported (Sahrmann and Norton 1977, Hammond et al. 1988). These findings may explain the slowness of movement and difficulty sustaining a limb position or grasp on an object commonly observable in patients.

Weakness of glenohumeral joint (GHJ) abductors, flexors and external rotators and of supinators has a significant effect on reaching actions, while weakness of wrist extensors, finger and thumb flexors and extensors, abductors and adductors affect the manipulation of objects. Sustaining and controlling grip force during grasping and lifting objects is a common problem. Force produced during gripping can be slow to build up, difficult to stabilize at the required level for a specific task and characterized by irregular force changes (Hermsdorfer and Mai 1996). Deficits in interjoint coordination are evident during reaching actions, with difficulty making smooth, continuous and accurate visually guided arm movements (Trombly 1992, Levin 1996, Cirstea and Levin 2000). Reaching movements are generally slower than in the able-bodied (Trombly 1992).

Clinical observation suggests that individual muscles appear weaker for some actions than for others, i.e. their activity seems to be task dependent (Carr and Shepherd 1987, Trombly 1993). There is some experimental evidence that this might be so, and that it might be due to the torques produced by other synergic muscles (Beer et al. 1999). Isometric strength curves in able-bodied subjects have been shown to change with different limb configurations (Winters and Kleweno 1993). It is likely, therefore, that biomechanical mechanisms that stem from segmental interactions may underlie the task- and context-specific differences in the force produced by a weak muscle post-stroke, particularly if it crosses more than one joint.

Patients have been shown to demonstrate superior motor performance when performing a concrete task involving meaningful interaction with an object compared to an abstract task with no object involved (van der Weel et al. 1991). In one study, performance was tested as patients either reached forward to take and drink from a cup filled with water (concrete) task, or performed the movement without interaction with the object (abstract) task. The movement was faster in the concrete task than in the abstract (van Vliet et al. 1995). Other studies have shown a significantly greater range of active supination during a dice game that was performed by rotating a handle (supination) compared to turning the handle as a rote exercise without the dice game (Sietsema et al. 1993), and superior kinematic performance has been reported during reaching to scoop coins off the table compared to the same movement without the coins (Wu et al. 2000).

Repeated practice of strengthening exercises and functional actions is critical after stroke as it is for anyone attempting to gain strength and skill in motor actions. However, the repetitive element is often lacking in physiotherapy practice (Butefisch et al. 1995) for several reasons, including fear of increasing spasticity. The primacy of spasticity as the impairment underlying motor dysfunction and therefore requiring focus in intervention is still stressed in rehabilitation, although this emphasis is not supported by clinical evidence. Although reflex hyperactivity, associated reactions and co-contraction may be present following stroke, they do not necessarily interfere with function (O'Dwyer et al. 1996, Ada and O'Dwyer 2001). Some currently used therapy approaches are based on the belief that resisted exercise is contraindicated as it increases spasticity. However, neither reflex hyperactivity nor muscle stiffness is increased by vigorous active exercise. Conversely, these phenomena can respond positively to vigorous task-specific exercise and training (Miller and Light 1997, Teixeira-Salmela et al. 1999).

Misconceptions about the clinical signs of spasticity have led to some counterproductive practices. For example, if the presence of muscle activity of finger flexors early after stroke is assumed to reflect the presence of spasticity rather than the presence of innervated motor units, active exercise and training may be avoided in favour of passive inhibitory techniques. In addition, what may appear on clinical testing to be spasticity (e.g. resistance to passive movement) may reflect adaptive muscle changes such as increasing stiffness and contracture. Clinical tests in use, most of which test resistance to passive movement of the upper limb, cannot distinguish between reflex hyperactivity and adaptive soft tissue changes such as stiffness (e.g. Ashworth scale, Fugl-Meyer scale).

Impairments in sensory perception (in particular tactile and proprioceptive inputs) and visuospatial impairments can also be major factors that interfere with reaching and manipulation in some individuals. Control of grip force depends on afferent inputs from thumb and fingers, and it has been shown experimentally that grip force regulation is impaired by loss of afferent input (by digital anaesthesia) to thumb and index finger (Johansson et al. 1992c).

Observational analysis

There are several valid and reliable tests that give objective and functionally relevant information about upper limb function. A selection is listed at the end of the chapter. As part of day-to-day motor training, however, therapists must rely on their own visual observation of motor performance for ongoing analysis and as a guide to intervention.

As soon as the person attempts to carry out a voluntary action, adaptive movements are evident. The pattern of adaptive movements reflects the pattern of muscle weakness, the degree of interjoint coordination, the biomechanical possibilities inherent in the segmental linkage, and lack of joint and muscle flexibility due to soft tissue length changes and increased muscle stiffness.

Some typical examples of adaptive movement during attempts at arm use are as follows.

- *Reaching for an object that is within arm's length*: flexion of the upper body at the hips instead of shoulder flexion (Cirstea and Levin 2000). This movement has been noted to decrease as shoulder flexion improves.

FIGURE 5.7   *(a) Adaptations to weakness or paralysis of shoulder muscles. He uses elevation of shoulder girdle, lateral flexion and rotation of spine to swing his arm forward. (b) The aim is to abduct the thumb to release the glass. Extension of the thumb and wrist flexion are attempts to substitute for weakness of abductor pollicis brevis.*

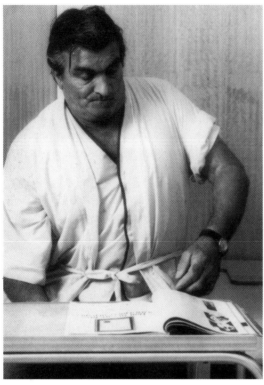

(a)

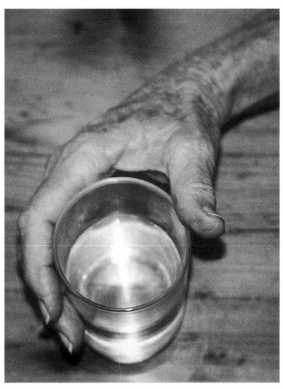

(b)

- *Reaching forward*: shoulder girdle elevation, lateral flexion of spine, abduction of shoulder with elbow flexion, internal rotation of shoulder and pronation of forearm (Fig. 5.7a).
- *Pre-grasp*: excessive opening of hand for grasp to compensate for potential inaccuracies.
- *Releasing objects*: finger extension with wrist flexed due to contracted long finger flexors, weak wrist extensors; extending thumb at carpometacarpal joint (CMCJ) and metacarpophalangeal joint instead of abducting at CMCJ (Fig. 5.7b).
- *Grasping*: excessive flexor force in compensation for poor control (see Fig. 5.13).

In addition, there are three common adaptive sequelae of stroke:

- use of the non-paretic limb preferentially when active movement is possible, and subsequent 'learned non-use'
- habitual posturing of the paretic limb, leading to adaptive length-associated changes to soft tissues including loss of extensibility and increased stiffness of muscle (Fig. 5.8a,b)

FIGURE 5.8	*(a) The webspace is reduced compared to normal and the glass forces the thumb into an unnatural flexed, abducted position at the metacarpal joint. Note the flexed wrist. (b) Compare the posture of the hand on the L to the normal posture on the R. The wrist is flexed with forearm pronated, and 4th and 5th fingers cannot make contact with the glass. Abnormal wrist–forearm joint relationships appear to have developed.*

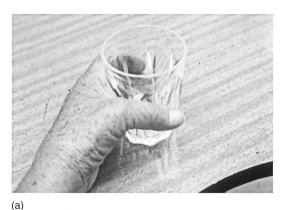

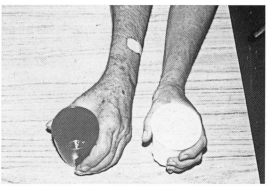

(a)

(b)

- joint stiffness and pain, particularly affecting glenohumeral (GH) joint and wrist.

Critical components of reach, grasp, manipulation

The complexity of upper limb movement arises from the number of potential interactions between the intention or goal, the object and the environment. It is, however, possible to identify components of movement, or sub-tasks, that are present in tasks that share similar dynamic features.

The simplifications inherent in listing critical components of complex actions are derived from scientific evidence for task- and activity-related groupings of fingers. Despite the apparently limitless variety of tasks performed daily, each task seems to represent ways of putting together in various combinations a relatively small number of component parts (Kapandji 1992). These components can be visualized as configurations, i.e. ways of putting together fingers and thumb to fit an object and what is to be done with it (Fig. 5.4). This is, of course, an oversimplification of dexterity, but it is a practical way of dealing with the extensive needs of the individual with a brain lesion (Carr and Shepherd 1998).

Support for this attitude comes from recent clinical studies which show functional improvements after simple wrist and finger exercises (Butefisch et al. 1995). For example, patients who practised repetitive finger and wrist flexion and extension against various loads twice daily for 15 minutes increased their grip strength, peak isotonic force of wrist extensions, speed of movement and functional motor performance. In contrast, a control group of patients who received neurodevelopmental therapy, with emphasis on decreasing tone

---

Box 5.1 Training of actions in upper limb function

Action	Movement
Reaching	Forward: flexion at GH joint*
	Sideways: abduction at GH joint*
	Backward: extension at GH joint* with
	— elevation of shoulder girdle
	— external rotation at GH joint
	— extension of elbow
	— supination and pronation of forearm
	— extension at wrist
Grasping	Extension of wrist and fingers, with abduction and conjunct rotation ('opposition') of the CMC joint of thumb and 5th finger
	Flexion of fingers and thumb around object
Releasing	Extension at wrist
	Extension at MCP joint of fingers
	Abduction and extension at CMC joint of thumb
Manipulation	Flexion and extension of MCP joints of fingers with wrist in extension
	Palmar abduction and conjunct rotation of CMC joint of thumb
	Combined flexion and conjunct rotation at CMC joints of 5th finger and thumb (e.g. cupping)
	Independent finger flexion and extension (e.g. tapping)
	Key grasp configurations, for example thumb–index; thumb–5th finger; 4th, 5th finger into palm; thumb + flexed MCP, extended interphalangeal (IP) joints of fingers (paper-holding grasp)

*These movements at the GH joint are accompanied by movement at shoulder girdle joints (ratio of glenohumeral to scapulothoracic movement in abduction is 6:1 before and 5:4 after 30° abduction) and, when reaching at arm's length and beyond, movement of the upper body.

---

without directly exercising the muscles, did not show improvement in functional movement (Butefisch et al. 1995).

Upper limb function basically comprises two groups of actions: reaching/pointing and grasping/releasing/manipulating. Since extending the distance that can be reached requires movement of the upper body in sitting and of the whole body in standing, balancing the body mass is part of upper limb action unless the individual is fully supported (Ch. 2).

Within these two groups there are key components which can provide a focus for training and a guide to analysis. Training of actions which comprise these components has the potential for some generalization to a variety of different functional tasks commonly performed. Strength training may need to focus on the muscles that produce these movements (Box 5.1).

In general, the types of action in which we need to be skilled can be compressed into a short list to aid us in focusing on what is most critical to emphasize in training. The list below is derived from clinical implications from the research findings described earlier.

- Pick up, grasp and release objects of different shapes, sizes, weights, textures.
- Hold and transport objects from one place to another.
- Move objects within the hand.
- Manipulate objects for specific purposes.
- Reach for objects in all directions in sitting and standing.
- Use two hands to accomplish specific tasks, e.g.
  — one hand holding and the other moving (unscrewing lid of jar)
  — both hands doing the same movement (rolling out pastry)
  — each hand doing two different movements (peeling an apple).
- Throwing and catching actions to regain the ability to time action and to respond quickly to the ball's speed, e.g. throwing ball, bouncing ball, hitting ball with bat.

GUIDELINES FOR TRAINING

It is now generally accepted that exercise and training need to be specific to task and context, i.e. related specifically to the tasks to be learned. Actions practised should be concrete rather than abstract, and involve an object (Wu et al. 2000). Support for task-specific and object-related training comes from several sources, including studies of constraint-induced training (Coote and Stokes 2001).

Given the complexity of upper limb functioning and the nature of the neural lesion, it is a challenge to develop effective methodologies. In individuals with some volitional motor function early after stroke, it is those interventions that require active participation and involve repetitive practice which have been shown to be effective, as Duncan (1997) has pointed out. The evidence so far supports the following methods of intervention:

- Repetitive exercise for wrist extensors, finger flexors and extensors (Butefisch et al. 1995)
- Forced use (with constraint of non-paretic arm) and intensive exercise and task training (Taub et al. 1993, Morris et al. 1997, Liepert et al. 2000, 2001)
- Bimanual training (Mudie and Matyas 1996, 2000, Whitall et al. 2000).

Exercise and training appear to be most effective under certain conditions:

- Presence of active wrist and finger extension (Wolf's 'Minimum Motor Criteria') (e.g. Taub et al. 1993)
- Sufficient intensity* of meaningful exercise (Sunderland et al. 1992, Kwakkel et al. 1997, 1999, Parry et al. 1999b, Taub and Uswatte 2000)

*There is some evidence that increasing the intensity of physiotherapy for the upper limb can be beneficial (e.g. Sunderland et al. 1992, 1994, Kwakkel et al. 1999). However, increasing the intensity of therapeutic methods which are not particularly effective is unlikely to improve outcome (Lincoln et al. 1999).

- Concrete practice using objects rather than abstract (van Vliet et al. 1995, Wu et al. 2000)
- Repetitive exercise (Taub et al. 1993, Butefisch et al. 1995, Duncan 1997, Dean and Shepherd 1997).

There is also evidence of the effectiveness under certain conditions of *electrical stimulation* (ES), including functional electrical stimulation (FES) (Faghri et al. 1994), *computer-aided training* (Sietsema et al. 1993), and specific *training of sensory awareness* (Yekutiel and Guttman 1993; Carey 1995).

The guidelines below include: soft tissue stretching to increase the extensibility of certain key muscles; simple exercises for patients with severe muscle weakness in the acute stage; and guidelines for organizing training and practice of everyday tasks involving reaching for and manipulation of objects, with some specially designed tasks which add interest and excitement to the practice session. Once patients are discharged, many will need to continue with exercise and practice. A computer printout with appropriate exercise suggestions can be supplied. Smits and Smits-Boone (2000) provide excellent advice on home exercises, including simple methods of measurement, developed by one of the authors after his stroke.

Occupational therapy is concerned with the practice of functional tasks involving the upper limbs in real-life environments including at home. Both physical and occupational therapists need to work together to ensure consistency in the interventions each provides to the patient.

Major recommendations

1. *Increased intensity of meaningful and task-oriented exercise.* Intensity of practice can be facilitated by: group practice, circuit training, work stations; use of assistants as well as physiotherapists to supervise and assist patients.
2. *Forced use by constraint of the non-paretic limb with task-specific exercise of the paretic limb.* The unilateral exercises and tasks below can be practised during constraint of the non-paretic limb in patients with some voluntary activation of wrist and finger extensors and who fail to use their affected limb outside therapy sessions despite having some functional use of the limb.
3. *Bimanual exercise.* Even when a patient has only minimal voluntary activation, bimanual practice (e.g. attempting to open a jar) may have a facilitating effect on muscle activation and coordination of the affected limb (Mudie and Matyas 2000). One of the reasons for the reported failure of individuals with a good level of function to use the limb at home (Broeks et al. 1999) may be difficulty using the two limbs together. Bimanual motor control differs from unimanual control, particularly in timing parameters, and needs to be practised for the necessary coordination to be trained. Repetitive arm training with rhythmic auditory cueing (BATRAC), using a custom-designed arm training machine, has been reported to improve

motor function, strength and active range of motion immediately after training and 2 months later (Whitall et al. 2000).

4. *Soft tissue stretching.* Patients with limited ability to move the limb voluntarily to extremes of range need to spend prescribed periods each day with the limb positioned with muscles at risk of shortening held in a lengthened position: GH joint internal rotators, adductors; forearm pronators; wrist and finger flexors; thumb adductor. Patients with the ability to move the limb voluntarily need to practise exercises which actively stretch these muscles.

Soft tissue stretching

Brief passive stretches are carried out immediately before an exercise session to decrease muscle stiffness and throughout exercises as needed (Box 5.2a). Active stretching occurs throughout active exercise. The thumb web space

Box 5.2a Brief passive soft tissue stretching	
Tissue	**Stretching procedures**
Long finger flexors, wrist flexors, thumb adductor	Brief stretch* with hand on wall, or table top, and manually
Forearm pronators	Brief manual stretch* with forearm on table top. Ensure pronator teres muscle is fully lengthened (Fig. 5.9a)
Adductors and internal rotators of GH joint	Brief manual stretch* in sitting (or supine) with hands behind head (Fig. 5.9b); in sitting with arm on table; in sitting with arm abducted, externally rotated, elbow extended

*Hold stretch for approximately 20 s, relax, repeat 4–5 times.

Box 5.2b Prolonged soft tissue stretching	
Forearm pronators	Positioning in mid-supination with forearm on gutter when in a wheelchair (Fig. 5.23)
Adductor pollicis and web space	Prolonged stretch† using a small plastic wrap-around thumb splint to hold the thumb in palmar abduction. This allows active grasping and may prevent contracture in patients with hand muscle weakness. Practising tasks with a large object in the hand actively stretches the web space
Adductors and internal rotators of GH joint	Prolonged stretch† in supine with hands behind head (Fig. 5.9b); with arm supported at 90° abduction on table top, elbow extended, forearm supinated (Fig. 5.9c)

†Hold prolonged stretch for 20–30 min.

(adductor muscle) is stretched during exercises that involve holding objects of different sizes – the larger the object the greater the stretch.

Patients with severe muscle weakness, particularly around the GH joint, require periods of more sustained passive stretching and positioning during the day (Box 5.2b).

Eliciting muscle activity

For patients with severe muscle weakness early after stroke, *simple exercises* may elicit muscle activity and increase force-generating capacity. The exercises may enable the individual to regain the ability to generate muscle force in a simplified context. Isolated repetitive movements or isometric contractions of a finger or the wrist may have a facilitatory effect on neuronal mechanisms (Hauptmann and Hummelsheim 1996).

FIGURE 5.9   *Stretching and positioning procedures. (a) Brief stretch to pronators before starting training. (b,c) Positioning to stretch GH adductor and internal rotator muscles.*

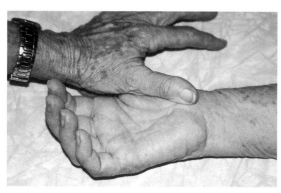

(a)

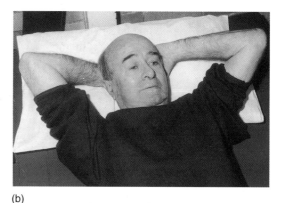

(b)

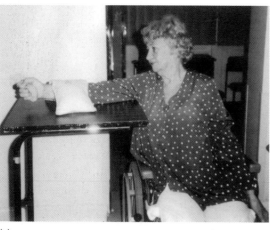

(c)

FIGURE 5.10 *Methods of eliciting muscle activity. (a) An EMG device monitors activity in deltoid muscle during attempts at passing the cup. (b,c) Demonstration of EMG-assisted functional electrical stimulation* of paretic wrist and finger extensors (b) showing the FES electrode over the motor point of wrist extensors with a reference electrode near the wrist. Between them is the EMG electrode that detects the signal. (c) The aim here is to push the weight (bean bag) off the table. For triceps brachii, the active FES electrode is on the R, reference electrode on the L, with the EMG electrode in the middle. For anterior deltoid the electrodes are similarly arranged but not visible here. (*Neurotrac 5, Verity Medical Ltd. Photographs by courtesy of Ruth Barker, University of Queensland, Brisbane.)*

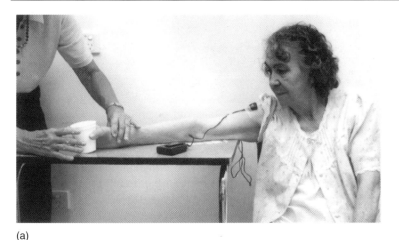

(a)

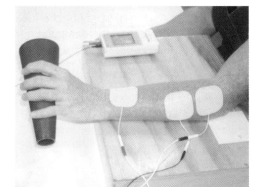

(b)

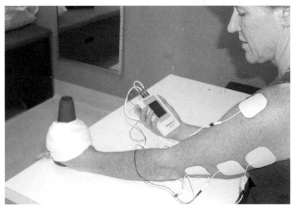

(c)

Electromyographic (EMG) *biofeedback* (Wolf et al. 1994) may be useful in the context of these exercises to assist the patient to activate a very weak muscle – the signal from muscles which are too weak to cause movement provides incentive (Fig. 5.10a). Periods of *electrical stimulation* (ES), preferably EMG-triggered, are carried out during the day to selected key muscles: wrist and long finger extensors (Fig. 5.10b), palmar abductor of thumb, deltoid, supraspinatus. ES can preserve muscle fibre contractility, and since it can be done with minimal supervision, it provides a way to increase time spent

FIGURE 5.11   *Simple exercises to elicit muscle activation. (a) In attempts at raising and lowering the glass, the therapist assists by keeping the forearm in mid-rotation so he can concentrate on activating his wrist muscles. Eccentric activity may be elicited initially by attempting to lower the glass. (b) Attempting to move the glass along the table may initiate activation of wrist extensors and flexors.*

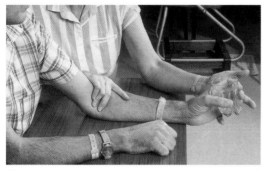

(a)

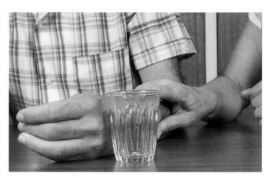

(b)

exercising muscles. *Mental practice* or imagery, in which simple physical actions are rehearsed 'in the mind', may assist some patients by focusing attention on the action to be performed (Page et al. 2001).

Simple active exercises

Simple exercises, by exploring the possibilities, may give the patient the idea of contracting muscles. Wrist extension is critical to grasping, manipulating and releasing objects.

Sitting with arm on table
Lifting and lowering an object held in palm and fingers over end of table
Lifting glass from table by radial deviation at wrist, forearm in mid-rotation (Fig. 5.11a), placing it to left and right by wrist flexion and extension
Sliding glass along table top to touch target by extending wrist (Fig. 5.11b)
Tapping table top with all fingers

Check
- Discourage wrist flexion unless it is required for the exercise.

Note
- Provide targets indicating how far to move, where to place glass.

The natural resting position of the forearm is in pronation. Exercises are necessary to enable practise of active supination and to retain the functional length of supinator muscle.

Holding a long ruler, supinate forearm to touch end of ruler to table
Make imprint in putty with knuckles (try for knuckle of index finger)
Encourage supination and cupping of hand by pouring seeds etc. with non-paretic hand into palm

FIGURE 5.12	*Independent practice of forearm supination and pronation on the Upper Limb Exerciser. The computer game linked to the manipulandum provides motivational and quantitative feedback. (Courtesy of Biometrics Ltd, PO Box 340, Ladysmith, VA 22501, USA.)*

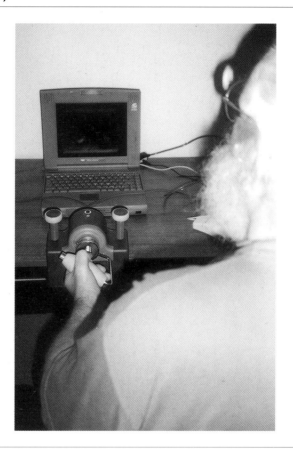

Beating a drum (by supinating)
Playing a computer game (Fig. 5.12)

Check
- Discourage lifting forearm off table.

Practice of certain tasks is used to train the control of force used in grasp. The following tasks are also likely to train dynamaesthesia when the patient pays attention to the shape of the cup.

Holding a polystyrene cup filled with water without deforming it (Fig. 5.13): transfer it to the other hand; place it on a target

Check
- As the cup is moved about, it must retain its shape.
- Encourage patient not to spill the water.

FIGURE 5.13   *Grasping a polystyrene cup gives feedback about excessive force generation. Therapist helps by holding forearm in mid-rotation while the patient tries to adjust muscle forces to avoid deformation of the cup.*

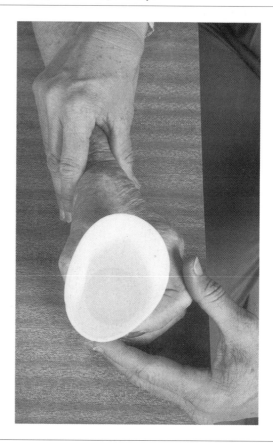

Simple exercises to elicit activation of muscles around the shoulder.

In supine. Therapist lifts arm and supports it in flexion, patient attempts various simple actions:

Reach up to touch target
Take palm of hand to head (eccentric activity of triceps brachii) (Fig. 5.14a)
Take hand above head to touch pillow (eccentric for triceps brachii, shoulder adductors/extensors)
Hand on forehead, move elbow down to pillow and up (Fig. 5.14b).

Check
- If patient experiences some pain when the arm is lifted into position passively, therapist can apply a minimal amount of traction to avoid nipping of stretched soft tissues between joint surfaces.

Shoulder girdle elevation is a critical part of arm movement and inability to do this action is implicated in poor recovery. The following exercise may enable the patient to get the idea of the movement.

FIGURE 5.14	*Simple arm exercises. (a) Eccentric and concentric activity of elbow extensors as she takes her hand down to her head and back. (b) Practise of eccentric and concentric activity of shoulder adductors (pectorals) as she takes her elbow down toward the pillow and back.*

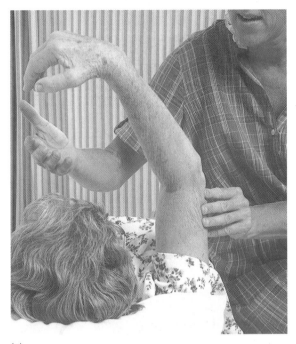

(a)

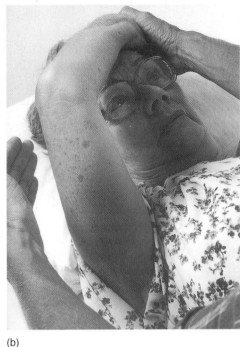

(b)

Sitting with forearm supported. Shoulder shrugging.

Check
- Do not allow trunk or head lateral movement as a substitute.

Simple reaching exercises are practised in sitting with arm supported on table top, for shoulder movement, elbow flexion and extension. These exercises may stimulate deltoid activity spontaneously in order to reduce friction of skin on table.

Glass of water in hand, arm on table top.
Slide glass forward in different directions (across the body, out to the side) to touch targets, keeping forearm in mid-rotation (Fig. 5.15).
Slide glass backward and forwards to touch targets by extending and flexing elbow.

Check
- In first exercise: elbow should not flex – draw two lines to indicate the 'track' the arm should take.

FIGURE 5.15   *He is able to reach out and pass the glass by sliding his arm along the table. A weak contraction of deltoid, which would normally reduce friction from the table, is elicited by this movement.*

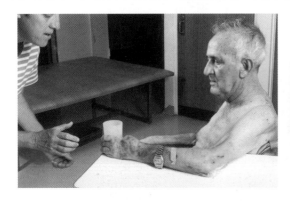 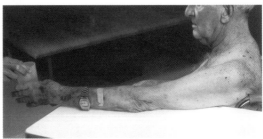

Note
- Table top is positioned against the body at shoulder height, shoulder at 90° starting position, varying between flexion and abduction.
- Reaching in a more lateral direction is important as it involves some GHJ external rotation.

When the patient has some muscle activity around the shoulder, reaching exercises are practised to exercise deltoid (and synergists such as upper trapezius) in small range movements.

Start with arm on table at 90° shoulder flexion. Reaching and pointing within controllable range above 90°, gradually increasing range, in forward and sideways directions.

Check
- Discourage excessive elevation of shoulder girdle as a substitute for flexion or abduction.
- Include reaching tasks that require mid-pronation or supination of fore-arm, not only pronation.
- Discourage overuse of non-paretic limb, such as shoulder elevation.

Note
- Objects are placed to 'force' a particular component of movement such as external rotation of shoulder (Fig. 5.16), mid-pronation of forearm
- All practice has a concrete goal, for example, 'Point to touch the target'.

Reaching and balancing practice

Sitting on stool: Reach forward, sideways or backwards to pick up an object, transport it to another place (e.g. the floor), pick it up again,

FIGURE 5.16   *Reaching to pick up a glass. Note glass is placed to 'force' external rotation of GHJ.*

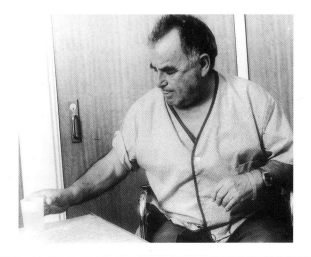

FIGURE 5.17   *Reaching to open cupboard doors and take out an object can be practised uni- and bimanually.*

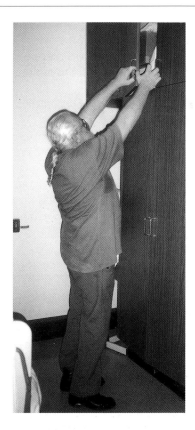

reach as far in one direction as possible then put it down. Also practise bimanually, reaching to pick up large objects that require both hands (see Fig. 2.10).

Point to different parts of a target, drawing on sheet of paper on wall.

Standing: Reach down to pick up and place objects on stool or floor, vary distance to be moved according to ability (see Fig. 2.9)
Reaching up to take object from shelf, vary height according to ability (Fig. 5.17).

Manipulation and dexterity practice

There are many activities that can be used to increase speed and precision of movement and, as a result, skill. The patient's help should be enlisted in thinking up tasks to practise that have relevance. Here are some examples*.

- *Tapping tasks*
  - touch each finger tip to thumb in sequence as rapidly as possible (do a given number of sequences within a given time)
  - tapping table with single fingers.
- *Hand-cupping tasks to train opposition of radial and ulnar sides of the hand*
  - hold seeds in palm and pour into dish
  - scooping coins from tabletop into palm of other hand (change hands).
- *Pick up different objects between thumb and finger(s), place them on various targets*
  - pick up objects between thumb and 4th, 5th fingers
  - pick up small objects from inside a cup with thumb and several fingers, thumb and forefinger (Fig. 5.18a)
  - pick up piece of paper from opposite shoulder
  - pick up pencil, put it down on table, turn it anticlockwise to point in opposite direction, then clockwise (Fig. 5.18b); use target lines on tabletop
  - stack dominoes
  - pick up and hold saucer or lid of large jar using 'spider' grip (Kapanji 1992) in which hand spans the whole diameter, thumb extended to the maximum, fingers stretched wide (Fig. 5.18c).
- *Pick up larger objects from one side of table and place to other side; vary weight, distance to be moved*
  - pick up glass of water and drink
  - pick up jug of water and pour into glass; vary amount of water, size of jug

*The items on this list can also be used as a training protocol for patients during constraint of the non-paretic arm.

FIGURE 5.18   *Manipulation and dexterity practice. These tasks train coordinated movements of fingers, wrist and forearm: (a) picking small objects out of a cup; (b) rotating the pen through 180°; (c) using the 'spider' grip; (d) tracing a circle without touching the lines; (e) punching in numbers on telephone key pad.*

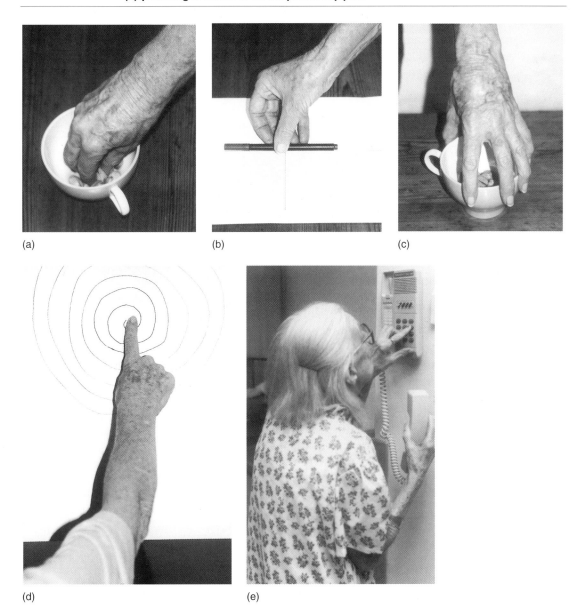

(a)   (b)   (c)

(d)   (e)

  — pick up mug of water and drink.
- *Use a stopwatch to time another member of the group.*
- *More difficult tasks (more complex, or requiring more muscle strength)*
  — type on a computer keyboard, play computer games using manipulandum

— drawing and writing
— tracing a circle without touching the lines (Fig. 5.18d)
— use telephone keypad (Fig. 5.18e)
— pegboard tasks, board games, playing cards
— turn door handles, knobs
— bounce and catch ball
— turn page of magazine
— lift and move saucepan of water, one handle, two handles
— walk while carrying a glass of water, teacup.

Check

- The pads of thumb and fingers are used for grasping, not the lateral surfaces.
- Wrist should be in extension in these tasks.
- All opposition movements should take place at CMC joints.

Bimanual practice

As soon as the patient has the ability to control simple movements with the affected limb, bimanual training should begin (Fig. 5.19). The first two exercises can be done with minimal muscle activity. If necessary, the hand can be bandaged to the handlebar.

- Arm cycling
- Bike riding (arms included)
- Push-ups against wall
- Pour water from jug to cup/glass and back
- Fold a towel
- Roll a rolling pin back and forth
- Scooping coins off table top into other hand
- Remove lids from jars, cans
- Pour from one polystyrene cup to another (do not allow deformation of the cup)
- Plunging action with coffee maker against water resistance
- Typing on a keyboard – start with two fingers, progress if previously skilled
- Remove small objects from pockets
- Hold newspaper – turn over pages with paper on table, progress to holding paper and page turning
- Reaching up to cupboard for box, different weights according to ability
- Reaching to pick up and place large objects of different shapes and weights
- Walking, walking up and down steps, standing up, holding a loaded tray
- Throwing and catching
- Manipulating a ball

For the patient to learn to manipulate a particular tool (toothbrush, comb, tools of trade or recreation) the therapist analyses the patient's performance of the action to establish what components are preventing

FIGURE 5.19   *Bimanual practice: (a) folding a towel; (b) removing the lid from a can requires a different action compared to unscrewing a lid; (c) pouring from one cup to another; (d) plunging action; (e) catching keys; (f) arm cycling; (g) rolling a ball between hands.*

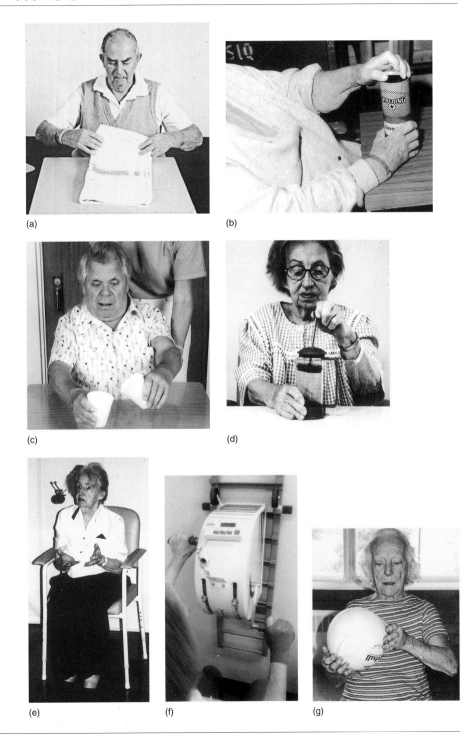

<table>
<tr><td colspan="2">Box 5.3 Bimanual training – use of cutlery</td></tr>
</table>

Task*	Action
Manipulating fork, knife, spoon into hand when it is picked up	Forearm in pronation, practise turning small objects over in the hand using fingers and thumb Pick up implement and move it into position
Holding fork, knife between ring, little finger and palm	Pick up and place small objects between thumb and ring or little fingers; supinate and pronate forearm while holding object Hold paper, putty, etc. between ring and little fingers and palm – try to pull paper out from grasp with other hand
Pressing down on fork, knife to hold or cut food	Forearm on table with three fingers in a fist, press down on putty with index finger. Keep finger extended at IP joints
Drinking from spoon†	Hold spoon and carry fluid to mouth. Practise moving hand while keeping fluid from spilling.

*After initial training, practice these tasks with food.
†This is a difficult task as the grasp has to be sustained and fluid kept level while the hand transports the spoon through space.

effective performance. How one might train a patient in the use of cutlery is described in Box 5.3 as an example.

Strength training

Upper limb muscle weakness is modifiable after stroke in patients with some muscle activity. It is likely that all patients who regain the ability to generate muscle force can benefit from strength training, particularly of muscles used in tasks performed with arms at 90° and above, and those involved in gripping and holding objects.

Note
- Amount and intensity (i.e. amount of resistance and number of repetitions) are graded to the individual's ability. As a guide, a maximum number of repetitions up to 10 should be attempted, performed in sets of three.
- Strength training can increase muscle strength without an increase in spasticity.
- Elastic band exercises are progressed by changing to a different coloured band. Start each exercise with band taut (slack taken up) (Ch. 7).

Some examples

- gripping exercises using grip force dynamometer, spring resisted gripping device or plastic putty

- elastic band exercises for GHJ flexors, abductors, external rotators, elbow flexors and extensors (Fig. 5.20)
- exercises with hand weights for wrist extensors and flexors, and muscles as above
- use progressively heavier objects in reaching, lifting and manipulating tasks.

FIGURE 5.20   *Elastic band exercises: (a) exercise for GHJ external rotators; (b,c,d) exercises particularly focused on GH and shoulder girdle muscles.*

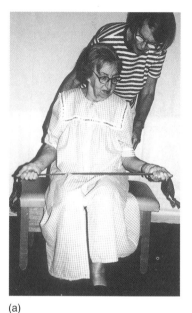
(a)

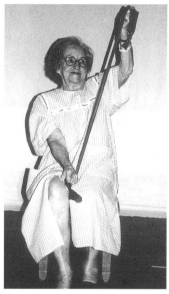
(b)

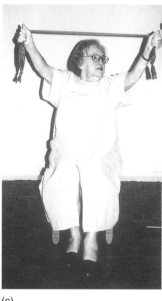
(c)

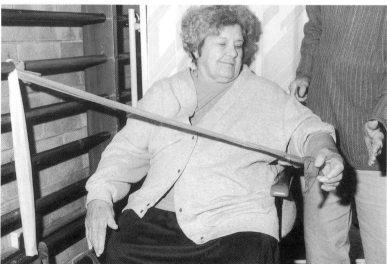
(d)

Shoulder pain prevention

As a consequence of weakness, joint immobility, disuse-provoked soft tissue and joint changes, adhesive arthritis, tendinitis and bursitis may develop, leading to pain in the shoulder and/or wrist. These inflammatory and painful conditions may be triggered by injury to the shoulder. Overextensibility of capsular structures of the GH joint, triggered by a prolonged period with the flaccid arm dependent, may lead to GHJ subluxation. Decrease in the pain-free range of movement may occur within the first 2 weeks of stroke (Bohannon and Andrews 1990), and subluxation within 3 weeks (Chaco and Wolf 1971). These are common sequelae after stroke and are discussed in detail elsewhere (Carr and Shepherd 1998, 2000).

Shoulder pain is known to have a negative effect on functional recovery, impeding rehabilitation (Bohannon et al. 1986, Wanklyn et al. 1996). A major cause of pain is the development of adhesive capsulitis (Ikai et al. 1998), which may develop due to immobility coupled with persistent maintenance of GHJ internal rotation and adduction. Muscle changes, particularly adaptive stiffness and shortening of internal rotator–adductor muscles, and weakness of GHJ external rotator and abductor muscles, are linked to the development of shoulder pain (Bohannon 1988). Although GHJ subluxation is assumed to be a cause of pain, there is no evidence that it is (Arsenault et al. 1991, Ikai et al. 1998, Zorowitz 2001). Pain may, however, be evident on passive shoulder movement in the presence of subluxation due to nipping of stretched soft tissues pinched between joint surfaces.

Passive range of motion exercises have been implicated in injury or activation of previously asymptomatic abnormalities of the paralysed shoulder (Kumar et al. 1990, Cailliet 1991). Adaptive shortening of muscles around the shoulder, particularly those linking scapula and humerus (Fig. 5.21), could interfere with scapulohumeral movement, resulting in small tears to soft tissues. Impingement of soft tissues may occur if the head of the humerus is compressed against the scapula when the shoulder is passively flexed or abducted without GHJ external rotation (Fig. 5.22).

Accidental trauma to the shoulder is implicated in shoulder pain (Wanklyn et al. 1996) and should be preventable. Patients who need most help in getting out of bed and standing up from a chair may be particularly susceptible to injury. Lifting the patient by pulling on the arm appears more common than one would expect given the likelihood of trauma to a shoulder unprotected by voluntary muscle activation, with a strong likelihood of tears to soft tissues due to their poor condition.

Any complaint of pain should be investigated and appropriate intervention given, as it would be in a non-stroke population. This enables treatment, such as joint mobilization, to commence. A standardized shoulder pain prevention programme, however, with particular emphasis on active exercise performed into external rotation, abduction and flexion–elevation, and periods of passive stretching, may be the best way to prevent a painful shoulder developing (Box 5.4).

FIGURE 5.21 *Muscles of the shoulder girdle and major forces acting on the shoulder joint. (Reproduced from Peat 1986, after Dvir and Berme 1978, with permission.)*

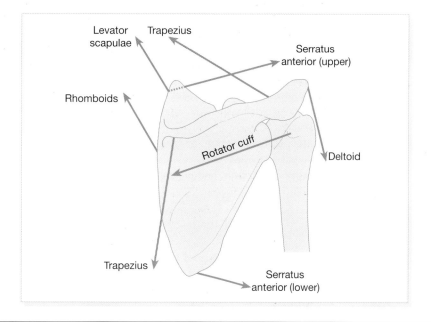

FIGURE 5.22 *(a) Scapulohumeral anatomical relationships. (b) External rotation of the humerus during abduction ensures that the greater tuberosity of the humerus is rotated out of the way of the acromion process.*

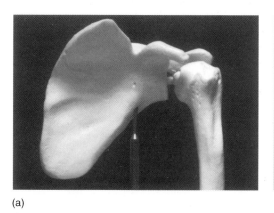 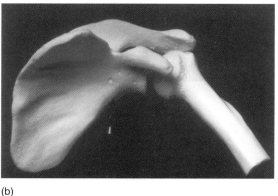

(a)   (b)

Subluxation is most commonly found in patients with extreme muscle weakness and lack of use of the limb, and must be largely due to the stretching effects of gravity on inactive soft tissues. It has been thought to be linked to downward rotation of the scapula positioning the glenoid fossa more vertically, but recent research suggests this is not the case (Culham et al. 1995). Decrease in subluxation is related to increases in range of shoulder abduction and significant motor recovery (Zorowitz 2001).

Box 5.4 Shoulder pain prevention protocol

- Positioning for at least 30 min each day
  — in supine: hands behind head (Fig. 5.9b)
  — at a table: GHJ in abduction, external rotation (Fig. 5.9c)
- Positioning in wheelchair: in mid-GHJ rotation, arm resting on gutter (Fig. 5.23). Arm must not be positioned in internal rotation for any more than brief periods during the day
- Pain-free active exercises for GHJ external rotators, abductors, flexors as in guidelines, with emphasis on GHJ between 90° and full elevation (Fig. 5.18d)
- Electrical stimulation: to anterior and posterior deltoid muscle
- Avoid activities likely to damage the shoulder, including passive range of motion exercises, and pulling the patient by the arm

FIGURE 5.23 *Arm gutter has been adjusted to ensure the GH joint and forearm are supported in mid-rotation and the hand is prevented from rolling over at the wrist. Note the increased tilt shown by the frame on the right which applies pressure against the wrist.*

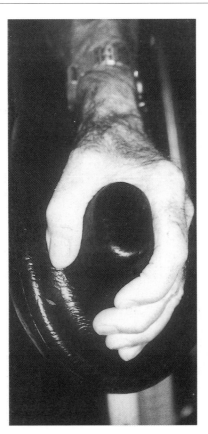
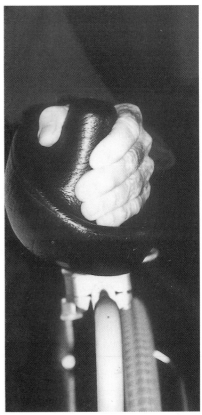

Slings for shoulder support

A variety of slings and supports are used in the clinic with the hope that they prevent subluxation and shoulder pain. Although some types of support may correct an existing subluxation to some extent, there is no evidence that they prevent subluxation. Most types of sling are contraindicated for two reasons of significance to the potential recovery of a functional limb: they promote learned non-use of the affected limb, and they provoke contracture and stiffness of the GHJ internal rotator and adductor muscles. For these reasons at least it should be mandatory that a triangular sling or any sling that holds the GHJ in internal rotation should not be worn. An exception is during assisted bathing in the early stages, to lessen the possibility of injury.

In the acute stage after stroke, arm support should only be considered when the limb is paretic, with little or no voluntary activity of muscles around the shoulder. A cuff-type sling, which allows the arm to hang naturally by the side, can be worn during sit-to-stand (STS) and walking practice if it makes the patient feel more comfortable. When sitting, the arm is supported on the table, or on an arm gutter when in a wheelchair. The arm gutter should be high enough to prevent the shoulder dropping, and the arm should be positioned to avoid shortening of the pronator muscles and pronation of the wrist in relation to the forearm.

Strapping to the shoulder, using non-stretch tape applied over a non-allergic tape to prevent skin reactions, can provide some support and comfort in patients who have some active use of the arm (Fig. 5.24).

| **FIGURE 5.24** | *Strapping to provide some support for the upper limb. (Courtesy of J McConnell.)* |

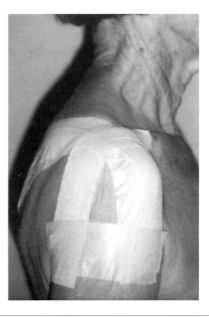

NOTES ON SPECIFIC METHODS

Forced use: 'constraint-induced movement therapy'

Taub (1980), after a series of primate studies, described a phenomenon called 'learned non-use' which he proposed may underlie the difficulty some patients have in using the affected upper limb when discharged home, despite the presence of a sufficient level of motor control and strength to demonstrate good scores on clinical tests. One way of forcing limb use in such patients, for which there is evidence of effectiveness, is a combination of intensive practice of meaningful motor tasks with constraint of the non-paretic limb (Taub and Wolf 1997). The rationale for this approach is that non-use of a limb is a learning phenomenon involving a conditioned suppression of movement (Taub 1980). Intensive repetitive practice and constraint may overcome this conditioned response by creating a real necessity to move. Contrast this with the typical hospital and rehabilitation setting, which makes only limited demands on a patient, therefore providing little incentive to use the affected limb. The patient can manage from day to day by using the non-affected limb and with the help of staff. Wheelchair mobility, achieved by single-arm propulsion, may be provided, despite the obvious emphasis on and over-use of non-paretic limbs, and it is still very common for patients to hold the affected arm in a sling for a large part of the day.

In several studies of small patient groups (Table 5.1), motor function was shown to have significantly improved after intensive practice plus constraint of the non-paretic arm in a sling (Taub et al. 1993, Kunkel et al. 1999, Miltner et al. 1999), with benefits lasting for at least 6 months (Miltner et al. 1999). Most importantly, many of these studies have shown dramatic improvements in the amount of use of the affected limb in real-world environments (e.g. Kunkel et al. 1999). Another study by Taub and Wolf (1997), in which a half glove (fingers free) was used, showed similar benefits, the patient being taught to use the glove as a cue not to use the non-paretic extremity. It is important to note that studies with more equivocal results (e.g. van der Lee et al. 1999) used constraint but without intensive task-oriented exercise and training.

Since therapists frequently express concerns about the application of constraint, it is interesting that a study of patients within 14 days of stroke reported that the patients tolerated the constraint well, and that no-one withdrew from the programme or lost independence as a result of not being able to compensate with the non-paretic limb (Dromerick et al. 2000).

The most compelling evidence in support of constraint plus intensive and meaningful exercise and practice comes from studies of brain reorganization after stroke. These studies showed an association between increased use of the affected limb, improved motor performance and brain reorganization. Liepert and colleagues, using focal transcranial magnetic stimulation, have reported significant brain changes including enlargement of the hand muscle output area in the affected cerebral hemisphere, suggesting recruitment of adjacent brain areas (Liepert et al. 1998, 2000). These changes remained 6 months later.

TABLE 5.1   *Upper limb function: clinical outcome studies*

Reference	Subjects	Methods	Duration	Results
Sunderland et al. 1992	132 Ss <5 weeks post-stroke Mean age 67.5 (range 32–92) yrs	Stratified randomized controlled design **ET**: Enhanced therapy (more intense + motor learning techniques) **CT**: Conventional (Bobath) therapy	**ET**: 10 weeks **CT**: 18 weeks ET group received > twice the amount of Rx per week	At 1 month: **ET** had significantly greater improvement on Extended Motricity Index (EMI) compared with **CT** $p < 0.01$. At 6 months: no significant difference between the groups; however, ET-mild subgroup had significantly better arm function on EMI, Nine Hole Peg Test $p < 0.01$ Frequency of arm pain in ET > CT
Sunderland et al. 1994	97 Ss			1-year follow-up: improvement not retained
Taub et al. 1993	9 Ss >1 year post-stroke Median age 65 yrs	Separate-groups design **1**: CIMT: constraint of unimpaired arm (splint and sling) + practice of tasks with impaired limb **2**: Attention-comparison group: no active training (procedures designed to focus attention on impaired limb + passive movements)	14 days Constraint: 90% of waking hours Training: 6 h, 5 days/week	**1**: Significant decrease in time on Emory Motor Function Test, in time taken to perform a series of tasks (Arm Motor Activity Test) **2**: No improvement on any test 2-year follow-up: gains were retained
Butefisch et al. 1995	27 Ss 3–19 weeks post-stroke Age range 35–80 yrs	Multiple baseline design **1**: Repetitive resisted exercises to wrist and fingers **2**: TENS for 2 weeks followed by training as above	Baseline: 3 weeks (45 min Bobath therapy) 8 weeks 15 min/twice daily	Baseline: no change in either group **1**: Significant increase in grip strength $p < 0.006$, peak isometric wrist extension force $p < 0.05$, peak acceleration of isotonic wrist extension $p < 0.05$ **2**: No improvement
Liepert et al. 1998	6 Ss 6 months post-stroke Mean age 51.9 ± 10.9 yrs	Pre-test, post-test design CIMT: constraint of the unimpaired arm (hand splint and sling) + intensive training of impaired limb	Constraint: no details Training: 2 weeks 6 h/day, 5 days/week	Motor function improved significantly on Amount of Use Test (AOU), Motor Activity Log (MAL). Significant increase in amplitude of motor-evoked potentials in affected hemisphere, and in size of cortical area capable of eliciting activity of abductor pollicis brevis $p < 0.05$

(Continued)

TABLE 5.1	(Continued)			
Reference	Subjects	Methods	Duration	Results
Lincoln et al. 1999	282 Ss recruited <5 weeks post-stroke Median age 73 yrs	Single blind randomized controlled design RPT: Routine Bobath therapy QPT: Additional Rx with qualified physiotherapist APT: Additional Rx with assistant	5 weeks RPT: 30–45 min, 5 days/week QPT and APT: 10 h additional Rx	99 Ss completed study No significant effect on arm function No between-group differences on Action Research Arm Test (ARAT), Rivermead Motor Arm Score (RMAS) at 3 and 6 months
Parry et al. 1999	As above	As above	As above	When outcome data in less severely impaired group were analysed, APT showed significant increase in ARAT and RMAS compared with QPT and RPT
Whitall et al. 2000	16 Ss >12 months post-stroke Age range 44–89 yrs	Single group design Bilateral repetitive arm training with rhythmic cueing (BATRAC)	6 weeks 20 min, 3 times/week	Significant improvements in Fugl-Meyer Upper Extremity Test, Wolf Motor Function Test $p < 0.05$ 2 months follow up: improvements retained
Blanton and Wolf 1999	1 S 4 months post-stroke	Single case design CIMT: constraint of unimpaired hand (mitten) + practice of tasks	14 days Constraint: all waking hours Training: 6 h/day, 5 days/week	Improvements on Wolf Motor Function Test (WMFT) at post-test. Amount of Use Test (AOU) on Motor Activity Log (MAL) at post-test 3-month follow-up: further improvements on WMFT and AOU
Miltner et al. 1999	15 Ss >6 months post-stroke Mean age 54 (range 33–73) yrs	Baseline, pre-test, post-test design CIMT: constraint of unimpaired arm (hand splint and sling) + training (shaping)	12 days Constraint: 90% of waking hours Training: 7 h/day for 8 days	No change between baseline and pre-test. WMFT time score significantly decreased. Increased use of impaired arm (AOU on MAL) 6-month follow-up: functional gains retained
Kunkel et al. 1999	5 Ss >3 years post-stroke Mean age 53 (range 47–66) yrs	Pre-test, post-test design CIMT: constraint of unimpaired arm (splint and sling) + training	14 days Constraint: 90% of waking hours Training: 6 h/day for 10 days	WMFT time score significantly decreased. Actual Amount of Use (AAUT) increased 98% 3-month follow-up: improvement retained

(Continued)

TABLE 5.1	(Continued)			
Reference	Subjects	Methods	Duration	Results
Liepert et al. 2000	13 Ss >6 months post-stroke Age range 42–68 yrs	Baseline, pre-test, post-test design CIMT: constraint of unimpaired arm (splint and sling) + training	12 days Constraint: 90% waking hours Training: 6 h/day for 8 days	Baseline: no change in Motor Activity Log (MAL) Pre-test to post-test: significant improvement on MAL ($p < 0.0001$). Transcranial magnetic stimulation (TMS) paralleled functional results 6-month follow-up: functional improvement retained Cortical area size became almost identical in both hemispheres
Liepert et al. 2001	9 Ss 4–8 weeks post-stroke Mean age 59.7 (range 50–72) yrs	Baseline t_0–t_1; 1 week 'conventional' therapy, no details Forced-use t_1–t_2: constraint of unimpaired hand (forearm splint) + 'conventional' therapy	1 week Constraint: duration fixed individually a priori	t_0 and t_1: no change in Nine Hole Peg Test. TMS: no change in motor output area t_1–t_2: Nine Hole peg test completed in significantly less time ($p < 0.02$), grip strength increased ($p < 0.00$). TMS: motor output area in affected hemisphere significantly larger than in unaffected hemisphere
Nelles et al. 2001	10 Ss <22.8 days post-stroke E: 68.0 ± 3.6 yrs C1: 63.0 ± 3.0 yrs	Randomized controlled design E: task-oriented training C1: passive movements, stretches, soft tissue mobilization C2: 5 age-matched healthy volunteers	3 weeks 45 min per session	E: Serial PET imaging revealed functional brain reorganization (relatively more activation bilaterally in the inferior parietal cortex (IPC) and in the contralateral sensorimotor cortex) C1: Weak activation of ipsilateral IPC C2: No change in age-matched healthy volunteers

C, control; CIMT, constraint-induced movement therapy; E, experimental; PET, positron emission tomography; Rx, treatment; Ss, subjects; TENS, transcutaneous electrical nerve stimulation.

Patients for whom this intervention should be provided include those who pass certain 'minimum motor criteria' (Taub and Wolf 1997) but who do not use the affected limb in daily tasks despite ability to move the limb voluntarily. This is the group of patients reported to benefit so far. It is not yet known whether patients without the minimum motor criteria would benefit. However, one patient in Taub and Wolf's investigations, who did not meet the minimum motor criteria, did not improve in activities of daily living.

Constraint of the non-paretic limb in almost all the studies reported so far involved a resting hand splint and sling worn for a large part of each day (90% of the waking day except for certain agreed upon functions) for 14 days. There is some evidence that wearing a mitt or glove may also provide effective constraint but it must be accompanied by staff actively discouraging use of the limb. The advantage of a mitt or glove is that it allows the limb to be used should safety be compromised. It should be noted that in these investigations patients attended for an intensive 6 h of task-oriented exercise and training. A shorter period may also be effective and future studies should address this question.

The Taub group ensure the patients' understanding and compliance with the constraint by:

1. teaching them to put on and take off the splint and sling independently
2. making a behavioural contract with each patient, working from the daily routine (whether in or outpatient) to decide which activities are to be carried out with constraint and which with two hands (see Morris et al. 1997 for details)
3. requesting a diary be filled in to enable monitoring of patient's activities outside therapy time.

In the protocol in Box 5.5 we have outlined a methodology following Taub and Wolf's research methodology. This protocol could be followed for 2 weeks initially and continued for longer if necessary.

Computerized training

Computer games controlled by a modifiable lever or manipulandum are likely to be increasingly used in the training of various aspects of upper limb movement. Efficacy has been reported in a training study of a 13-year-old boy with Erb's palsy (Krichevets et al. 1995). Use of a game in this manner focuses attention on outcome of movement rather than the movement itself, and the motivating effects of being an active participant in an interesting task may be powerful facilitators. A computer is also used in strength training for particular muscle groups. A hand-strengthening device is connected to a computer so that particular magnitudes of force production are required to operate the game (Pashley 1989). There have been several encouraging reports showing efficacy (King 1993). Figure 5.25 shows the clinically significant changes in active supination range of movement after a period of computer-assisted training in one individual (shown in Fig. 5.12) following stroke.

Box 5.5 Recommended protocol in constraint-induced movement therapy

Criteria for inclusion	Wolf's minimum motor criteria: ability to voluntarily extend wrist at least 20°, IP and MCP joints of fingers at least 10° Willingness of a patient to attend initially for a training programme 5 days/week for 2 weeks
Constraint	Hand splint with wrist of non-paretic arm in some extension + sling, or mitt/glove + reminders not to use the non-paretic limb Wear for a prescribed number of hours on each weekday for 2 weeks
Behavioural contract	Seek agreement with patient about activities to be performed without constraint (e.g. bathing, parts of dressing, activities where balance may be an issue) and with constraint (e.g. eating, grooming, toileting, some domestic tasks)
Programme of exercise	Prescribed number of hours of task-oriented training and practice for the affected limb + home practice
Measurement	Before and after 2 weeks

FIGURE 5.25 *The results for one individual (see Fig. 5.12) after 6 weeks' training of supination with a computerized system. (Unpublished data courtesy of Dr S Kilbreath.)*

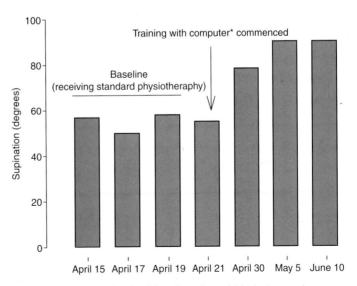

*Computer-assisted training: 2 sessions of 14 minutes per day

Electrical stimulation

There is increasing interest in the potential of electrical stimulation (ES) to reduce secondary adaptive changes in muscle, to initiate muscle activity, and to prevent stretching of rotator cuff muscles and the GHJ capsule. ES enables repetitive muscle exercise in those individuals who have little active movement in the early stages (Chae et al. 1998, Chae and Yu 2000). This repetitive exercise provides a means of retaining the contractility of muscle fibres.

According to two comprehensive reviews (Chae and Yu 2000, Price and Pandyan 2001), the evidence of increases in pain-free range of passive external rotation of GHJ and reductions in severity of subluxation supports the use of neuromuscular ES for short-term goals. Functional electrical stimulation (FES) – the use of multiple contraction sites to evoke a particular pattern of muscle activity – has shown positive results following stroke. For example, stimulation of supraspinatus and posterior deltoid muscles prevented shoulder pain and subluxation, and improved external rotation of GHJ when stimulation was administered for several hours a day (Faghri et al. 1994, Chantrain et al. 1999). Intramuscular electrodes implanted into supraspinatus and posterior deltoid have been reported to have similar effects (Yu et al. 2001). Improvements in active wrist and finger extension have been reported and decreases in resistance to passive movement and co-contraction (Chae and Yu 1999, Powell et al. 1999, Cauraugh et al. 2000). However, evidence of generalization into improved functional activity remains limited. Although arm function may improve in the short term there may be no long-term maintenance effect (Sonde et al. 2000). It is also noteworthy that beneficial effects of ES are maintained after cessation of treatment only when patients have regained some functional use of the limb (Yu et al. 2001).

Combining afferent biofeedback from an EMG signal with ES can be effective (Francisco et al. 1998, Cauraugh et al. 2000). For example, improvements in manual dexterity and on the Motor Assessment Scale have been reported in individuals with some voluntary wrist extension (Cauraugh et al. 2000). However, another study compared EMG-triggered ES and repetitive hand exercises in individuals with some active limb use. It found no improvements in grip strength or maximum isometric and isotonic wrist extension force after the 2 weeks of ES but improvements in all tests after the 2-week hand exercise programme (Hummelsheim et al. 1997). The authors pointed out that ES required no cognitive engagement which is a critical factor in motor learning. This may partially explain the fact that the latter study found repetitive voluntary exercise of hand muscles superior to EMG-triggered ES. Few studies have addressed a combination of task-oriented training and ES to enhance motor learning but the results are promising (Mackenzie-Knapp 1999).

Further clinical research will clarify the patients who may benefit, what these benefits may be and optimal dosages. In the future, neuromuscular ES using active repetitive movement training mediated by cyclic and EMG-triggered ES may prove to be effective as an aid to task-specific motor training and repetitive exercise in promoting motor learning in certain patients.

TABLE 5.2	*Tests for upper limb function**	
Test	Reference	Testing method
Functional tests		
Motor Assessment Scale: upper limb items	Carr et al. 1985, Poole and Whitney 1988, Malouin et al. 1994	The test consists of 8 separate motor items, each measured on a 7-point scale. Three items measure upper limb function: upper arm function, hand movements, advanced hand activities. Administration is strictly standardized. For patients who achieve top scores, additional tests of dexterity need to be performed such as the NHPT below
Nine-hole Peg Test (NHPT)	Mathiowetz et al. 1985	A measure of dexterity. Time taken to complete the test is measured as the patient grasps 9 pegs and places them in holes on a board
Grip force	Mathiowetz 1990, Bohannon et al. 1993, Hermsdorfer and Mai 1996	Grip-force dynamometer
Spiral test	Verkerk et al. 1990	A measure of coordination. Patient draws a line as quickly as possible between two spirals, separated by a distance of 1 cm, without touching either spiral. Particularly useful for a patient with cerebellar ataxia
Arm Motor Mobility Test (AMAT)	Kopp et al. 1997	Measures ability to perform 13 activities of daily life composed of 1–3 component parts. The time taken to perform each task is measured with a stopwatch; the actions are videotaped and rated on 6-point scales
Action Research Arm Test (ARA)	van der Lee et al. 2001	The ability to grasp, move, release objects of different size, weight and shape is tested by measuring three sub-tests (grasp, grip, pinch) on a 4-point (0–3) scale. Points 2 and 3 are qualitative in the original scale but subjectivity can be overcome by setting time limits for each item
Measures of real-life arm use		
Motor Activity Log: Amount of Use Scale (AOU)	Taub et al. 1993	Provides information about actual use of the limb in life situations. Patient reports at semi-structured interview whether and how well, on a 6-point (0–5) scale, 14 daily activities were performed during a specified period
Actual Amount of Use Test (AAUT)	Taub et al. 1993	Measures actual use of the limb on 21 items using a 3-point rating scale. Patients are videotaped
Biomechanical tests	See Trombly 1993	Kinematic analysis of reaching
Shoulder range of motion tests	Mngoma et al. 1990	Isokinetic dynamometry: LIDO Active System[†], a valid and reliable measure of resistance to passive external rotation of the GH joint. Goniometer plus hand-held dynamometer (to standardize force)
Tests of isometric strength		Hand-held dynamometry; grip force[‡] dynamometry; pinch force[‡] dynamometry
Tests of sensation	Lincoln et al. 1998	Nottingham Sensory Assessment
	Carey 1995	Tactile Discrimination Test
		Proprioceptive Discrimination Test

*Conditions of testing must be standardized.
[†]Loredan Biomedical Inc., 3650 Industrial Boulevarde, West Sacramento, CA, 95691, USA.
[‡]Digital Pinch/Grip Analyser, MIE Medical Research (see Sunderland et al. 1989).

MEASUREMENT

There is a large number of tests for upper limb function (see Wade 1992, Carr and Shepherd 1998). Table 5.2 provides a selection of commonly used functional measures which are valid and reliable, and some biomechanical testing methods.

3 Appendices

SECTION CONTENTS

6 **Impairments and adaptations**   **209**

7 **Strength training and physical conditioning**   **233**

8 **Overview**   **259**

6 Impairments and adaptations

CHAPTER CONTENTS

- **Introduction**
- **Motor impairments**
  - *Muscle weakness*
  - *Loss of dexterity*
  - *Spasticity*
- **Adaptive features**
  - *Physiological, mechanical and functional changes in soft tissues*

  Adaptive motor patterns
- **Sensory impairments**
  - *Somatosensory impairments*
  - *Visual impairments*
  - *Perceptual–cognitive impairments*

INTRODUCTION

Following an acute upper motoneuron (UMN) lesion, it is generally recognized that the major impairments interfering with functional motor performance are paralysis and weakness (decreased muscle force) and loss of dexterity (disordered coordination) (Landau 1980). In addition, adaptations occur in response both to the neural lesion and to subsequent disuse (i.e. to joint immobility and lack of muscle contractility). Common soft tissue adaptations to disuse which have the potential to impact severely and negatively on the potential for regaining functional motor performance include increased muscle stiffness and muscle shortening or contracture.

Although spasticity – defined as velocity-dependent stretch reflex hyperactivity or hyperreflexia (Lance 1980) – can be demonstrated in some patients following stroke from 4–6 weeks onwards (Chapman and Weisendanger 1982, Thilmann et al. 1991a, Thilmann and Fellows 1991), its significance for functional performance and the causative mechanisms of the hyperreflexia remain equivocal. There appears to be no evidence that a relationship exists between spasticity (reflex hyperactivity) and degree of disability in voluntary movement (Fellows et al. 1994), and the contribution of spasticity to motor disability following stroke may therefore be smaller than previously thought (Pierrot-Deseilligny 1990). The contribution of increased resistance to passive muscle lengthening (called hypertonia) may, however, be considerable.

In clinical practice, the relevance of spasticity remains controversial. Clinical research findings are often difficult to interpret due to:

- the use of different measurements
- confusion arising from the persistent use of the word 'tone', a concept with no clear meaning (Niam et al. 1999)

- the synonymous use of the terms hypertonus (resistance to passive movement) and spasticity (reflex hyperactivity).

It is important that future clinical studies define the terms used so it is clear what is actually being tested.

What is not controversial, however, is that, despite a long-standing focus on spasticity in both research and rehabilitation, recent findings indicate that the major impairments in terms of their effects on motor performance and functional activity are muscle weakness and loss of motor control, and that adaptive changes to muscles and other soft tissues are major factors impacting negatively on recovery. Somatosensory impairments and disorders of perceptual–cognitive function can also impact on functional activity in some individuals. In the following discussion, we present some recent research-based information on impairments and adaptations which has relevance to clinical practice and which clarifies the direction of physiotherapy intervention at the present state of our knowledge.

MOTOR IMPAIRMENTS

It has been typical to classify the features of the 'upper motor neuron syndrome' as positive and negative (Jackson 1958, Burke 1988) (Fig. 6.1). Since it is becoming clear that certain adaptations follow on from the lesion-induced features, Figure 6.1 includes a third set of features which can be identified from experimental studies as adaptive (Carr and Shepherd 1998). This classification has some explanatory value for clinical practice in providing guidance as to mechanisms underlying clinical signs. However, in reality the human system is so naturally flexible and adaptive that it is difficult to draw a line between the primary impairments and some of the secondary adaptations. Historically, the

FIGURE 6.1   *Classification of the positive and negative features of the upper motoneuron lesion (UMNL) and their relationship with the adaptive features.*

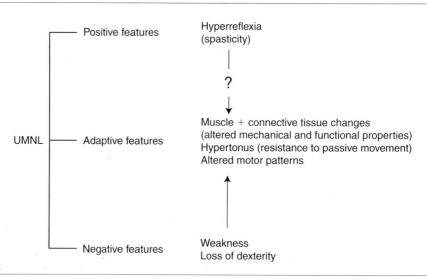

negative and positive features have been considered relatively independent phenomena, related to site and amount of tissue damage and spontaneous recovery processes (Landau 1980). However, it is now considered that many of these features are adaptations to lesion-induced impairments compounded by adaptations to disuse subsequent to the lesion. Further research will no doubt enable a more cogent set of descriptors.

Muscle weakness

Following stroke, muscle weakness arises from two sources: primarily from the lesion itself, as a result of a decrease in descending inputs converging on the final motoneuron population, and hence a reduction in the number of motor units available for recruitment. Since skeletal muscle adapts to the level of use imposed upon it (Lieber 1988), secondary sources of weakness arise as a consequence of lack of muscle activity and immobility (Cruz-Martinez 1984, Farmer et al. 1993). Contrary to previous opinion, weakness in agonist muscles is not due to spasticity (reflex hyperactivity) in an antagonist muscle group (Sahrmann and Norton 1977, Gowland et al. 1992, Newham and Hsiao 2001) but is a direct result of reduction in descending motor commands, compounded by disuse and adaptive muscle changes.

Normally the production of muscle force is dependent upon the number and type of motor units recruited and the characteristics of both the motor unit discharge and the size of the muscle itself. Muscle force is augmented by increasing the number of active motor units and the firing rates and frequencies of those units. The structural features of muscle (e.g. cross-sectional area) also contribute to the potential force which can be produced. Strength is therefore a neuromuscular phenomenon. As a result, a neural lesion in which motor commands to the muscles are deficient results in a decrease in strength, even paralysis.

Intact descending inputs are necessary for shaping complex movements by graded activation of coordinating muscles and for bringing motoneurons to the high frequency discharge necessary for sustained contraction strength (Landau 1988); i.e. for muscles to produce the force required to carry out a goal-directed action, a necessary number of muscle fibres must contract simultaneously and the various muscles involved in the action must coordinate their force production specific to the task and context. The interruption of descending pathways following stroke results in a decrease in the number of motor units activated, decreased firing rate of motor units and impaired motor unit synchronization (Rosenfalck and Andreassen 1980, Gemperline et al. 1995). These factors cause disorganization of motor output at the segmental level and underlie the motor control problems exhibited by patients even when they are able to generate some force.

The distribution of muscle weakness varies among individuals, probably reflecting such factors as lesion location and size. Colebatch and Gandevia (1989) examined arm muscle weakness in two individuals, one with a greater distal than proximal weakness, the other with a similar degree of involvement of all muscles tested (Fig. 6.2). Another study (Adams et al. 1990) examined the distribution

FIGURE 6.2   *Distribution of muscle weakness in two subjects with hemiparesis. The subject shown in the top bar chart shows greater distal than proximal weakness; the subject in the lower chart shows similar involvement in all muscles tested. Ad, adduction; Ab, abduction; Fl, flexion; Ex, extension; FDI, first dorsal interosseus. (Reproduced by permission of Oxford University Press from Colebatch JG and Gandevia SC 1989. The distribution of muscular weakness in upper motor neuron lesions affecting the arm. Brain, 112, 749–763.)*

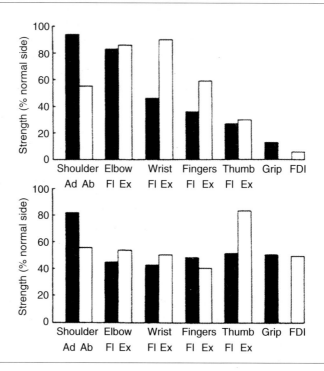

of weakness in the lower limb in 20 individuals and found the distribution did not conform to a common pattern in different subjects, nor was any single muscle group always the most severely affected. With the group overall there was a tendency for greater weakness of muscles crossing the ankle than those crossing the hip and knee, with no significant difference between degree of weakness of flexors compared to extensors. A second study of 31 individuals supported these findings (Andrews and Bohannon 2000). Several studies have reported weakness of muscles of the limb ipsilateral to the lesion (Adams et al. 1990, Desrosiers et al. 1996, Harris and Polkey 2001).

The above findings demonstrate that, contrary to the common clinical view, muscle weakness does not follow a particular typical pattern following stroke. There was no evidence of consistently greater distal weakness than proximal or of flexion versus extension weakness, and no difference between severity of weakness in upper versus lower limb (Duncan et al. 1994, Andrews and Bohannon 2000). There is relative sparing of muscles of the trunk (abdominals and erector spinae) after stroke, in part due to their bilateral innervation (Kuypers 1973), and several clinical studies have reported minimal reductions in strength of trunk muscles (Dickstein et al. 1999). Weakness of trunk muscles does not, therefore, appear to be the major problem following stroke as suggested in some therapy literature (e.g. Davies 1990).

After an UMN lesion, weakness is demonstrated by deficits in generating force and sustaining force output (Bourbonnais and Vanden Noven 1989, Davies et al. 1996). However, the reduction in peak muscle force (torque) is compounded by a decrease in the rate of force development (Canning et al. 1999). In experimental work on muscle activation, impaired initiation and cessation of muscle activity as well as inability to sustain a contraction have been reported (Hammond et al. 1988). Control problems may vary among different muscles. For example, in a study of nine subjects following stroke, delayed recruitment and inability to sustain a contraction were found in extensor carpi radialis while flexor carpi radialis had delayed recruitment but could maintain a contraction (Hammond et al. 1988).

Slowness of movement and in building up tension during the initiation of movement can have a major effect on functional performance, are more evident in fast than in slow movements (Hammond et al. 1988, Farmer et al. 1993), and appear to be associated with impaired motor unit synchronization. Canning and colleagues (1999) cite a patient who could generate a peak elbow flexor torque of 9 Nm, sufficient to lift her forearm and carry a small object. However, since it took her 7 s to reach peak torque, the muscle's apparent strength was of limited functional use. Several clinical studies have reported slower-than-normal performance of actions such as walking and sit-to-stand (Giuliani 1990, Ada and Westwood 1992).

An interesting phenomenon, which is clearly observable in the clinic, is the presence of differential degrees of muscle weakness according to joint position and task. For example, a person may be able to generate sufficient muscle force to bear weight in standing without knee collapse when the knee is flexed a few degrees but not be able to hold the knee extended to 0° (Winter 1985, Carr and Shepherd 1987). One inference is that the knee extensor muscles are able to generate sufficient force when the muscles are at one length but not at another.

The above example may be explained by findings from research into muscle function. In normal muscles it has been shown that strength is affected by the length at which the muscle is contracting. The muscle's length affects actin and myosin overlap and the length of the moment arm (Zajac 1989, Winters and Kleweno 1993). Strength–torque measures show that most torque is normally generated at mid-length and least at the shortest length (Herzog et al. 1991a,b). A differential effect of length on strength, with selective weakness of elbow flexors and extensors at shorter lengths, has been found experimentally following stroke (Ada et al. 2000).

Measurement

Tests of muscle strength (Ch. 7) include tests of isometric strength using a dynamometer (van der Ploeg et al. 1991, Andrews et al. 1996, Andrews and Bohannon 2000) or the modified Medical Research Council muscle tests, called the Motricity Index (Collin and Wade 1990). The Lateral Step-up test (Worrell et al. 1993) provides an indication of functional lower limb strength. Use of such tests requires close observance of standardization procedures.

Loss of dexterity

Loss of dexterity appears to result from deficits in the sustained and rapid transfer of sensorimotor information between cerebral cortex and spinal cord (Darien-Smith et al. 1996). According to Bernstein, dexterity is the ability to carry out any motor task precisely, quickly, rationally and deftly (cited in Latash and Latash 1994). He suggested that dexterity is not present in the motor act itself but rather in its interaction with the changing environment. Although the term 'dexterity' is commonly associated with the hand, Bernstein's definition enables its use to encompass all skilled motor activity.

Loss of dexterity appears to involve the loss of coordination of muscle activity to meet task and environmental requirements through an impaired ability to fine tune coordination between muscles (Kautz and Brown 1998). Although impaired dexterity is typically considered in its association with weakness and slowness to contract muscle, there is some evidence that they may be independent phenomena (Canning et al. 2000).

Lack of consistency in timing and modulating muscle activation may be a cause of the decreased coupling between muscle activation and target movement reported when stroke patients attempted a flexion–extension elbow movement to track a target with a low friction manipulandum (Canning et al. 2000). Impaired fine tuning of muscle coordination has also been noted during ergometer peddling (Kautz and Brown 1998). Since rate of transmission from cortex to spinal cord affects dexterity (Darien-Smith et al. 1996), individuals following stroke may have difficulty adapting to the reduced number of corticospinal inputs, having to rely also on slower and less direct corticobulbar channels for relaying information (Canning et al. 2000).

At the neurophysiological level, the relationship between muscle strength (generation of appropriate force) and dexterity (coordination of muscle activation) is unclear. However, even if they are independent phenomena, in a functional sense it is likely that they are linked, being both task and context specific and necessary for skill. Control of synergic linkages (i.e. timing, generating and coordinating the necessary forces for a particular context) is probably the necessary factor that underlies dexterity. There is physiological evidence that, for the forearm, cortical motoneurons can project to the motoneuron pools of more than one muscle.

A relationship has been reported between increased muscle strength in lower limbs and improved standing balance (Bohannon 1988) and walking speed (Sharp and Brouwer 1997, Teixeira-Salmela et al. 1999, 2001), and between hand muscle strength and functional hand movements (Butefisch et al. 1995). Such results may reflect improved coordination after exercise, and demonstrate that improved force production and coordination of muscle activity according to task and contextual requirements are both required for effective motor performance.

Box 6.1 provides a summary of muscle weakness and loss of dexterity.

> **Box 6.1** Summary of muscle weakness
>
> - Muscle strength is normally dependent on the number and type of motoneurons (MN) recruited and characteristics of MN discharge. Structural features of muscles contribute
> - Muscle weakness after UMN lesion is due primarily to a decrease in descending inputs converging on spinal MN and secondary disuse
> - Dexterity is the ability to perform a motor task in a coordinated manner
> - Decreased number of MN activated, decreased firing rate and impaired motor unit synchronization lead to disorganization of motor output at segmental level and underlie motor control problems (including loss of dexterity)
> - Note:
>   — weakness is not due to spasticity of an antagonist muscle
>   — there is no typical pattern of weakness, no consistent difference between proximal and distal muscles, upper and lower limb, flexors and extensors
>   — trunk muscles are relatively spared

Spasticity

A widely accepted definition of spasticity is that of a motor disorder characterized by a velocity-dependent increase in tonic stretch reflexes with exaggerated tendon jerks, resulting from hyperexcitability of the stretch reflex (Lance 1980). However, the term 'spasticity' is typically used in the clinic in a more generic sense to cover a disparate collection of clinical signs including hyperreflexia or reflex hyperactivity, abnormal movement patterns, co-contraction and hypertonia. The term 'hypertonia' is usually reserved for a perceived resistance to lengthening of muscles by passive movement.

This imprecise use can create a problem in reading clinical studies, since it may not be clear whether it is stretch reflex hyperactivity that is being measured or physiological and mechanical changes to muscles such as increased stiffness. Since the measurement and intervention methods used in clinical practice reflect the clinician's understanding of the mechanisms underlying a clinical sign, it is important to attempt some clarification. The ensuing discussion examines the possible mechanisms underlying the clinical phenomena traditionally considered to be indicative of spasticity, in an attempt to more usefully guide treatment planning.

Reflex hyperactivity

It is not clear to what extent hyperreflexia is present in patients after stroke, or what its contribution to functional disability might be. Although there are several studies that report hyperreflexia some time after the lesion (Thilmann et al. 1991a), others have reported stroke subjects with no significant increase in tonic stretch reflexes during velocity-controlled stretch (O'Dwyer et al. 1996, Ada et al. 1998), and no electrical activity in muscles of limbs in which there was resistance to passive movement.

Increased reflex activity may not be evident clinically for 4–6 weeks after stroke (Chapman and Wiesendanger 1982), and some studies have demonstrated that it can increase progressively over time. These findings suggest that reflex hyperactivity may be an adaptive response (Burke 1988, Brown 1994). Muscle extensibility and tonic stretch reflex hyperactivity appear to be closely linked (Gracies et al. 1997). The tonic stretch reflex is modified not only by the velocity of stretch but also by the length of the muscle at which stretch occurs (Burke et al. 1971). The activation of tonic stretch reflexes may occur earlier in range (at a shorter length) than usual, even if hyperreflexia is not present (O'Dwyer et al. 1996, Ada et al. 1998). It is theoretically possible therefore that the gradual development of stretch reflex hypersensitivity could be influenced by increasing muscle stiffness and contracture in patients who are relatively immobile; i.e. hyperreflexia may occur as an adaptive response to non-functional, contracted and stiff muscles (Gracies et al. 1997) which are persistently activated at short lengths over a long period. A report that reflex hyperactivity could only be elicited toward the end of range in a muscle with contracture suggests the presence of contracture may be a potentiator of the stretch reflex (O'Dwyer et al. 1996). It is also suggested that increased stiffness in connective tissue that attaches to muscle spindles may increase sensitivity (Vandervoort et al. 1992). An interesting clinical observation is that muscles most at risk of shortening (e.g. shoulder adductors, internal rotators, ankle plantarflexors) are also those traditionally thought to develop spasticity.

Resistance to passive movement

The classic view is that increased resistance to passive movement (also called hypertonia) is indicative of spasticity, and arises as a result of exaggerated stretch reflex activity (Lance 1980). Theoretically, the mechanisms underlying this clinical sign have been considered to include reflex hyperactivity and peripheral factors such as changes within the musculoskeletal system, including increased muscle stiffness and decreased muscle length. It has been assumed that velocity-dependent stretch reflex hyperactivity can contribute to resistance to passive movement because the two (resistance and hyperreflexia) occur together in some patients (Thilmann et al. 1991a).

It is becoming increasingly evident, however, that factors other than reflex hyperactivity (e.g. adaptive increases in muscle stiffness, changes in muscle length, structural reorganization of connective tissue) may be major contributors to resistance (Dietz et al. 1981, Hufschmidt and Mauritz 1985, Ibrahim et al. 1993, Sinkjaer and Magnussen 1994, Malouin et al. 1997). The issue of adaptive changes is discussed in more detail later in this chapter.

The assumption that increased resistance to passive movement is an indicator solely of spasticity can be confusing, particularly when reading the results of clinical research. For example, tests commonly used in the clinic which are said to measure spasticity, such as the Ashworth scale (Ashworth 1964), directly measure resistance to passive movement (Pandyan et al. 1999) and any reflex component is not distinguishable. This is demonstrated by the report of a significant relationship between Ashworth scale scores and muscle stiffness (Becher et al. 1998). The pendulum test, also used to measure spasticity, similarly does not distinguish between reflex hyperactivity and muscle stiffness (Fowler et al. 1997). Since such tests do not differentiate between the two phenomena, they cannot identify the cause of the resistance (Neilsen and Sinkjaer 1996).

Lack of resistance to passive movement ('hypotonia') may be largely the result of weakness preventing voluntary muscle activation (van der Meche and van Gijn 1986). The historical explanation that the presence or absence of resistance is due to increased or decreased tone does not add to our understanding since the concept of tone has itself no clear meaning (Niam et al. 1999).

Excessive and redundant muscle activity

Clinical signs such as abnormal movement patterns, muscle co-contraction and associated movements have been assumed to reflect spasticity. However, recent research has made it clear that there could be other explanations. Several studies of elbow flexors have shown no association between reflex hyperactivity and unnecessary muscle activity (Bourbonnais and Vanden Noven 1989, Canning et al. 2000, Ada and O'Dwyer 2001). There is some evidence that excessive muscle activity may be related to abnormal electromyography–torque relationships (Dietz et al. 1981, Bourbonnais and Vanden Noven 1989) and reflect adaptive changes in synergic relationships (Carr and Shepherd 1998, 2000). Abnormal muscle activation may also result from altered descending central nervous system (CNS) influences, such as an increase in facilitatory input to alpha motoneurons, or from secondary peripheral changes such as increased sensitivity of alpha motoneurons to synaptic input due to changes in neurotransmitter concentration (Singer et al. 2001).

Excessive muscle activity is frequently apparent in muscles that act unopposed due to weakness of their usual synergists. For example, the way in which the patient moves when attempting a task with the upper limb illustrates the effects of unopposed muscle activity on the dynamics of the segmental linkage. A commonly observed adaptive movement pattern seen in individuals with muscle weakness as they attempt to reach forward for an object illustrates this point (Fig. 6.3). In the presence of marked deltoid weakness, the patient may flex the shoulder by contracting biceps brachii. If so, the elbow may also flex because the biarticular biceps imposes a force on the forearm which is normally countered by activity of biarticular triceps. If triceps is paretic, it cannot act effectively as an antagonist. It is pertinent to note that electromyography (EMG) of two-joint muscles in able-bodied individuals is maximal when a muscle is acting as an agonist over both joints. In the clinical example above, biceps – since it is unopposed by its antagonist – is acting concentrically as an agonist over both shoulder and elbow. It is particularly common to see repetitive and excessive activity of this muscle.

Co-contraction of muscles

This is not itself an abnormal phenomenon in motor control. Muscle co-contraction and stiffening of a limb can illustrate lack of skill and is found in able-bodied individuals attempting a novel task, or moving at fast speeds, and in children. Excessive muscle activation following stroke may therefore be a manifestation of lack of skill in reorganizing task-specific muscle activation patterns in the presence of inadequate motor unit recruitment and weakness.

A decrease in motor unit firing rate (Gemperline et al. 1995) results in decreased tension, and additional motor units have to be recruited to enable greater force

FIGURE 6.3   *Biceps brachii flexes the elbow as well as the shoulder when triceps brachii is paralysed.*

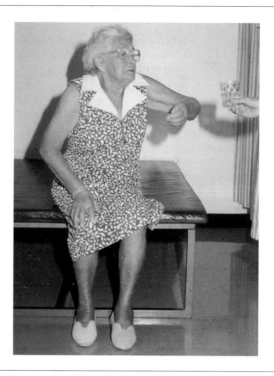

development. The result for the patient can be an increased sense of effort at low levels of activation (Tang and Rymer 1981). Stiffening the lower limb in stance may illustrate difficulty in controlling muscle contraction when bearing weight through the limb. A patient may stiffen the limb, generating excessive force in several muscles in order to prevent limb collapse. Functionally inappropriate co-contraction can also be due to prolonged activation of a muscle, for example, carried over from agonist phase to antagonist phase in a reciprocal movement such as elbow flexion and extension. Nevertheless, several studies have found no co-contraction (Davies et al. 1996) in stroke subjects performing simple actions.

Associated movements

Also called synkinesis or overflow, these movements are frequently seen in able-bodied individuals under conditions of stress. They are recognized as redundant movements or increases in muscle activity which are also evident in children younger than 5 years (Abercrombie et al. 1964). In adults they are associated with lack of skill when performing complex tasks or when generating maximum force levels (Carey et al. 1983). They have been defined as unintentional movements which may accompany volitional movement, resulting from irradiation or overflow of neuronal excitation in the cortex or spinal cord during voluntary movement.

Associated movements are also seen in patients after stroke during stressful activities, most noticeably in the upper limb. The term 'associated reactions' may be used when the redundant movements occur in the presence of pathology (Walshe 1923) and are defined in some physiotherapy literature as pathological movements indicative of spasticity and occurring in the presence of spasticity with increased effort (Bobath 1990, Stephenson et al. 1998). As a result, when such movements are observed during strong muscle contraction in another limb, they may be considered by the therapist to be contraindications to exercising against resistance for fear of eliciting associated reactions and thereby increasing spasticity.

A recent report found associated movements in the affected biceps brachii in 7 out of the 24 patients tested (Ada and O'Dwyer 2001). The amount of muscle activity was related more to the the amount of torque produced during 50% maximum voluntary contraction (MVC) of the contralateral quadriceps femoris than to contraction of the contralateral biceps brachii. There was no relationship between associated movements and spasticity (tonic stretch reflex hyperactivity). It is notable that other studies reporting a relationship between associated movements and spasticity (Dickstein et al. 1996, Dvir et al. 1996) have measured resistance to passive movement (Ashworth scale) and not tonic stretch reflex activity.

Persistent limb posturing

Persistent posturing such as the sustained flexion of the elbow observed in some individuals after stroke with no signs of soft tissue shortening or hyperactive stretch reflexes (O'Dwyer et al. 1996), may be due to neural and/or mechanical factors as yet not understood. These factors may include length-dependent facilitation of elbow flexors related to increased stiffness or shortening of muscle fibres associated with an adapted resting length of biceps caused by prolonged positioning of the elbow in flexion. There has been little investigation of muscle resting length and it is not well understood, although it seems likely that different muscles normally have different resting lengths.

Muscle inactivity with persistent joint (limb) posturing can be associated with changes in spindle sensitivity, muscle activation being triggered at a shorter length than normal (Gioux and Petit 1993). It is possible that the signal for limb position may be provided by the resting discharge of muscle spindles (Gregory et al. 1988). If the sense of the limb's position is affected, this could account for the altered resting position ('abnormal posture') noticeable, particularly at the elbow, in some patients following UMN lesion. It is possible that in some individuals chronic hyperactivity of muscles at a shortened length may have a compounding effect on stretch reflex hypersensitivity (Gracies et al. 1997).

Since there is no evidence of a relationship between persistent limb posturing and spasticity, such posturing is more likely to reflect the history of the muscles, such as gravitational effects, limb immobility, soft tissue disuse changes and functional adaptations to spindles and to muscle resting length. The distorted dynamic posturing seen in some individuals – termed 'dystonia' (Fig. 6.4) – may, however, result from a different mechanism.

The role of stretch reflexes in functional actions is therefore unclear and if hyperactive reflexes are present after stroke they do not necessarily constitute a major impairment (O'Dwyer et al. 1996, Becher et al. 1998). Reflex hyperactivity does not appear to be a major contributor to tension development in muscles during active movement (Dietz and Berger 1983, Berger et al. 1984),

FIGURE 6.4   *Dystonic movement evident during a reach to pick up a glass. Note the pronated forearm, flexed wrist and extended metacarpophalangeal joints.*

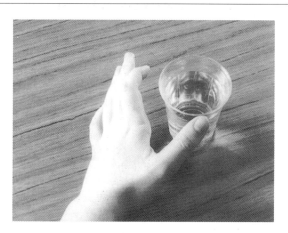

although it may contribute to muscle stiffness when the joint is moved passively (Vattanasilp et al. 2000). It is also not clear to what extent spasticity is adaptive nor to what extent muscle (and muscle spindle) changes impact on the neural system and contribute to stretch reflex hyperactivity. However, clinical signs such as increased stiffness, hyperreflexia and abnormal movement patterns may reflect, at least in part, adaptation of the system to the neural lesion and to subsequent inactivity and disuse.

It has been shown recently that sustained passive stretching for 10–15 min can decrease motoneuron excitability (Hummelsheim and Mauritz 1993), with the effect lasting longer when stretch is prolonged to 48 h with plaster casting. However, an isolated reduction in stretch reflex hyperactivity is not necessarily followed by improved motor performance or by the ability to learn a new motor skill. Exercise and motor training, however, can have positive effects on functional performance whether or not spasticity is present (Wolf et al. 1994), and active exercise can itself cause a reduction in muscle stiffness, co-contraction and associated reactions as well as an improvement in functional performance (Butefisch et al. 1995). Muscle strength can be increased by resisted repetitive exercise without an increase in resistance to passive movement or associated reactions, but with improvements in functional performance (Miller and Light 1997, Sharp and Brouwer 1997, Teixeira-Salmela et al. 1999). Botulinum toxin, administered by injection directly into stiff muscles, can reduce resistance to passive movement where this is severe. However, as with any technique that has a local effect, it is likely that the benefits achieved in the short term can only be maintained by ongoing stretching, strength training and task practice.

Measurement

Whether or not a focus on measuring reflex hyperactivity is valid after stroke is being questioned (Vattanasilp and Ada 1999, Pomeroy et al. 2000). Tests in clinical use that are purported to measure spasticity (Ashworth scale, pendulum

> **Box 6.2** Summary of spasticity
>
> - Spasticity is characterized by a velocity-dependent increase in tonic stretch reflex activity
> - Reports of the presence of reflex hyperactivity in individuals after stroke are inconsistent
> - Spasticity may be an adaptive response. It is evident 4–6 weeks post-stroke, increasing over time. It is modified by muscle length
> - Spasticity appears unrelated to functional disability in stroke and its contribution to motor disability may be minimal
> - Major causes of resistance to passive movement are adaptive muscle stiffness and contracture. The role of reflex hyperactivity (spasticity) is unclear – it may contribute in some individuals
> - Abnormal patterns of movement, co-contraction and redundant muscle activity may be, at least in part, adaptations to muscle weakness, changes in motoneuron firing patterns and soft tissue contracture
> - Note: Abnormal movement patterns, excessive and redundant muscle activity (associated movements, co-contraction) are not necessarily indicative of spasticity but reflect adaptations to muscle weakness. Strength training is not contraindicated by the presence of these phenomena

test, Fugl-Meyer scale) do not measure reflex hyperactivity but resistance to passive movement, and no relationship has been found in studies comparing the Ashworth scale with instrumented tonic stretch reflex evaluation in calf muscles (Vattanasilp and Ada 1999). Measures of velocity-dependent reflex activity require equipment generally available only in a laboratory.

Resistance to passive movement, however, is an indication of such mechanical factors as stiffness and contracture. It can be tested by the modified Ashworth scale, which is reported to be reliable if a standardized protocol is used (Bohannon and Smith 1987). The modified Tardieu scale (Tardieu et al. 1954, Gracies et al. 2000) also evaluates resistance to passive movement. It specifies the velocity of movement, and grades the muscle reaction by measuring the angle at which the catch response is detected. It also quantifies clonus.

Range of motion and muscle stiffness can be measured using a dynamometer and goniometer with a standardized protocol. This has been described for the ankle (Moseley and Adams 1991), using a specially designed instrument which allows standardization of the magnitude and angle of applied force (see Fig. 7.4).

Box 6.2 provides a summary of spasticity.

ADAPTIVE FEATURES

Physiological, mechanical and functional changes in soft tissues

Adaptation can occur at all levels of the neuromusculoskeletal system from muscle fibre to motor cortex (McComas 1994). The potential of adult skeletal muscle fibres to change their biomechanical properties in response to functional demands is remarkable (Dietz et al. 1986). Lack of muscle activity and of joint movement results in adaptive anatomical, mechanical and functional changes to the neural and musculoskeletal systems. These include loss of functional motor units (McComas 1994), changes to muscle fibre type, physiological changes in muscle fibres and changes in muscle metabolism, and increased muscle stiffness. Changes in joints include proliferation of fatty tissue within joint space, cartilage atrophy, weakening of ligament insertion sites and osteoporosis (Akeson et al. 1987). Malalignment of joints can also occur when muscles are weak and a limb is not in active use. Malalignment of the wrist seems to be common. Figure 5.8b illustrates the rotation of the hand into a pronated position at the wrist, which can develop into a change in bony alignment of the hand in relation to the forearm.

Paretic muscles have reduced oxidative capacity and decreased overall endurance (Potempa et al. 1996). Compared to the less affected leg, the paretic limb after stroke shows reduced blood flow, greater lactate production and a greater utilization of glycogen plus a diminished oxidative capacity (Landin et al. 1977). Changes to muscle fibre type include severe atrophy of type II muscle fibres and predominance of type I fibres (also atrophied) during later stages (Edstrom and Grimby 1986). There are suggestions that changes in muscle discharge pattern may cause the muscle fibre transformations (Dietz et al. 1986).

Weakness and fatiguability can arise secondarily from disuse, especially if the person spends much of the day sitting down. Secondary changes are particularly evident in antigravity postural muscles since their previous roles are no longer practised. Quadriceps atrophy has been reported as early as 3 days after immobilization in non-stroke individuals (Lindboe and Platou 1984), with a 30% reduction in cross-sectional area within 1 month (Halkjaer-Kristensen and Ingemann-Hansen 1985). Disuse accentuates fatigue by further reducing the ability of motor centres to recruit motoneurons maximally (McComas et al. 1995). Impaired motor drive can be a result both of the lesion and disuse, loss of motor drive also being reported in individuals without brain damage (McComas 1994). Adaptive changes to the cardiovascular system arise from lack of physical activity, and fatigue can be a sign of a low level of aerobic fitness as well as of low muscle endurance.

Increased muscle stiffness and contracture

Imposed immobility after stroke is associated with changes to muscle occurring within a few days. Increased passive stiffness*, due to adaptive mechanical and morphological changes in muscle fibres, appears to be a major cause of disability in many individuals following stroke (Sinkjaer and Magnussen 1994), and is a major contributor to the increased resistance to passive stretch found on clinical testing. Patients themselves complain of 'stiffness' interfering with their attempts at active movement. Clinical and laboratory tests have demonstrated

---

*Stiffness can be defined as the mechanical response to a tensile load on a non-contracting muscle (Harlaar et al. 2000). It is the ratio of the tension developed in the muscle when it is stretched to the length of the muscle (Herbert 1988).

the functional interference imposed by increased stiffness (Sinkjaer and Magnussen 1994). Increased stiffness in paretic plantarflexors has been reported by 2 months post-stroke (Malouin et al. 1997), although it is likely to occur much earlier as has been shown in animal experiments (Herbert and Balnave 1993). Severe stiffness has been reported more than 12 months following stroke (Sinkjaer and Magnussen 1994, Thilmann et al. 1991b). Postural muscles with a large proportion of slow twitch fibres (e.g. soleus) appear particularly vulnerable. Stiffness and contracture of soleus can have significant functional effects, interfering with walking, standing up and balancing in standing.

There is increasing evidence that stiffness results primarily from adaptive changes in mechanical fibre properties of muscle and tendon (Hufschmidt and Mauritz 1985, Thilmann et al. 1991b, Carey and Burghardt 1993) as well as a build-up of connective tissue (Williams et al. 1988). These changes occur due to lack of contractile activity. The length of immobilized muscle affects the changes that occur over time. Muscles subjected to prolonged positioning at a short length, and which are rarely exposed to active or passive stretch, undergo changes in crossbridge connections, lose sarcomeres and become shorter (develop contractures) and stiffer. Arthrogenic structures appear to play an increasing role in limiting joint motion, particularly if immobility extends beyond 2 weeks. Changes in connective tissue contribute both to stiffness and contracture (Williams et al. 1988), since water loss and collagen deposition also occur in response to disuse (Carey and Burghardt 1993). Increased stiffness is also found in the absence of contracture (Malouin et al. 1997).

The phenomenon of thixotropy is a possible contributor to stiffness and resistance to passive movement (Hagbarth et al. 1985). A substance is called thixotropic if it can be be changed from a stiff gel to a fluid solution after stirring; i.e. stiffness of a substance such as muscle is reduced by motion but is re-established some time after motion ceases (Walsh 1992). Results from a recent study of 30 individuals with stroke suggest that thixotropy may not be a major contributor to long-term stiffness but confirmed that contracture was a significant contributor (Vattanasilp et al. 2000).

Whether or not there is a neural contribution to passive muscle stiffness is unknown. Sinkjaer and Magnussen (1994) describe stiffness in a contracting muscle as the sum of the non-reflex features, i.e. the properties of fibres contracting prior to the stretch (intrinsic properties) and the response from passive tissues, together with the reflex response from stretch-mediated reflex contraction. They tested a group of nine individuals post-stroke by stretch to the calf muscles imposed on top of a maintained contraction and found that the reflex and intrinsic contributions to stiffness were within the range of the healthy subjects tested, while the passive stiffness was significantly greater.

Adaptive motor patterns

Adaptive motor patterns are evident after stroke (Carr and Shepherd 1987, O'Dwyer et al. 1996), and are usually (except when there is dystonia) functional

---

Box 6.3 Summary of adaptive features

- Decreased muscle activity and joint movement leads to adaptive anatomical, mechanical and functional changes in the neuromuscular system
- Changes to muscle resulting from weakness and disuse include altered muscle fibre type and length, atrophy and altered metabolism. Functional sequelae are increased stiffness and weakness, decreased endurance and fitness
- Increased muscle stiffness is a major contributor to resistance to passive movement and a major cause of disability
- Adaptive motor patterns reflect muscle weakness, imbalance, stiffness and length

---

adaptations seen during attempts at goal-directed movement. These motor patterns appear to reflect an individual's best attempt at an action given the state of the neural and musculoskeletal systems and the dynamic possibilities inherent in the musculoskeletal linkage (Figs 5.7, 6.3) (Carr and Shepherd 1998). Adaptive movements during attempts at functional actions illustrate the muscle imbalance caused by paralysis or extreme weakness in some muscles and not in others, i.e. by the unopposed activity of stronger muscles. Soft tissue contracture also has an impact on performance, preventing the required range of movement at a particular joint.

Box 6.3 provides a summary of adaptive features.

Concluding this section, at the present time the research literature supports the current shift in emphasis in physiotherapy toward addressing weakness, loss of dexterity (lack of coordination) and the adaptive changes occurring to muscle and connective tissue. The former require exercise and training to increase strength (force generation) and promote motor (re)learning; the latter require passive stretching, active stretching in exercise and training, with, if necessary, electrical stimulation, splinting or botulinum toxin injection. There is evidence that such an emphasis can have positive effects on muscle contractility, strength and functional motor performance. Definitive studies of the effects of stretching, exercise and training on the development of adaptive muscle changes such as stiffness, contracture and stretch reflex sensitivity have yet to be carried out. There seems to be no evidence that the prevailing emphasis in physiotherapy on decreasing spasticity has any effect on functional performance, nor that it is necessary to inhibit hyperactivity before exercise and training (Wolf et al. 1994).

SENSORY IMPAIRMENTS

Partial or complete loss of discrete sensation (tactile or proprioceptive) and perceptual–cognitive disorders (visuospatial impairments, inattention) impact upon motor behaviour to varying degrees. Difficulties with discriminating and interpreting sensory inputs have the potential to affect in particular the recovery of hand function and balance. For example, poor feedback from the glass while taking a drink, the knife slipping in the hand when eating, or unsure whether or not the knee will collapse while going up a step, contribute to lack of confidence and may result in a decrease in activity and, in the case of the hand, an adaptation to one-handed living.

For the purposes of this book we include only a brief résumé of this topic. The reader will find more information in an earlier publication (Carr and Shepherd 1998) and in the references cited below.

Somatosensory impairments

Loss of discrete sensation represents a failure of sensory impulses to reach the relevant areas of the brain from the various sense organs of skin, joints, muscles, ears, eyes and mouth (see Carey 1995 for review).

Light touch, *pin prick* and *temperature* are usually recognizable, although the qualitative element may be only crudely appreciated. A lesion of the brain stem may result in *hemianaesthesia* and/or *hemianalgesia* on the contralateral or ipsilateral side, depending on the lesion site. Spontaneous *pain* (sometimes acute) down the opposite side of the body may result from sub-thalamic lesions.

Although *impairment of joint position and movement sense* may for some patients result in a failure to recognize that movement is occurring, others may be able to recognize limb movement but not the position of the limb or direction of movement. *Tactile impairments* include difficulty with localization and discrimination of tactile inputs causing astereognosis (inability to identify a common object by its physical properties with eyes closed), poor two-point discrimination (inability to recognize two points when simultaneously applied with eyes closed) and inability to recognize bilateral simultaneous stimuli.

Sensation functions in both regulatory and adaptive modes (Gordon 2000), guiding movements during their execution and correcting movements in order to improve the next attempt. Recent experimental work has focused on the relationship between motor and sensory function during the performance of real-life tasks and there is now a substantial body of knowledge of relevance to physiotherapists, enabling the development of strategies for testing and for specific training of sensory discrimination and motor performance. Of particular interest is work on the relationship between sensation and functional motor output in the hand. For example, Johansson and Westling (1984) have shown in healthy subjects that grip force varies according to the friction properties of the object being handled, in that the more tendency there is for the object to slip the more force is generated by the finger flexor muscles.

There have been several studies of individuals with neural lesions that illustrate the impact sensory impairments can have on functional performance, particularly on hand use. A study of 21 people following stroke found a high correlation between perception of joint position and the ability to produce coordinated limb movements (Lee and Soderberg 1981). Other studies of individuals with a sensory impairment associated with a cortical lesion have described motor impairments including slowed movements, difficulty in performing coordinated finger movements, difficulty in sustaining a constant level of force and poor spontaneous use of a limb, particularly of the hand (Jeannerod et al. 1984, Dannenbaum and Dykes 1988).

Training specific somatosensory perceptions can be effective (Carey et al. 1993, Yekutiel and Guttman 1993). Whether or not this improvement in sensory perception generalizes into more effective functional motor performance is currently unclear. It is likely that the task-specific training practices described in this text also impact on sensory discrimination since the nervous system is selective in utilizing those sensory inputs that are most relevant to the action. Practice of meaningful tasks and specific exercises may give the damaged system the opportunity to regain the ability to recognize, select and use those sensory inputs that are relevant to the action being practised. For example, practice of standing up and sitting down provides the opportunity to attend to and utilize inputs from tactile receptors in the soles of the feet.

Challenging and meaningful problems posed to the hand as a sense organ may be addressed by the patient attending to and concentrating on the form of sensory inputs and their relationship to the task being attempted (Yekutiel and Guttman 1993). Training can involve cueing the individual into the sensory information required for the task. Encouraging the patient to pay attention to the relevant sensory cues (e.g. visual, tactile, muscle force), setting up an environment appropriate to the task, and providing verbal and visual feedback as reinforcers may not only affect motor performance but may also improve sensory awareness. Paying attention appears critical. Animal studies have shown that focusing attention increases the responsiveness of cells in sensorimotor cortex (Hyvarinen et al. 1980).

The impairment that the system needs to overcome involves the interpretation of signals from the sense receptors that are reduced or distorted by the brain lesion. This is why providing arbitrary sensory stimulation (icing, brushing, sensory bombardment) to which a patient need not attend is unlikely to result in improved use of sensory inputs during motor functions. Such stimulations may be seen by the system as mere noise (Yekutiel and Guttman 1993).

Where there is a specific sensory impairment, such as inability to recognize bilateral simultaneous tactile stimuli, or astereognosis, specific training can be provided to assist the person to regain the maximum sensitivity possible. Such training may not need to be modality specific (Wynn-Parry and Salter 1975), which may result in poor generalizability, but rather may require the solving of meaningful sensory-identification problems.

Several studies illustrate the potential for sensory retraining involving cognitive manipulation of sensory information. One controlled trial of the training of sensory function involving the hand demonstrated that somatosensory impairments could be improved even years after stroke (Yekutiel and Guttman 1993). The authors supported the incorporation of systematic sensory retraining as well as motor training into rehabilitation. Sensory training involved 45-minute sessions three times a week for 6 weeks based on the following principles.

- The nature and extent of sensory loss was explored with the patient.
- Emphasis was on sensory tasks the patient could do and each session started and ended with these.
- Tasks which interested the patient were chosen.
- Use was made of vision and the non-paretic hand to teach tactics of perception.
- Frequent rests and changes of task were used to maximize concentration.

Tasks to practise included: identification of number of touches or lines, and of numbers and letters drawn on the arm and hand; 'find your thumb' when blindfolded; discrimination of shape, weight and texture of objects or materials placed in the hand. Subjects were tested on location of touch, sense of elbow position, two-point discrimination and stereognosis. Only patients in the treatment group made large gains on the sensory tests. Further research is needed to examine whether or not improved sensory awareness is associated with improved functional performance, particularly whether patients were using their affected hand more spontaneously.

Another study (Carey et al. 1993) examined a programme of task-specific training carried out by a small number of subjects 5–26 weeks following stroke, using attentive exploration and quantitative feedback. The results showed a marked improvement in tests of tactile and proprioceptive discrimination which was maintained in most subjects for several weeks.

It is not known if specific sensory training can affect reorganization processes within the brain itself. Animal experiments have shown that somatosensory cortical representations of skin surfaces are remodelled by use throughout life and, following cortical damage, cortical maps have been shown to reorganize following training (Jenkins et al. 1990).

Visual impairments

Vision is a major source of information about the environment and our place in it. Reaching out to pick up an object involves complex interactions between head, eye and hand movements. The action is guided by visual information about the location of both object and arm, and about the relationship between wrist, finger and hand movements just prior to and while grasping the object (Mountcastle et al. 1975, Jeannerod 1988). Visually selective neurons are driven by particular object properties such as shape and orientation (Taira et al. 1990). Vision is also crucial for identifying and negotiating critical features of the environment as we walk about, features such as obstacles to be stepped over, and traffic lights which require us to time our walking across the street.

Visual impairments can have a negative impact on the patient's ability to engage actively both in rehabilitation and in daily life. Impairments can include pre-existing retinal dysfunction, and problems with visuocognitive manipulations of inputs to the retina manifested by such clinical signs as visual field loss or visuospatial agnosia.

Perceptual–cognitive impairments

Perceptual–cognitive function enables the processing and interpretation of sensory information. Perceptual–cognitive impairments reflect a breakdown in the interactive links between perceptual and cognitive processes. These impairments include inattention, disorders of right–left discrimination, or body image and lack of awareness of one (usually the left) side of space. There are a number of manifestations of the last two. In 1953, Critchley classified nine types of impairment, pointing out that they are not clearly circumscribed but fuse into one another. These impairments include unilateral spatial neglect, lack of concern over the existence of hemiplegia, denial of hemiplegia with delusions (anosognosia) and loss of awareness of one body half (autotopagnosia). The agnosias are taken to reflect not only a failure of sensory perception but also of cognitive awareness.

Unilateral spatial agnosia or 'neglect'

Individuals who do not identify, respond to, or orient toward meaningful stimuli which are contralateral to the lesioned hemisphere, but whose deficit cannot be attributed to sensory or motor impairment, are said to demonstrate neglect of the body and extrapersonal space contralateral to the lesion site (Ladavas et al. 1994). This agnosia is most commonly reported following a lesion of the right hemisphere; however, it is evident that some degree of visuospatial malfunction may also exist with left hemisphere lesions (Wilson et al. 1987).

Spatial disorders can involve impairments of perception, attention, memory and executive function (Calvanio et al. 1993). Neglect may be accompanied by discrete sensory impairment (tactile, proprioceptive and stereognostic), muscle weakness or paralysis, impaired coordination and visual field deficits. Patients frequently exhibit reduced general arousal and inability to sustain attention.

Reported incidence of unilateral spatial agnosia varies from 29–85% of patients (Wilson et al. 1987), probably depending on tasks tested and on the definition of neglect. Agnosia may be transitory, with individuals making a spontaneous recovery within a few weeks (Wilson et al. 1987). However, it may persist in some individuals despite lack of obvious behavioural indications. Severe and persistent neglect is considered to have serious effects on rehabilitation and recovery (Kinsella and Ford 1980, Calvanio et al. 1993), which may reflect the co-occurrence of neglect with large severe strokes. There have been few systematic investigations and no clear consensus on the evaluation of neglect.

Neglect can be manifested as a 'directional hypokinesia', in which the impairment appears to be a defective organization of arm movement toward the left side of space (Bottini et al. 1992). Spatial and temporal kinematic analyses of reaching have shown that patients may use a similar pattern of movement to able-bodied controls but need more time to determine the spatial location of the target (Fisk and Goodale 1988). Hemispatial neglect can be a subtle deficit, showing up only in the temporal and spatial form of movement detected on kinematic analysis (Goodale et al. 1990).

Neglect is most commonly seen in visually guided activities. The individual with a spatial impairment may not dress or wash the left side of the body or shave on the left (autotopagnosia), eat food only on the right side of the plate, brush teeth on one side only, start reading a sentence from the middle of the page and fail to attend to objects and people on the left side. Walking through a doorway, the individual may veer to one side or bump into the door frame. The person may deny the left arm or leg belongs to them, or deny the existence of hemiplegia (anosognosia). Difficulties with writing, reading and drawing also come under this general heading, together with impairments of line orientation and verticality perception. Clinical features regarded as making up the syndrome of neglect may, however, have nothing more in common than the fact that there is involvement of the left side of space (Halligan and Marshall 1992).

It has been proposed that the inferior and posterior parietal cortex may be critically involved in monitoring and directing attention within the visual environment, with more anterior lesions resulting in impaired initiation and execution of movements within the contralateral side of space (Coslett et al. 1990). However, neglect phenomena cannot be explained in terms of a single mechanism (Halligan and Marshall 1992, Riddoch and Humphrey 1994) since a brain lesion, even a relatively discrete one, disrupts an entire functional system.

Three main hypotheses have emerged in attempts to explain the impairment (Ladavas et al. 1994):

- a *representational* hypothesis which considers the impairment to be an inability to form a whole representation of space (Bisiach and Vellor 1988)
- an *arousal* hypothesis in which the impairment is viewed as a selective loss of orienting responses to space (Heilman et al. 1987)
- a *selective attention* hypothesis in which there is an imbalance in the attentional system which favours shifts to the opposite side (Ladavas et al. 1990).

Attention to one side to the exclusion of the other seems very compelling to the affected individual. For example, stimuli in the right visual field may provide a strong magnet, making it difficult to disengage attention once it is visually captured (Posner et al. 1987). For patients to be able to shift visual attention they need to be able to disengage their attention from one target, shift it to another, then focus attention on this new target (Herman 1992). A patient may report difficulty turning the eyes toward the left side without also moving the head. Different components of attention may be affected (Ladavas et al. 1989, Humphreys and Riddoch 1992):

- arousal–activation mechanisms, the physiological readiness to respond to stimuli wherever they are located (Heilman and van den Abell 1980)
- orientation and selective attention to a space (Posner et al. 1987)
- shifting attention from one target to another (Mark et al. 1988)

- intention, the motor activation necessary to respond to a stimulus (Verfaelli et al. 1988).

Outcome for individuals with neglect may be affected by the state of the individual's brain pre-stroke. In a small study of patients with large right hemisphere lesions, the degree of recovery was inversely related to the amount of pre-stroke cortical atrophy, i.e. recovery was greatest in those whose pre-stroke atrophy was least (Calvanio et al. 1993).

The term 'pusher syndrome' is used by therapists (Davies 1985, Ashburn 1995) in an attempt to explain a puzzling behaviour in some individuals who lean toward the hemiplegic side, resisting strongly any attempt at passive correction of posture that would move weight toward or across the midline of the body to the non-affected side. There has been little investigation of this phenomenon and it is not certain whether the behaviour observed by therapists represents a separate syndrome or is an adaptive or learned behaviour in a person who has some of the impairments described above under unilateral spatial agnosias.

A Danish study (Pedersen et al. 1996) examined the incidence of ipsilateral pushing in an attempt to establish whether or not there is such a syndrome and to determine the effect of pushing on functional recovery. The incidence was found to be 10% of the 327 subjects studied and the diagnosis of 'pusher' was provided by therapist observation and not by any standardized or reliable measure. All patients with unilateral pushing had the more severe strokes, were no more likely to suffer neglect or anosognosia than the non-pushers, were distributed evenly between left- and right-sided lesions, and spent longer in rehabilitation. The authors concluded that there was, therefore, no support for the so-called 'pusher syndrome', in the sense of a syndrome encompassing both physical and neuropsychological symptoms.

There is some evidence that individuals with this problem have an impairment in verticality perception. Misperception of verticality has been reported to be associated with falling in elderly individuals, including those with stroke (Tobis et al. 1981). Lateropulsion has been described by Dieterich and Brandt (1992) as part of Wallenberg's syndrome, which includes poor visual perception of the vertical. It has been hypothesized that the midline of the trunk and/or head serves to divide space into a right and a left sector, i.e. the body's midline serves as a physical anchor for the calculation of internal egocentric coordinates for representing the position of the body relative to external objects (Karnath et al. 1991). The relationship with verticality perception needs further investigation.

Anecdotally, the tendency to lean toward the affected side and to resist strongly attempts by the therapist to shift the person toward the other side seems to disappear after a short period of active and intensive balance training, and as patients regain their ability to move about voluntarily in sitting and standing. If patients have experienced a change in their perception of the midline of the body, this would explain the anxiety and fear expressed if they are moved passively by the therapist (e.g. into a more 'symmetrical' sitting position). It is possible that some passive techniques used in therapy, which involve the patient being moved about by the physiotherapist rather than moving actively, may reinforce the abnormal behaviour and cause it to persist for longer. If an individual's subjective midline has shifted to one side, being moved by another person to the opposite side could be perceived as a large excursion away from the midline. Affected patients are clearly distressed when attempts are made to move them to the unaffected side since they seem to think their appropriate position in space is to the left of true centre (Bohannon 1996). They appear to cope much better when they practise tasks such as reaching for an object which requires active movement of the body to both sides, with visual cueing and feedback provided by the success or otherwise of their performance. It can be helpful to point out that they are being misled about the nature of vertical and to encourage them to look at objects they 'know' to be vertical (the leg of a bed, a door frame); i.e. to intellectualize the 'idea' of vertical and to try to align themselves with known vertically oriented objects. There is some evidence that this approach involving active practice of specific tasks can be effective (Bohannon 1998).

In conclusion, it is evident that somatosensory impairments can improve significantly following specific sensory retraining. However, there is little evidence of carryover from methods which are not aligned to meaningful tasks. It is likely that specific sensations are improved by the natural ongoing sensory inputs occurring during active training and practice of tasks. Task-oriented training provides the opportunity for the lesioned system to put together sensory inputs and appropriate motor outputs. Neuropsychological methods of intervention include repetitive visual scanning, cueing and sustained attention training.

Measurement

For training to be rationally planned, sensation must be tested. Although many of the tests used in the clinic are subjective, recently tests have been developed which, if performed under standardized conditions and with the appropriate

---

Box 6.4 Summary of sensory and perceptual–cognitive impairments

- Somatosensory impairments include partial or complete loss of discrete sensations, including impairment of joint position and movement sense and tactile sensation
- Visuocognitive impairments include visual field loss and visuospatial agnosia
- Perceptual–cognitive impairments include disorders of body image and impaired awareness of one side of space (usually the L) as in unilateral spatial agnosia (neglect)
- Lateropulsion (the 'pusher syndrome') may be associated with a disorder of verticality perception
- Therapists should avoid moving passively a person who leans persistently to one side but instead should encourage active balancing exercises
- Specific sensory retraining appears effective in improving sensory discrimination but carryover into improved function needs to be investigated

equipment, enable a quantification of the individual's ability to perceive specific sensory inputs (Yekutiel and Guttman 1993, Carey 1995, Winward et al. 1999). Where facilities are available, afferent projections from limbs to cerebral cortex are studied using somatosensory evoked potentials (Burke and Gandevia 1988, Kuzoffsky 1990). Perceptual–cognitive impairments are tested by a clinical neuropsychologist.

Sensory and perceptual–cognitive impairments are summarized in Box 6.4.

7 Strength training and physical conditioning

CHAPTER CONTENTS

- ■ **Introduction**
- ■ **Increasing muscle strength**
  - *Type of exercise*
  - *Specificity of strength training*
  - *Eliciting activity in very weak muscles*
  - *Efficacy of muscle strength training after stroke*
  - *Exercise prescription*
  - *Maximizing skill*
  - *Measures of muscle strength*

- ■ **Preserving muscle length and flexibility**
  - *Stretching prescription*
  - *Measures of joint range*
- ■ **Physical conditioning**
  - *Exercise prescription*
  - *Measures of exercise response*
- ■ **Conclusion**

INTRODUCTION

The major goal of physiotherapy in neurological rehabilitation is the optimization of functional motor performance. Major impairments limiting motor performance are muscle weakness or paralysis, soft tissue contracture, lack of endurance and physical fitness.

This appendix provides some general guidelines for strength training in relation to the optimization of motor control and skill, training to increase physical fitness and endurance, and methods of decreasing stiffness and preserving soft tissue length.

INCREASING MUSCLE STRENGTH

The physiological factors which affect strength are structural and functional. Structural factors include the cross-sectional area of the muscle (its size), the density of muscle fibres per unit cross-sectional area and the efficiency of mechanical leverage across joints. The functional factors include the number, type and frequency of motor units recruited during a contraction, the initial length of muscles and the efficiency of cooperation between synergic muscles involved in the action. In addition, biomechanical factors also affect strength. For example, the viscoelastic properties of the contractile and non-contractile tissues absorb energy when an active muscle is stretched and this can be used to increase the concentric force of the contraction. Strength is therefore a function of the properties of muscle and depends on intact neurological function (Buchner and de Lateur 1991).

It follows that strength training is necessary after stroke to improve the force-generating capacity and efficiency of weak muscles and to improve functional motor performance. The relationship between strength and performance is complex. The amount of strength required depends on the person's physical size (weight of hand, total body weight) – i.e. relative as opposed to absolute strength (Buchner and de Lateur 1991) – and on the action to be performed (walking on a flat surface vs stair climbing). Skilled motor performance, however, requires the following:

- each muscle involved in the action has to generate peak force at the length appropriate to the action
- this force has to be graded and timed so synergic muscle activity is controlled for task and context
- the force has to be sustained over a sufficient period of time
- peak forces must be generated fast enough to meet environmental and task demands such as increasing walking speed to cross the road at traffic lights.

Although reductions in muscle force production and its control cause major motor dysfunction after a lesion of the neuromotor system, strength training has been eliminated from many therapy programmes over the past five decades, to a large extent due to the continuing influence of certain physiotherapy beliefs. First, weakness has been thought to be due to inhibition from spastic antagonists and 'low tone' of agonists rather than a direct result of the reduction in descending inputs to spinal motoneurons; second, exercises causing effort are therefore contraindicated as they are expected to increase spasticity, co-contraction and abnormal movement patterns.

These views are still being taught and many clinicians are therefore maintaining an approach to rehabilitation that is no longer supported either by scientific theory or clinical evidence. Clinical research has shown that effort applied in strength training does not increase spasticity (reflex hyperactivity), associated movements, co-contraction or resistance to passive movement* (Butefisch et al. 1995, Davies et al. 1996, Sharp and Brouwer 1997, Brown and Kautz 1998, Smith et al. 1999, Teixeira-Salmela et al. 1999, Ada and O'Dwyer 2001, Bateman et al. 2001). On the other hand, not only does strength training result in increased muscle strength following stroke, but also improved functional performance and decreased spasticity, for example decreases in resistance to passive movement, stretch reflex hyperactivity and co-contraction (Butefisch et al. 1995, Miller and Light 1997, Smith et al. 1999, Teixeira-Salmela et al. 1999). The dynamic stretching that occurs during active exercise may play a part in decreasing reflex hyperexcitability and increasing muscle compliance (Otis et al. 1985, Hummelsheim et al. 1994). The evidence is mounting that repetitive, task-oriented strength training is effective following stroke, as is also being

---

*Variously tested by resistance to passive movement on the Ashworth scale, response to pendulum test, presence of abnormal movement patterns, or inappropriate muscle activity or co-contraction on EMG.

shown following cerebral palsy and traumatic brain injury. It is also likely that practice and training, by improving aspects of motor control such as timing of muscle activations, would result in decreased co-contraction (Carr and Shepherd 1987). There seems little doubt that active exercise and training provoke efficacious changes in motor control.

There is another consideration when planning intervention. Many individuals who have stroke are elderly. For some, their pre-stroke physical condition may have been poor due to ill health, excessive weight, or a sedentary lifestyle. Consequently, reductions in muscle strength due to the lesion, together with pre-existing reductions in joint flexibility, strength, endurance and physical fitness, combine to impact severely on the patient's ability to regain the necessary functional motor skills. Poor physical condition and being elderly are not barriers to strength and fitness training post-stroke but are instead imperatives. It is known that regular moderately vigorous exercise has positive effects on muscle mass and strength, postural stability and prevention of falls, joint flexibility, bone density, psychological function and cardiovascular responses to exercise (read Mazzeo et al. 1998 for review and recommendations). The avoidance of strength training in patients with muscle weakness who are also lacking in fitness is very likely, therefore, to have a significant negative impact on functional outcome after stroke (Miller and Light 1997).

Factors associated with the nature of the lesion, the patient's pre-stroke physical condition and subsequent physical inactivity provide, therefore, several compelling reasons for emphasizing strength training following a stroke, summarized as follows.

1. Muscle weakness is a major impairment to effective functional performance
   — a stroke usually results in some degree of muscle weakness, including paralysis, primarily as a direct result of a reduction in descending inputs on spinal motoneurons and of the number of motor units activated
   — the immobility which ensues results in mechanical and functional changes to the muscles and connective tissue, and predisposes to further reductions in strength
   — elderly individuals may have had varying degrees of muscle weakness and reduced endurance and cardiovascular responses pre-stroke due to a decline in physical activity.
2. There is mounting evidence that strength training is effective following stroke
   — muscle strength is increased
   — increased strength can be associated with improved functional performance
   — when incorporated into an intensive activity programme, exercise capacity and endurance are also improved.
3. There is no evidence that spasticity (hyperreflexia) or hypertonus (resistance to passive movement) increase, and some evidence that they decrease, after strength training.

The mechanisms underlying the improvement of muscle strength and motor control reported following stroke may be similar to those after strength training in able-bodied individuals. Neuromuscular adaptations associated with muscle strengthening and task acquisition are described by several authors (e.g. Sale 1987, Rutherford 1988, Moritani 1993). It is generally accepted that a large part of any early increase in muscle strength in the able-bodied is due to neural adaptations, including task-specific adaptations to neural drive, which are both quantitative (increased neural drive to target muscles) and qualitative (reduced co-contraction and improved coordination among synergists) (Hakkinen and Komi 1983, Rutherford and Jones 1986, Carolan and Cafarelli 1992, Yue and Cole 1992). Muscle hypertrophy or an increase in cross-sectional area plays a part in later increases in strength. Furthermore, neural adaptations appear to be specific to the training action or task. Strength training effects are, therefore, both neural and structural, and include:

- *stimulation of neuromuscular changes* due to reorganized drive from supraspinal centres. Changes include enhanced muscle excitation, improvements in recruitment of motoneuron pool, inhibition of antagonist muscles, motor unit activation and synchronization of the firing pattern of motor units (Hakkinen and Komi 1983, Sale 1987)
- *stimulation of metabolic, mechanical and structural muscle fibre changes* that result in larger and stronger muscles due to an increase in actin and myosin protein filaments (Sale 1987, Thepaut-Mathieu et al. 1988).

These effects are reported from studies of able-bodied individuals but their relevance to individuals with motor impairments is obvious. It has been shown with able-bodied young men on an 8-week progressive strength training programme that an increase in maximal force produced by the lower limb extensors was accompanied by increases in neural activation (integrated EMG) of those muscles (Hakkinen and Komi 1993). It is likely that increased strength following stroke also results from increased mechanical efficiency of the muscles themselves, improved limb control and motor learning (Rutherford and Jones 1986, Rutherford 1988). Increased strength occurs in muscles not directly strengthened but which, since they act as stabilizers and synergists during the exercise, are also affected positively (Fiatarone et al. 1990).

There may be some advantageous effect of increase in muscle size after stroke (Hakkinen et al. 1998, Harridge et al. 1999), since it is likely that muscle atrophy can become a factor in disuse weakness after stroke as it is during other conditions of imposed limb immobility. In animal experiments, quadriceps atrophy has been reported as early as 3 days after immobilization (Lindboe and Platou 1984) with 30% reduction in cross-sectional area within 1 month (Halkjaer-Kristensen and Ingemann-Hansen 1985). One study has reported that muscle weakness and atrophy due to disuse are essentially preventable by exercise that activates high threshold motor units such as sit-to-stand, stair walking and eccentric knee extension training (Hachisuka et al. 1997). In the very elderly (85–97 years) an increase in quadriceps cross-sectional area, measured at mid-thigh with magnetic resonance imaging, has been demonstrated after 12 weeks of isotonic knee extensor strength training without any change in muscle activation. The authors suggest that increased muscle mass may have functional and metabolic benefits for the very elderly (Frontera et al. 1988, Harridge et al. 1999).

Some of the improvements in activity levels reported after strength training may also be due to improved psychological state, self-concept (McAuley and

FIGURE 7.1	*(Left) Hip, knee and ankle muscles contract in synchrony in kinetic chain exercises such as step-ups. (Right) An exercise for quadriceps femoris that isolates movement to the knee joint.*

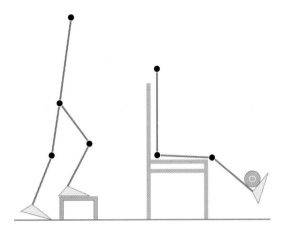

Rudolph 1995) and/or energy levels. The effects of 12 months of bicycle ergo-meter training included improved self-concept and functional status in chronic stroke (Brinkman and Hoskins 1979). Improvements in functional status are also attributed to positive feedback from success in training, and social enjoyment.

Type of exercise

There are several methods of strength training in use in rehabilitation:

- *Isometric exercise*: a muscle contraction is performed with little movement or change in muscle length
- *Isotonic exercise*: an exercise in which the resistance remains constant; includes active gravity-eliminated exercise, free weights*, weight-loaded machines and elastic band exercise
- *Isokinetic exercise*: exercise that uses an isokinetic dynamometer in which the speed is kept constant and the variable resistance matches the force applied.

Single joint and kinetic chain exercises

Isotonic and isokinetic exercises may be performed by isolating one segment (sometimes called open-chain exercise). In these exercises, the limb moves against resistance with the distal segment free, as in the seated knee extension exercise in Figure 7.1. Functionally, however, in many everyday actions, the foot, shank and thigh behave as a linked segmental chain (Fig. 7.3). The term lower limb kinetic chain (or 'closed-chain') exercise (Palmitier et al. 1991) is used to describe exercises that recruit all three links together. Movement at one joint, of necessity, produces movement of the other joints.

*Free weights are not purely isotonic since muscle tension varies according to gravity and segmental relationships.

FIGURE 7.2   *(a) Modified leg press exercise (affected leg) performed independently on a tilt table. He uses a counter to keep track of number of repetitions. (b) Leg press exercises for weak right leg using pneumatic strength training equipment. Note that a more reclined position can be used to increase the range of hip extension. (Courtesy of Keiser Sports Health Equipment Inc., Fresno, CA.)*

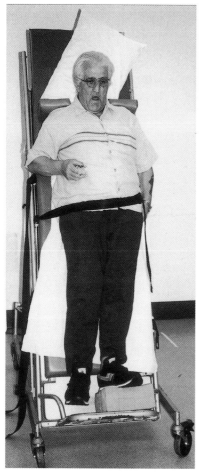

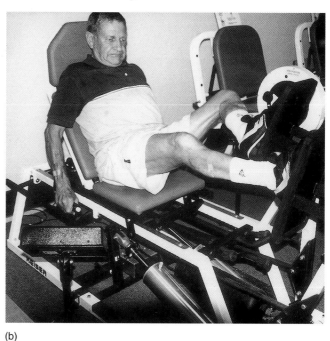

(a)   (b)

Kinetic chain weightbearing exercises are typically given to strengthen lower limb extensor muscles using body weight and other forms of resistance, and include exercises in which the body mass is lowered and raised over the feet, for example, step-ups (see Fig. 3.22), modified squat to stand (see Fig. 2.17), heels raise and lower (see Fig. 3.24), and leg press exercises (Fig. 7.2).

These exercises take advantage of the specificity principle in that muscles are exercised concentrically and eccentrically in a movement pattern that shares some of the dynamic characteristics of commonly performed motor actions such as sit-to-stand, bending down to pick up objects in standing, stair climbing and descent (Palmitier et al. 1991) (Fig. 7.3). Exercises such as these not only enable

FIGURE 7.3   *Diagram showing lower limb segments and eight muscle groups affecting segmental rotation during flexion and extension of the lower limbs over a fixed foot. g max, maximum gravity; gastroc, gastrocnemius; hamstr, hamstrings; rect fem, rectus femoris; tib ant, tibialis anterior; tib post, tibialis posterior. (Reprinted from Journal of Biomechanics, Vol. 26, AD Kuo and FE Zajac, A biomechanical analysis of muscle strength as a limiting factor in standing posture, p. 139, copyright 1993, with permission from Elsevier Science.)*

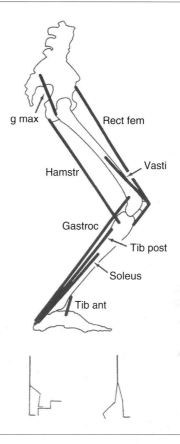

practice of lengthening and shortening contractions of muscles spanning several joints (e.g. biceps femoris, gastrocnemius), they also have the advantage of training the complex neural control involved in these actions (Pinniger et al. 2000), and place functional stresses on the limb which are similar to those in many weightbearing activities (Shelbourne and Nitz 1992). It is apparent on clinical observation that individuals can have difficulty after stroke with actions that involve switching from concentric to eccentric muscle activity, particularly when weightbearing. This has been observed also in elderly individuals. Exercises involving actions that require a switch from one mode of contraction to the other, such as step-ups, can provide a focus for training coordination while also providing an action-specific strength training stimulus.

In weightbearing kinetic chain exercises, synergistic muscle activity plays a large part in the action. Consequently, the individual is not only increasing the strength of a group of muscles but is being trained to control the muscle forces produced across the segmental linkage. There is some clinical evidence that weightbearing exercises for the lower limb can improve strength and functional performance in individuals with disability. For example, a programme of this type of strength training was followed by improved isometric strength, gait and sit-to-stand (STS) performance in children with cerebral palsy (Blundell et al. 2002), and practising step-up exercises was associated with improved gait after stroke and in elderly subjects (Nugent et al. 1994, Sherrington and Lord 1997).

It is likely that in patients with very weak muscles – say, Motricity Index (MI) score < 3 – any method of strength training, including exercises performed with the distal segment free, may be of value. There is some theoretical support for the view that, in this situation, any exercise that stimulates muscle activation and requires the muscle to work eccentrically, concentrically or isometrically will transfer into improvements in functional motor performance. Isokinetic exercise, where available, may be particularly useful in patients who have difficulty sustaining appropriate levels of muscle activation through range. However, when muscles are stronger, i.e. above a certain threshold (unknown at this time but let's say MI score > 3), that strength training should consist of exercises that are dynamically similar to the actions being trained in order to train motor control and maximize carryover into function.

Exercises are progressed by increasing the number of repetitions, the range of movement (e.g. height of step) and the amount of resistance or load.

Concentric and eccentric exercise

The force-producing capacity (tension regulation) of muscle differs during lengthening and shortening contractions (Pinniger et al. 2000). Voluntary eccentric contractions produce greater muscle force than concentric muscle contractions (Komi 1973) yet appear to involve lower rates of motor unit discharge than concentric contractions (Tax et al. 1990), i.e. lesser levels of muscle activation are needed for greater levels of force (Westing et al. 1990). Eccentric exercise has greater mechanical efficiency (Komi and Buskirk 1972). At comparable work loads, the cost in terms of metabolic energy is less than in concentric exercise (Asmussen 1953).

In an able-bodied population, utilizing both concentric and eccentric muscle contractions in strength training has been shown to produce better gains in strength than concentric contractions alone (Hakkinen and Komi 1981). When the muscle is actively stretched in an eccentric contraction, tension in the series elastic component increases and the stored elastic energy is used in the subsequent concentric action (Asmussen and Bonde-Petersen 1974, Svantesson et al. 1999). In patients with neuromotor impairment, it is possible that, at the neural level, concentric activation of weak muscles may be facilitated by the enhanced muscle spindle activity occurring as a result of the rapid switching from eccentric to concentric muscle activity (Burke et al. 1978). It is known from studies of the able bodied that, if an eccentric muscle contraction immediately precedes a concentric contraction, as in the brief flexion counter-movement of the lower limbs which immediately precedes the extension phase of the vertical jump, the concentric phase generates more force due to the effect of the stretch-shortening cycle (Asmussen and Bonde-Petersen 1974, Bosco et al. 1982, Svantesson et al. 1994). This mechanism seems to play a significant role in many everyday actions including sit-to-stand (Shepherd and Gentile 1994) and walking (Komi 1986).

Elastic band resistance exercise

Elastic bands provide an inexpensive and simple means of exercising which can be carried out by patients on their own. Examples of such exercises are given in the chapters on walking and upper limb function. The bands are provided in a range of resistance levels which enables prescription to suit an individual's strength level. Tests of these bands have provided details of the approximate amount of resistance provided by the particular colours. For example, for Theraband* at 100% deformation: yellow = 13 N, green = 25 N, black = 36 N (Simoneau et al. 2001). There are several other colours, however, and recent work has shown that the red band provides resistance between the yellow and green bands. The silver band provides the largest amount of resistance, approximately double that of the green band (Patterson et al. 2001).

Each exercise should start with the slack of the elastic band taken out. One advantage of the elastic band over hand weights is its ability to provide variable resistance throughout the range of movement. Simoneau and colleagues (2001) describe the properties of elastic bands and factors to consider in their use.

There is some difficulty in controlling the exact amount of resistance offered by elastic bands (Hintermeister et al. 1998). Nevertheless, for individuals following stroke the use of these bands is recommended as a means of increasing muscle strength, preserving or increasing joint range and muscle extensibility, and encouraging unsupervised exercise for both upper and lower limbs. Progression involves increasing intensity of exercise (number of repetitions), load (using band colour to increase resistance) and frequency (number of times per day).

There is evidence that exercises using elastic band resistance to isotonic movements can be effective in increasing strength in elderly individuals (Mikesky et al. 1994, Skelton et al. 1995), with some carryover into improved balance and gait (Topp et al. 1993, 1996). It is yet to be investigated, however, whether or not muscle strength is increased by such exercise in individuals following stroke, or if there are other benefits such as improved motor performance, increased activity levels and, in the case of the upper limb, a decreased tendency to develop adhesive capsulitis with painful shoulder.

Specificity of strength training

The conventional approach to atrophy and muscle weakness in individuals following musculoskeletal trauma is to increase strength and restore muscle bulk by high resistance strength training exercise (Rutherford 1988). The assumption is often made that improved strength will transfer automatically into improved

*Theraband, The Hygenic Corporation, Akron, Ohio.

functional ability. This may not, however, be the case. The body adapts specific-ally to the demands imposed upon it, and research over many years has shown that exercise effects tend to be specific to task and context (Rutherford 1988, Morrissey et al. 1995), with the greatest changes occurring in the training exer-cise itself. For example, increases in strength of a muscle appear to be specific to such factors as joint angle (muscle length), subject's posture (standing or supine), velocity of movement and muscle contraction type. Muscle length specificity is of particular interest, with the greatest increases in maximum vol-untary contraction consistently found at the training angle after isometric exer-cise. Results of one study showed that the shorter the muscle length at which training was carried out the more the gain in maximum voluntary contraction was limited to the training angle (Thepaut-Mathieu et al. 1988).

The principle of specificity is usually explained with reference to such factors as the structure and function of particular muscles, biomechanical constraints such as length of moment arm, and the nature of synergic cooperation. Functional actions are made up of complex movements of the multisegment linkage which require strength, coordination and balance. The relationship between muscles that span one joint and those that span two (or many) joints is particularly complex and little understood (Bobbert and van Soest 2000).

The extent to which the intrinsic strength of stabilizer and other synergic muscles influences the strength of a prime mover muscle has been little investigated. However, a recent analysis of a task that involved pushing a heavy object (Kornecki et al. 2001) drew attention to the importance of muscles acting as sta-bilizers to 'stiffen' the degrees of freedom not involved in the action. The study found that the ability to stabilize a key joint influenced muscle activation patterns. Stabilizing the wrist joint was associated with decreased EMG in the upper arm muscles (triceps brachii, deltoid), the prime movers for the pushing movement.

After stroke, when muscle weakness is part of a more general motor control impairment, it may be critical that strength training is oriented toward specific tasks and designed to ensure the greatest transfer possible into improved func-tional motor performance. Strength training may need to focus on exercising muscles through a specific part of the range (e.g. calf muscles from fully length-ened to mid-range for stance phase of gait). It is therefore critical that a close examination is made of the patient's ability to generate and sustain force as active motor tasks are practised, and that this is followed up by exercise and training specifically targeting the muscles in which weakness is evident and apparently affecting function.

Transfer from strength to function

It is intuitive that a relationship should exist between strength and function; however, the nature of the relationship appears complex and dependent on the degree of muscle weakness. An hypothesis put forward by Buchner and de Lateur (1991) suggests that the relationship between strength and function is curvilinear and activity specific. In a study of elderly individuals, Buchner and colleagues (Buchner et al. 1996) showed that a curvilinear relationship exists between lower limb strength and walking velocity. They pointed out that this relationship reflects a mechanism by which small changes in strength may produce relatively large changes in performance in very weak adults, while large changes may have little or no effect in able-bodied adults. When muscles are beyond a certain task-dependent threshold (a threshold that for most everyday tasks is well below normal strength values), exercises are required that are task oriented. Buchner's hypothesis may explain the discrepant results in studies reporting a relationship between strength and function.

A recent study illustrated the beneficial transfer effects of task-oriented strength training in an able-bodied group. Glenohumeral internal and external rotation exercises (incorporating elastic band and hand weight resistance) performed by tennis players in standing, with shoulder at 90° abduction, resulted in significant increases in force production of the actions practised, with a transfer into increased speed of serve (Treiber et al. 1998). Transfer is unlikely to occur, however, unless subjects are also practising the task to be learned (in the above case, the tennis serve), even in some modified context.

Transfer from single joint exercise to kinetic (weightbearing) actions may be limited except where muscles are very weak. It has been shown that open-chain knee extension exercise can increase strength of quadriceps in terms of the weight that can be lifted through range (the exercise), with no improvement in maximum power output measured in isokinetic cycling (a closed-chain action in the pedal-pressing phase). Some studies have produced more equivocal results. This may be due to the relevance of the exercises to the functional action being learned or to the individual's strength level.

Variations in body position also affect muscle activity patterns. An early experiment showed that strength training of elbow muscles carried out in standing resulted in greater increases in strength than the same exercises carried out in supine (Rasch and Morehouse 1957). The strength increases found in standing were in large part the result of learning to coordinate all the muscles involved in the movement, which included those controlling balance.

Strength training that involves repetitive practice of the action being learned can improve strength and endurance if load is progressively increased in some way. For example, walking on a treadmill (and overground) can be progressed by increasing speed and slope; STS can be practised repetitively from increasingly lower seat heights, and at increasing speed. If done repetitively with sufficient load, such training provides a means of strengthening lower limb muscles and increasing endurance, as well as control over the dynamics of the particular action to be regained.

Also critical to the regaining of effective performance is the development of flexibility of performance, which is achieved by practising the action under a variety of different conditions, i.e. in different environmental and task contexts. Repetitive practice of the action to be learned can therefore have dual benefits, enabling the patient to practise the action as well as increasing muscle strength (Rutherford 1988). Strength training for individuals following stroke should be considered to have as its main effects improved performance in actions required in daily life and prevention of falls.

It may follow that when individuals have a marked degree of weakness, i.e. below a certain threshold of strength relative to a particular activity such as walking, several types of strength training may be effective. Any increase in strength is likely to result in some improvement, such as the ability to at least attempt walking: i.e. any exercise that requires a muscle to contract and lengthen its fibres against even a small amount of resistance is likely to be beneficial initially when muscles are very weak. Above a particular activity-specific threshold of strength, however, strengthening exercises may have minimal effect if they do not share similar dynamic characteristics to the action being trained.

Eliciting activity in very weak muscles

Following stroke, exercises to strengthen muscles are selected according to the degree of weakness. An estimation of muscle strength is gained by simple testing using the Medical Research Council (MRC) grades or the Motricity Index (MI) which is based on the MRC grades. If muscles can be voluntarily activated but are very weak (say, grade 2–3), strength training can include partial body weight resistance, or resistance through a small range of movement (e.g. STS from a high seat), lifting small weights through a limited range, elastic band exercises, and concentric and eccentric exercise on an isokinetic dynamometer.

Training may require an exploration to find the conditions under which a very weak or paralysed muscle (grade 0–1) can be stimulated to contract. Figure 5.14a shows a method of eliciting eccentric activity in triceps surae in an individual who had severe weakness of this muscle. Since lower levels of muscle activation are required for the same force effect in eccentric compared to concentric exercise, attempts at eccentric contraction may enable an individual with very weak muscles to improve activation of those muscles. For example, if a person is unable to contract quadriceps, a voluntary contraction may be elicited eccentrically by attempting to lower the shank slowly with an isokinetic dynamometer (see Fig. 3.26).

Biofeedback may be combined with exercise to spur the individual on to greater efforts (Wolf et al. 1994). Mental practice may also be useful in some individuals (Page et al. 2001). Early after stroke, electrical stimulation (ES) or electromyography-triggered ES may give the person the idea of muscle activation if a voluntary contraction appears impossible. It has been suggested that repetitive motor training via neuromuscular ES may facilitate motor learning by modifying the excitability of specific motor neurons (Chae and Yu 1999). There is some evidence that ES can have a positive effect on joint movement, muscle strength and functional performance (Baker et al. 1979, Lieber 1988, Dimitrijevic et al. 1996, Glanz et al. 1996, Chae et al. 1998, Sonde et al. 1998). These methods are discussed further in the context of upper limb training (Ch. 5).

Efficacy of muscle strength training after stroke

Information on physiological responses to exercise in an individual with a brain lesion is limited (Lexell 2000). However, there is a rapidly growing body of knowledge about the effects of exercise on strength and function in the elderly, and following stroke. It is increasingly evident that muscle weakness after stroke is modifiable through strength training of an appropriate intensity, even in very elderly individuals (Sharp and Brouwer 1997, Mazzeo et al. 1998, Teixeira-Salmela et al. 1999, Ng and Shepherd 2000).

Studies have reported the following changes after periods of strength training and physical conditioning:

- Increases in muscle strength, improved postural stability and reduction in falls in the elderly (Aniansson et al. 1980, Aniasson and Gustafsson 1981, Sauvage et al. 1992, Fiatarone et al. 1990, 1994, Judge et al. 1993, Tinetti et al. 1994, Campbell et al. 1997, Gardner et al. 2000)
- Increases in muscle strength after stroke (Sunderland et al. 1992, Engardt et al. 1995, Sharp and Brouwer 1997, Sherrington and Lord 1997, Brown and Kautz 1998, Duncan et al. 1998, Teixeira-Salmela et al. 1999, 2001, Weiss et al. 2000).

Many of these studies also document a positive relationship between increased strength and functional performance. For example, increased strength of lower limb muscles (hip and knee flexors and extensors, ankle dorsi- and plantarflexors) is associated with improvements in aspects of:

- gait performance (Nakamura et al. 1985, Bohannon and Andrews 1990, Nugent et al. 1994, Lindmark and Hamrin 1995, Sharp and Brouwer 1997, Krebs et al. 1998, Teixeira-Salmela et al. 1999, 2001, Weiss et al. 2000)
- ability to balance (Hamrin et al. 1982, Weiss et al. 2000)
- stair climbing (Bohannon and Walsh 1991).

A single case study of static dynometric strength training with computer-driven visual feedback of force showed an increase in the amount of static direction-specific force produced through the lower limb plus improvement on the Timed 'Up and Go' test, comfortable gait speed and endurance (Mercier et al. 1999). Furthermore, a significant level of improvement was maintained 6 weeks later. This study was designed to test a novel method of repetitive resisted exercise in which the subject was required to control the direction of force, responding to feedback on both direction and amplitude.

In another study of lower limb strength training, increases in quadriceps and hamstring muscle strength were accompanied by increases in gait velocity following a 6-week programme of exercise which included stretches and isokinetic strengthening for quadriceps and hamstrings (Sharp and Brouwer 1997). A 10-week programme of strength training for hip, knee and ankle muscles plus physical conditioning exercises resulted in gains in the Human Activity Profile and the Nottingham Health Profile, both of which reflect the ability to perform household tasks and recreational activities, and increases in gait speed and performance. After training, patients were able to increase power generation by ankle plantarflexors and hip flexors and extensors (Teixeira-Salmela et al. 2001). In another study, 15 patients increased force output in their paretic lower limb after a period of pedaling against various loads (Brown and Kautz 1998).

The role of peak muscle power (the product of force and velocity of muscle shortening) in functional independence has been examined in elderly individuals (Bassey et al. 1997), with the suggestion that power may be more directly related to impaired physical performance than strength in the elderly. This is of interest in neurorehabilitation, given the reported deficits in power production reported after stroke (Olney and Richards 1996). In the elderly, the velocity with which force can be generated declines along with muscle strength itself, power decreasing to a greater degree than strength. Recent studies have reported that peak lower limb muscle power, tested on a leg press device is a predictor of self-reported functional status in older women (Foldvari et al. 2000), and there is some evidence that lower limb strength and power can be improved by high velocity power training in this population (Fielding et al. 2002).

Treadmill exercise can increase muscle strength and endurance. A recent study of task-oriented aerobic treadmill training carried out three times a week for 3 months showed increased strength of quadriceps measured on an isokinetic dynamometer (Smith et al. 1998).

There are few studies of strength training for upper limb muscles after stroke. However, a strength training programme involving repetitive hand and finger flexion exercises performed against various loads showed increases in strength of hand grip, wrist extension strength and speed of wrist extension (Butefisch et al. 1995). Another study reported a relationship between increased grip strength and improved hand function (Sunderland et al. 1989).

Whether or not increases in muscle strength and function in individuals with stroke are maintained after a training programme has concluded is not clear. Nevertheless, it is likely that the opportunity for long-term, periodic exercise training at home and in community classes, and attendance at a specialized gymnasium, is necessary for many individuals after stroke.

Exercise prescription

There are certain basic considerations in planning a muscle strengthening programme. The exercise dosage can be increased by increasing the number of repetitions, the number of sets, and the resistance provided. In general, in able-bodied subjects, muscles should be exercised to the point of fatigue but not pain in order to obtain some change (Wajswelner and Webb 1995). Patients should be warned that they may experience a small degree of delayed muscle soreness. The exercise should be as specific as possible to the functional actions being trained to ensure carryover (Morrissey et al. 1995). In the case of patients with very weak muscles, however, any type of exercise which results in the generation of some force can be practised.

Strength training in the able-bodied appears to produce greatest strength increases when subjects train at high but submaximal loads. As a general guide, the patient should attempt 10 repetitions of 80% of the maximum possible load that can be lifted in one attempt. Ten repetitions is called the 10 repetition maximum (10 RM). This is set as a goal, although a very weak person may start at

50% of the maximum load and with fewer than 10 repetitions (Fiatarone et al. 1990, Teixeira-Salmela et al. 1999). It should be noted that the repetition maximum is the maximum number of repetitions that can be performed maintaining good form (Wajswelner and Webb 1995). The weight or load for a given RM (in this case 10) is the load that can be lifted 10 times without gross error.

A recent study provides guidelines for exercise prescription. Teixeira-Salmela and colleagues (1999) investigated the effects of a strengthening and physical conditioning programme in 13 individuals with chronic stroke. Each session consisted of:

- 5–10 min warm-up (calisthenics, stretching, range of motion exercises)
- aerobic exercises (graded walking, stepping or cycling)
- strength training (hip, knee and ankle flexors and extensors)
- 5–10 min cool-down (muscle relaxation, stretching).

Strength training consisted of isometric, concentric and eccentric exercises as described by Fiatarone et al. (1990). Initial load was set at 50% of 1 RM for 3 sets of 10 repetitions, increasing to 80%. Resistance was provided by body weight, sandbag weights and elastic bands. Maximum repetitions were reassessed every 2 weeks and training adjusted to keep the load at 80%.

It appears that greater strength gains may be achieved when repetitions are carried out without a rest between each repetition (Rooney et al. 1994). Each group of 10 repetitions comprises a set and the goal should be to repeat the set three times with a short rest between each set. This dosage for strength training applies whether the exercise utilizes free weights, elastic bands or practice of sit-to-stand. Load is increased in STS by decreasing seat height by prescribed increments. A person with very weak lower limb muscles can start with three sets of a few repetitions from a higher than usual seat, increase number of repetitions to 10, then progress to 10 repetitions from a lower seat.

The relationship between number of repetitions and amount of resistance is different when the goal is endurance. In this case, high repetitions are practised at low levels of resistance. For individuals following stroke, improving endurance is important for a return to the community, so part of the exercise session should involve this type of exercise, and can include treadmill walking and stationary cycling. For the latter, the hand or foot can be bandaged to the handlebar and pedal if necessary.

The individual's exercise programme should include variation in methods as there is some evidence in the able-bodied that variation of stimulus has more effect than repetition of the same movements under the same conditions (Hakkinen and Komi 1981). Variation can involve a group circuit class, with patients moving between work stations set up for specific types of exercise: step-ups, heels raise and lower, stationary cycling, treadmill walking with or without harness, free weights, elastic band exercises, exercises on an isokinetic dynamometer, and leg and arm press machines. Pneumatic strength training equipment such as the Keiser* enables concentric and eccentric exercise including the leg press,

*Keiser Sports Health Equipment Inc., Fresno, CA.

Box 7.1 Summary of strength training

- Strength training is carried out with sub-maximal loads – as a general rule 10 repetitions at 50–80% of maximal possible 1RM load, with a goal of 3 sets
- Strength training utilizes resistance from body weight, free weights, elastic bands, isokinetic dynamometry, exercise machines, treadmill walking
- Exercise dosage is increased by increasing repetitions, number of sets, load
- Strength training is task specific or oriented towards characteristics of tasks to be learned
- For endurance, high repetition numbers are practised at low levels of load, and include stationary cycling, arm cycling and treadmill walking
- For very weak muscles, the methods used are those which best facilitate force generation for that individual and may include simple exercises, biofeedback, mental practice, electrical stimulation
- Strength training can be carried out under supervision, independently and in group circuit training classes

---

with variations in position as required. The class is made enjoyable by the company of others and the opportunity for socialization, two factors identified as key components of successful programmes (Barry and Eathorne 1994). In addition, exercise classes can provide increased levels of mental stimulation. The class can be supervised by therapists and aides and is a time-efficient way of organizing intensive training. Some patients will need close supervision, others will not. Provision of harness support may alleviate fear of falling and facilitate practice.

Adequate recovery time needs to be allowed so that muscles can adapt without breaking down. A patient can, within a circuit training class, for example, intersperse lower limb exercises with strengthening exercises for the upper limb or practice of manipulation tasks, in this way exercising different muscles but transferring energy and attention immediately from one action to another.

Patient participation and enthusiasm for exercise and training is encouraged by the display of graphs of progress, videotapes of their motor performance and photographs of performance to be achieved. Interest is sustained by ensuring participants are always pushing toward their optimum performance, never practising what is already easily achievable.

A summary of strength training is provided in Box 7.1.

Maximizing skill

Emphasis in training is on regaining optimal skill in particular functional motor actions. Methods of maximizing skill in motor performance are based on research into motor learning carried out with able-bodied subjects. In skilled performance the goal is achieved successfully on most occasions, i.e. the action is flexible enough to be performed under different environmental conditions, with minimal energy cost.

Following a brain lesion affecting the motor system, an immediate need is to help the patient regain the ability to activate paretic muscles and generate force. Strength training involves many repetitions under constrained conditions as a means of increasing muscle contractility and strength and laying down a pattern of coordination. Repetitive exercise may be as critical to motor learning following stroke as it is for healthy individuals learning to play the piano (Butefisch et al. 1995). It is assumed that repetitive practice of a particular movement may drive brain reorganization by what appears to be a process of motor learning (Asanuma and Keller 1991). However, repetitive practice of the same movement may not be sufficient for promoting skill. While repetition is necessary for increasing strength when muscles are weak, what Bernstein (1967) called 'repetition without repetition' is preferable when skill is to be acquired.

Strength training oriented toward the motor tasks in which competence must be regained has the advantage of addressing both the reduced force generating capacity and the regaining of skill. An example is the use of repetitive standing up and sitting down (STS) as a strengthening exercise which also involves practice of the action itself. Other examples illustrate the transfer effect of repetitive practice of an action that shares similar dynamic characteristics with other actions. Repetitive practice of reaching to objects beyond arm's length in sitting was found to improve not only reaching performance but also STS (Dean and Shepherd 1997). In this example, STS may have improved because the patients repetitively practised reaching beyond arm's length, which involves controlling upper body movement forward over the feet, a characteristic also of the initial phase of standing up.

Methods of facilitating motor learning and skill training are described briefly in Chapter 1 and in more detail elsewhere (Gentile 2000).

Measures of muscle strength

Dynamometry (grip force, hand-held, isokinetic dynamometers).   A measurement of peak isometric muscle force. In hand-held and isokinetic dynamometry the subject does a maximum muscle contraction against a known force in a standardized position (Mathiowetz et al. 1985, Bohannon et al. 1993, Murphy and Spinks 2000). Isokinetic dynamometry can also be used to test multijoint and more functional movement.

Other measures include:

- *Lateral Step Test* (Worrell et al. 1993)
- *Medical Research Council (MRC) grades or Motricity Index* (Medical Research Council 1976, Wade 1992)

PRESERVING MUSCLE LENGTH AND FLEXIBILITY

In able-bodied individuals, the length of muscles and other soft tissues is normally sufficient for the activities regularly performed. Typically we spend some time stretching (e.g. hip flexors, calf muscles) in order to increase our 'flexibility' when we exercise or plan to engage in an unaccustomed sport. However, flexibility declines with age (Roach and Miles 1991), partly due to changes in collagen, a component of the fibrous connective tissue of ligaments and tendons. Length-associated changes can also occur after any prolonged period of immobility, such as after an acute neural lesion. Stretching exercises are therefore a critical part of a rehabilitation programme.

Increased range of motion after stretching may involve biomechanical, neurophysiological and molecular mechanisms. Certain basic biomechanical properties influence the muscle–tendon unit's response to stretch (Taylor et al. 1990). Tension in muscle comprises passive and active components. Stretch can affect the active component by altering neural activity and the passive mechanical component by affecting viscous and elastic properties of the muscle. The mechanisms of increasing muscle length and range of motion are not well known, but may be found eventually in the cellular and adaptive mechanisms of a muscle fibre (De Deyne 2001).

One characteristic of viscoelasticity is that the tissues respond to stretch and to being held at a constant length with a decrease in tension, i.e., the stress or force produced by the tissues at that length gradually declines, called 'stress relaxation' (Duong et al. 2001). During stretch, soft tissues undergo progressive deformation and they can be progressively extended with a constant force which is called 'creep'.

Application of a passive stretching force affects an individual muscle according to its anatomy, individual fibres receiving various amounts of stress depending on their orientation relative to the longitudinal axis of the muscle (De Deyne 2001). Short-term increase in range of motion following a brief passive stretch is explained by the viscoelastic behaviour of muscles and short-term changes in muscle extensibility (Best et al. 1994). Longer term adaptive changes (Halbertsma et al. 1996) that occur after sustained passive stretch produce a longer muscle. The biological and molecular mechanisms by which this occurs are not well understood; however, increase in sarcomere number has been reported from animal experiments (Williams 1990).

Both decreased muscle length (contracture) and increased muscle stiffness are common sequelae of stroke, appear to develop quickly and have potent negative effects on the person's ability to exercise, train and regain effective performance of motor actions. Contributors to loss of extensibility are disuse, degenerative processes associated with ageing, and the effect of the stroke on the motor system. Loss of extensibility of calf muscles in particular can potentially have negative effects on the ability to balance in standing, on walking, particularly up and down stairs, and on standing up (Vandervoort 1999), and is said to predispose the elderly to falls (Studenski et al. 1991).

Since contracture alters the resting limb position, it affects the resting length of muscles crossing the joint and the lever torque angle relationship at the joint (Lieber 1992). This alters the muscle's force output and can lead to muscle imbalance (Vandervoort 1999). In some elderly subjects, joint limitation and stiffness in the shoulders and spine, and some calf muscle shortening may have been present before stroke.

Patients need to be monitored with diligence from immediately after a stroke, since prevention of increased soft tissue stiffness and contracture is critical if the negative effects are to be prevented. Intervention must be proactive and a matter of routine within the hospital and rehabilitation centre. Patients who are able to do unsupervised stretching and exercise should be advised to stretch for a few minutes several times a day, particularly before and during training sessions, and when they are practising on their own. Practice of simple exercises with elastic bands is one method of actively stretching muscles. Practice of STS with the feet placed well back provides a simple method of actively stretching the soleus muscle, provided weight is borne through that foot.

For patients who cannot voluntarily move a limb, passive means such as positioning a limb or a joint are necessary. It has been shown that connective tissue accumulation, a major contributor to increased muscle stiffness in shortened muscles, can be prevented by passive stretching when muscles are inactive. For example, short-term stretch (30 min daily) in animals prevented serial sarcomere loss, muscle atrophy and reduced range of motion (Williams 1990). In humans, brief stretch of calf muscles can produce a decrease in stiffness (Vattanasilp et al. 2000) and increased muscle compliance (Otis et al. 1985), and is thought to 'precondition' a muscle prior to training (Taylor et al. 1990). Although passive stretching may change the length of the muscle, it is active stretching during dynamic task-oriented practice that affects the dynamic range of a movement. One of the advantages of treadmill training is likely to be the dynamic and task-specific stretch imposed on muscles in the stance limb such as soleus, gastrocnemius and rectus femoris.

There is some evidence that passive stretching affects the active (neural) component of muscle tension, with a reduction of motoneuron excitability (Odeen 1981, Kukulka et al. 1986, Hummelsheim and Mauritz 1993). It is unlikely, however, that decreasing reflex hyperexcitability by passive stretching has any more than a short-term effect on reflex status, nor that it will be followed by any improvement in motor control or function, if it is not also accompanied by active stretching as part of functional training.

It is likely that the early institution of active stretch (through exercise and task practice) may be a major factor in preventing the development of the adaptive reflex hyperactivity associated with stiff, short and inactive muscles. There is evidence that repetitive exercise and strength training can increase range of motion and decrease resistance to passive movement (Blanpied and Smidt 1993, Butefisch et al. 1995, Miller and Light 1997, Teixeira-Salmela et al. 1999).

Nevertheless, in patients with minimal active movement, muscles that can be predicted to shorten and stiffen due to persistent maintenance of their resting posture (e.g. calf muscles, long finger flexors, shoulder internal rotators and adductors) need to be positioned for short periods of the day to preserve length. Where contracture is present, progressive stretching by serial casting is necessary (Moseley 1997). Injections of botulinum toxin may also be effective

---

Box 7.2 Summary of stretching

- Prolonged passive stretching (15–30 min) via positioning during the day if a limb cannot be actively moved, to prevent predictable muscle shortening and stiffness (plantarflexors, shoulder adductors, internal rotators, elbow flexors, forearm pronators, thumb adductors, long finger flexors). Daily passive stretch (15–30 min) prevents atrophy and loss of sarcomeres in animals (Williams 1990)
- Short (20 s) stretch to a stiff muscle(s), done manually by patient or therapist, just prior to and during exercise. This can have the effect of preconditioning the muscle(s) through stress relaxation and decreasing stiffness (Vattanasilp et al. 2000)
- Prolonged stretch to contracted soft tissues using serial casting (Moseley 1997), combined with exercise and training carried out while casting is in place, with follow-up exercise and training

---

in decreasing stiffness where it is extreme and accompanied by reflex hyper-activity. These methods must be combined with active exercise if the effects are to be associated with functional improvement. So far there has been little research into methods of prevention in stroke.

Stretching prescription

There is little basic information to guide the rational use of passive stretching (Taylor et al. 1990). Although the optimal dosage for stretching is not clear, there is evidence to suggest that holding a stretch for approximately 20 s and repeating the stretch 4–5 times can be effective at lengthening the muscle–tendon unit by inducing some stress relaxation and a reduction in the individual's perceived stiffness (Taylor et al. 1990). Prolonged stretch of 30 min has been reported to decrease passive restraint in ankle plantarflexors in individuals with paraplegia (Harvey and Herbert 2002). Passive joint mobilization may be necessary for individuals with spinal, glenohumeral or wrist joint pain and/or stiffness. Stretching to preserve muscle length and flexibility is summarized in Box 7.2.

It should be noted that, although commonly used in some clinics, there is little experimental support for the use of splinting (e.g. hand splints) to prevent or correct length changes. The negative effects in terms of promoting learned non-use and altering the biomechanics of actions may outweigh any possible positive effects. A splint worn at night may, however, be useful for those who do not regain active use of the hand.

Measures of joint range

Dynamometer and goniometer.　A known torque is applied to produce movement in a standardized testing position. Range of movement is calculated from skin surface markers. The use of polaroid photography, a calibrated spring-loaded device and a goniometer have been found to be reliable for testing ankle range of motion (Moseley and Adams 1991, Moseley 1997) (Fig. 7.4).

| FIGURE 7.4 | *A torque controlled measurement procedure. Ankle angle is measured using skin surface markers and photography. (Reproduced from Moseley 1997, with permission.)* |

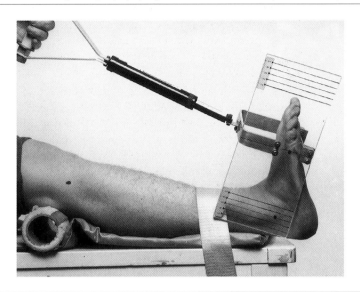

PHYSICAL CONDITIONING

Many individuals post-stroke are left with residual neurological deficits and physiological changes in muscle fibres and muscle metabolism that are likely to continue to impair function and impose excessive energy demands during the performance of common daily activities, particularly walking. Metabolic changes include decreased muscle blood flow, increased lactate production, increased utilization of muscle glycogen and decreased capacity to oxidize free fatty acids (Landin et al. 1977). In addition, muscle fibre changes leading to a decrease in oxidative metabolism and low exercise endurance can include a decrease in proportion of type I muscle fibres due to the transformation of high oxidative (type I) fibres to low oxidative (type II) fibres.

It is well documented that cardiovascular limitations lower exercise tolerance to work capacity. A sedentary life-style leads to a further decline in muscle strength and cardiovascular fitness. Complaints of fatigue attributed to disease process are equally likely to be due to the demonstrably low levels of aerobic fitness and endurance. Several studies have reported that stroke subjects have less energy, and experience increased social isolation and emotional distress when compared with individuals of a similar age (Ahlsio et al. 1984, Ebrahim et al. 1986). However, until recently, there have been relatively few studies examining the exercise (aerobic) capacity of those affected by stroke. Individuals post-stroke do not have the same functional capacity as healthy individuals due to loss of physiological muscle mass. It is therefore difficult to use normative data from healthy populations to predict capacity and guide training programmes (Potempa et al. 1996).

In a discussion of the rationale for aerobic exercise after stroke, Potempa and colleagues (1996) summarize cardiovascular responses to exercise testing in individuals after stroke, taken from available studies in chronic stroke. They include:

- lowered peak exercise responses
- reduced oxidative capacity of paretic muscles
- decreased endurance.

Reduced functional capacity after stroke is therefore likely to be due, to varying extents, to reduction in the number of motor units recruitable during dynamic exercise, reduced oxidative capacity of weak muscles and low endurance, compounded in some individuals by the presence of comorbid coronary artery disease and physical inactivity.

In spite of evidence that after stroke individuals are physically deconditioned, aerobic exercise is not routinely prescribed for stroke patients, either early in rehabilitation or after discharge (Smith et al. 1999). One of the reasons for this may be that therapists have restricted any activities involving intensive effort, in part because of a belief that effort increases spasticity, in part because many patients are elderly. Neither point appears valid according to the evidence. Effort applied in exercise does not increase spasticity or muscle stiffness. Elderly individuals are capable of increasing their cardiovascular fitness, and improving lifestyle and self-efficacy, with moderately vigorous exercise (Hamdorf et al. 1992, Mazzeo et al. 1998). In addition, aerobic exercise has the potential to minimize secondary effects on muscle fibre transformation by enhancing motor unit recruitment and favouring development of high oxidative fibres (Potempa et al. 1996). Appropriate exercise may increase endurance capacity and minimize symptoms of cardiovascular disease (Hamm and Leon 1994). Exercise and physical activity are known to have positive psychological effects in the able-bodied young and elderly, and in disabled individuals. There also appears to be a relationship between physical fitness and cognition (Rogers et al. 1990, Spirduso and Asplund 1995).

Recent studies have shown the benefits of physical conditioning programmes following stroke, including improvements in both aerobic capacity and functional abilities (Potempa et al. 1995, 1996, Macko et al. 1997, Teixeira-Salmela et al. 1999). There are reports of improved aerobic capacity with appropriate training such as bicycle ergometry (Potempa et al. 1995, Bateman et al. 2001), with graded treadmill walking (Macko et al. 1997) and with a combination of aerobic and strengthening exercises (Teixeira-Salmela et al. 1999). Supervised aerobic training programmes have been shown to improve VO_{2max}, with the improvement significantly related to improvements in motor function (Potempa et al. 1995). The evidence so far suggests that aerobic exercise on a bicycle ergometer, treadmill walking or with graded walking significantly improves physical fitness when individuals are tested on the training exercise (Table 7.1). As might be expected, the effects are exercise specific. Generalization occurs, however, in the improvements noted in general health and well-being. Any generalization to performance of other actions probably depends on the patient's level of impairment (Bateman et al. 2001).

TABLE 7.1		Conditioning: clinical outcome studies		
Reference	Subjects	Methods	Duration	Results
Potempa et al. 1995	42 Ss >7 months post-stroke Age range 21–77 yrs	Randomized controlled trial E: adapted cycle ergometer (training load was gradually increased from workload at 30–50% of maximum effort to the highest level attained by the subjects) C: passive ROM	10 weeks 3 days/week, 30 min	Only E showed significant improvements on maximum oxygen consumption, workload and exercise time, lower systolic blood pressure at submaximal workloads during graded exercise test. Aerobic capacity was related to improvement in function (Fugl-Meyer Scale)
Macko et al. 1997	9 Ss >6 months post-stroke Mean age 67 ± 2.8 yrs	Pre-test, post-test design Low intensity aerobic exercise (graded treadmill training at 50–60% heart rate reserve; warm up, cool down period)	6 months 3 days/week, 40 min	Significant reduction in energy expenditure ($p < 0.02$), exercise-mediated decline in oxygen consumption ($p < 0.02$) and respiratory exchange ratio ($p < 0.01$) during standardized 1mph submaximal effort treadmill walking
Smith et al. 1998	14 Ss >6 months Mean age 66 ± 3 yrs	Pre-test, post-test design Low intensity aerobic exercise (graded treadmill training at 50–60% heart rate reserve; warm up, cool down period) Resisted or strengthening exercises on isokinetic dynamometer (at 4 angular velocities 30°, 60°, 90°, 120°/s)	3 months 3 days/week, 40 min	Significant increases in quadriceps torque ($p < 0.01$) generated across all angular velocities in eccentric and concentric modes bilaterally. Affected limb: eccentric mode 51%; concentric mode 38% Non-affected limb: eccentric mode 25%; concentric mode 17%
Silver et al. 2000	5 Ss >6 months post-stroke Mean age 60.4 ± 2.7 yrs	Pre-test, post-test design Aerobic exercise (graded treadmill walking at approximately 60–70% heart rate reserve)	3 months 3 days/week, 40 min	Significant reduction in time taken to perform modified Get Up and Go Test ($p < 0.05$), increased gait velocity ($p < 0.01$) and cadence ($p < 0.05$). No change in gait symmetry during Get Up and Go Test

C, control group; E, experimental group; ROM, range of movement; Ss, subjects.

Since aerobic training has the potential to enhance the development of high oxidative muscle fibres and motor unit recruitment, it is interesting that there is promising evidence that strength training and physical conditioning programmes result in significant improvements in performance of functional activities. For example, Silver and colleagues (2000) reported that an aerobic treadmill training programme, three times a week for 3 months, resulted in an increase in gait velocity and cadence, and a decrease in the overall time required to perform a modified 'Get Up and Go' test. Exercise intensity was individualized and advanced to 40 minutes' training at approximately 60–70% of maximum heart rate reserve. Teixeira-Salmela et al. (1999) assessed subjects' general level of physical activity on the Human Activity Profile, a survey of 94 activities including transportation, home maintenance, social and physical activities, which are rated according to their required metabolic equivalents. The results indicated that subjects were more able to perform household chores and recreational activities after strengthening and aerobic training. These subjects also reported an improved quality of life, as previously reported some years ago (Brinkman and Hoskins 1979).

Although clinical evidence of cardiovascular disease may limit exercise and training initially, Potempa and colleagues (1996) suggest that a monitored aerobic training programme may improve endurance and functional ability and have the following physiological benefits:

- increased work capacity
- decreased resting and sub-maximal heart rates and blood pressure
- weight loss
- improved lipoprotein profile
- decreased platelet aggregation
- delay in onset of angina.

A recent study has shown the early deconditioning that occurs within the first 6 weeks after stroke (Kelly et al. 2002) and illustrates the need for exercise of greater intensity than is typically provided. The study also shows that, for the patients investigated, exercise testing was well tolerated at this early stage. Patients performed incremental maximal effort tests on semi-recumbent cycle ergometers (see Fig. 3.26), with continual monitoring of heart rate and blood pressure by a physician.

Exercise prescription

Once intensive exercise can begin, patients can work on a cycle ergometer, with adaptive devices as necessary (e.g. foot can be strapped to pedal) (Potempa et al. 1995), on a device such as the Motomed Leg Trainer*, or on a treadmill. As an example of exercise prescription suitable for this patient group, Potempa et al. (1996) adapted the criteria of the American College of Sports Medicine for patients with low functional capacity (Kenney et al. 1995) for their conditioning programme:

- Initially patients train at a workload equivalent of 40–60% of VO_{2max} progressing up to 30 min, 3 times/week.
- When 30 min is reached, intensity is progressively increased to the highest workload tolerable without symptoms.
- 10 min warm-up and cool-down periods of unloaded cycling.

Another study describes a similar programme of graded treadmill walking (Macko et al. 1997).

Changes in muscle function, particularly in the elderly, are not maintained without ongoing training (Fiatarone et al. 1990). Ongoing post-discharge exercise

*MOTOmed Pico Leg Trainer, Reck, Reckstrasse 1–3, D-88422, Betzenweiller, Germany.

programmes, either home based, in which case they need monitoring at regular intervals, or gymnasium or health centre based, need to be available for individuals following stroke, particularly when they are elderly. Commenting on programmes for the healthy elderly, Mazzeo and colleagues (1998) point out that exercise programmes for strength and fitness should consist of scientifically based strategies rather than the non-specific 'movement' programmes typically offered.

As a general health precaution it is advisable for older individuals to have a medical check prior to starting a moderately vigorous exercise and fitness programme. This should also occur after stroke. The contraindications to exercise training appear to be few, even in the very old (Mazzeo et al. 1998). Certain conditions such as febrile illness or unstable chest pain need investigation. Patients with arthritis can also tolerate strength training well (Lyngberg et al. 1988). Exacerbation of joint pain from underlying arthritis may necessitate modification of exercise; for example, closed-chain exercise may be preferable to open-chain exercise for those with infrapatellar pain.

Measures of exercise response

Maximal effort exercise testing

Standardized maximal treadmill or cycle ergometer test.   After stroke, exercise testing is typically carried out using a treadmill or bicycle ergometer. A stationary cycle is considered by some to be preferable to treadmill or arm-mobilized ergometer for testing after stroke (Potempa et al. 1995). A cycle ergometer makes it easier to quantify external workload. A standardized methodology, such as the Balke Protocol (Fletcher and Schlant 1994), is used (Macko et al. 1997). Maximal testing requires simultaneous electrocardiograph monitoring and is carried out by specially trained staff. Tests of VO_2 peak and O_2 consumption per kilogram body weight at a given power output while cycling, graded walking or treadmill walking provide a means of evaluating cardiovascular response to exercise (Jankowski and Sullivan 1990).

Submaximal effort exercise testing

Standardized submaximal treadmill test.   Macko and colleagues (1997) describe a treadmill test (1 mph, no incline) representative of the slow walking typical after stroke, performed with open circuit spirometry to measure oxygen consumption (VO_2) under steady state conditions. Patients wore a nose clip and breathed through a mouthpiece, or were fitted with a non-rebreathing mask to collect expired air. All procedures must be standardized.

Monitoring exercise level during training

Standardized heart rate test.   A simple measure of heart rate (HR) gives an indication of intensity of exercise. It can be used to monitor level of exercise to ensure it is sufficiently vigorous and as a simple test of whether or not the patient's cardiovascular system is adapting to exercise. The target HR is determined using a HR monitor:

Calculate maximum age-predicted HR by subtracting the patient's age from 220

Maximum age-predicted HR = 220 − age

Calculate target HR as between 60 and 80% of maximum age-predicted HR

Target HR range = 60−80% × maximum age-predicted HR

Endurance can be tested specifically for walking by the 6-minute or 12-minute walk tests (Guyatt et al. 1985), in which the distance walked in 6 or 12 minutes is measured.

CONCLUSION

Participation in exercise programmes designed to increase strength and fitness and preserve soft tissue length and flexibility can result in significant improvements in strength, functional motor performance and physical fitness in individuals following stroke. There may be additional benefits in terms of attitude, self-concept, self-efficacy, cognition, and confidence in engaging in physical actions, together with recognition of functional potential and the ability to deal with disabilities more effectively (Mazzeo et al. 1998, Teixeira-Salmela et al. 1999). The regaining of skill in critical tasks requires specific training, with intensive practice of actions in the appropriate contexts. The individual must, however, be fit enough to perform the tasks of daily life.

Mazzeo et al. (1998) in their position paper on exercise in the elderly comment that 'sedentariness' appears a far more dangerous condition than physical activity in the elderly. They point out that a large amount of data dispels myths of futility of exercise and provides reassurance about the safety of exercise in the oldest adults. Following discharge from rehabilitation, the potential for negative effects from immobility and inactivity following stroke should be an ongoing public health issue.

One focus of future research needs to be on the retention of gains after the completion of exercise programmes. It is likely that older individuals with stroke need to continue with both home-based and periodic supervised group exercise in order to retain functional gains and reduce the functional declines associated with ageing. Exercise for this group, as is advocated for the healthy elderly, appears critical to offset loss of muscle mass, improve bone density, decrease likelihood of falls and reduce the risk factors associated with, for example, diabetes and cardiovascular disease.

8 | *Overview*

If individuals are to make their best possible recovery from the effects of stroke, they should initially be in a ***stroke unit*** with specially trained staff. In this environment they can receive appropriate diagnostic and medical interventions to reduce the likelihood of complications. Stroke unit care has been shown to be associated with a reduction in death and dependency which was independent of such factors as patient age and sex (Indredavik et al. 1997, Stroke Unit Trialists' Collaboration 1997). A stroke unit provides opportunities for early active intervention. A specialized unit can offer support, encouragement and education programmes for patients and their families with staff trained to coordinate multidisciplinary rehabilitation.

Immediately after stroke it is difficult to predict the extent of eventual recovery. After about 2 weeks post-stroke, good prognostic signs include urinary continence, younger age, mild stroke, rapid improvement, good perceptual abilities and no cognitive disorders. Significant predictors of poor outcome appear to be persistent incontinence and poor premorbid functioning (Cifu and Stewart 1996). However, there are patients who improve unexpectedly and others who do poorly despite having a good prognosis.

Early and proactive physiotherapy can reduce the likelihood of negative sequelae such as soft tissue contracture, learned non-use and persistence and habituation of perceptual–cognitive impairments. Active training in sitting in the acute phase is critical to prevent complications associated with the supine position and bed rest. It is well established that early mobilization can itself reduce secondary thromboembolic events, pneumonia and mortality in stroke. Getting the person upright and active is also necessary to activate the patient's attentional state. It is possible that the longer the delay in starting active training of balancing in sitting, the more likely it is that the patient will become fearful and apprehensive in any attempt at dealing with gravity. Even a very weak patient can be assisted to turn to one side, to sit up over the side of the bed, and to actively practise balancing in sitting (Fig. 8.1). Rehabilitation starts, therefore, in the acute phase.

The rate and extent of mobilization depend on the patient's condition. However, active training in sitting and standing is commenced as soon as vital signs are

FIGURE 8.1   *Lateral neck flexion is encouraged as he is assisted to sit over the side of the bed. Ensure that there is a firm surface for him to put his feet on if they do not reach the floor.*

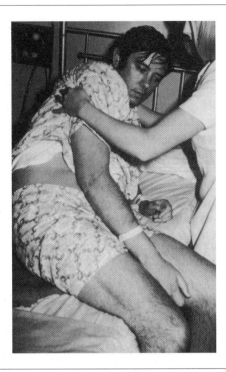

stable (Fig. 8.2). If medical complications preclude sitting out of bed and active mobilization, regular and frequent turning is required to maintain skin integrity, prevent aspiration and pooling of secretions in the lungs. While the patient is confined to bed, positioning of the limbs with repetitive passive and active range of motion exercises are instituted with the aim of preventing stiffness. Care should be taken when passively moving the shoulder. Any movement into elevation should include external rotation.

Patients and their families are given information and provided with the opportunity to learn about the stroke, the process of rehabilitation and their role in this. Since the patient and family will be distressed and anxious in the early stages, the opportunity to gain information needs to be ongoing. Members of stroke support groups, who have themselves experienced a stroke, can be helpful in talking with the patient.

The impact of stroke on many body systems is particularly evident in the very early stages. Since rehabilitation is carried out by a multidisciplinary team, it is necessary for all members to understand these complications and their overall management. Five common complications are discussed briefly below. The reader should refer for more detailed information about the management of these and other complications associated with stroke (Gresham et al. 1995, Carr and Shepherd 1998).

FIGURE 8.2   *In her room, both bed and chair are adjusted to a suitable height to enable practice of standing up and sitting down. (a) Therapist stabilizes the foot. (b) Stand-by assistance.*

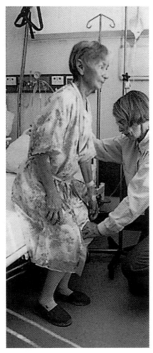
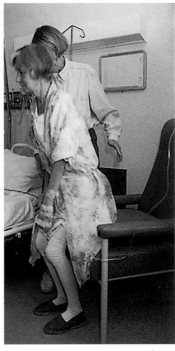

(a)   (b)

Dysphagia, or difficulty swallowing, is a relatively common problem following stroke and may lead to aspiration of saliva, food or liquids. The prevalence is hard to determine. Early detection and treatment is important in preventing both aspiration and dehydration. Primary deficits are incoordination of the oral and pharyngeal phases of swallowing, and delayed or absent triggering of the swallow reflex, or both. Specific training of orofacial musculature to assist chewing and swallowing safely should be commenced in sitting as soon as dysphagia is identified. A modified diet the consistency of mashed potato may aid the re-establishment of control of swallowing. Nasogastric tube feeding may be required where dysphagia is severe. Videofluoroscopy using a modified barium swallow may be used to evaluate the pharyngeal phase of swallowing and the mechanism of aspiration in patients whose dysphagia persists beyond the early stage of recovery.

Urinary incontinence is common but usually transient following stroke. It can be related to motor and sensory impairments, difficulty communicating (which interferes with making the need to void known to others) and immobility, as well as to cognitive deficits and inability to recognize the need to void. There is some evidence of neurological deficits leading to retention or overflow or both (e.g. Gelber et al. 1993) and a catheter may be required. Early assumption of standing and early ambulation usually help the individual to overcome incontinence. If it does not, a bladder training programme can be instituted. Persistent incontinence may be secondary to poor cognitive function (Wade et al. 1985) and suggests a poor prognosis.

Communication deficits. The aphasias (usually dysphasia, since there is rarely a total loss of language) are disturbances of language. They are distinct from motor disorders of speech resulting from weakness and incoordination of the muscles controlling the vocal apparatus, which is classified as dysarthria. Communication deficits isolate the patient and may, not surprisingly, lead to anger and frustration as attempts to communicate fail. It is critical to establish communication with the patient through gesture, situational cues, visual prompts, facial expression, short simple sentences and eye contact. Care should be taken not to exclude the patient from the conversation. Individuals with language impairment usually experience some degree of spontaneous improvement (Wade et al. 1986). A speech and language professional identifies the type and severity of the problem and can provide advice on the best methods of communication.

FIGURE 8.3	*Two slide sheets (Hemco MFG Industries, Ballarat, Australia) are used to move the patient up in the bed so she will be sitting upright when the top of the bed is elevated.*

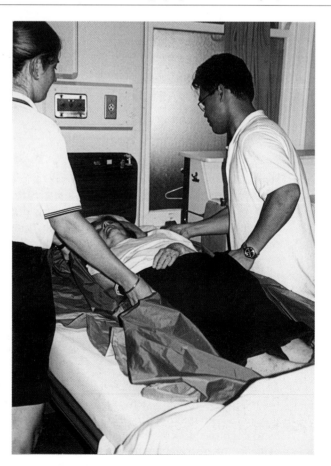

Injury to the paretic, unprotected shoulder can occur through lifting the patient under the arms or pulling on the paretic arm. These lifting methods should be replaced by use of slide sheets to move the patient up in the bed (Fig. 8.3), a hoist when sitting a very weak patient out into a chair, and a slide board (Patboard) to move a patient from hospital bed to exercise table (Fig. 8.4a). Positioning the shoulder is particularly important when the patient is sitting in a chair (see Fig. 5.23).

Excessive attentional focus to the right side occurs in patients with visuospatial agnosia (neglect). This disorder is complex (Ch. 7). The head and eyes may be strongly deviated to the right with an apparent inability to turn the head and eyes to the left. It appears that the person pays attention only to right-sided cues. The patient's deficit is brought to their attention in a way that motivates attempts to offset the deficits, rather than covering up for what they cannot understand. Strong, consistent cues are required to orient the patient to turn the head and eyes and pay attention to the left. Features of a task and the relevant

FIGURE 8.4	*(a) Slide board and sheets are used to move an acute patient on to a firm height-adjustable surface to practise sitting balance. (b) Sitting practice: therapist prevents his L foot from sliding forward. He could only hold his head up momentarily – a soft collar would provide a more erect head position to facilitate spatial orientation and eye contact with the person in front of him. Here he is trying to move the upper body forward by flexing at the hips and sliding hands forward on the table. During previous attempts to sit on the more compliant surface of his bed, two people were needed to prevent him from falling. Here, the firmer surface and the table enable him to be trained by one person.*

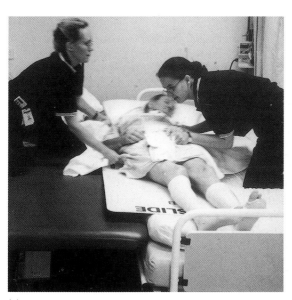

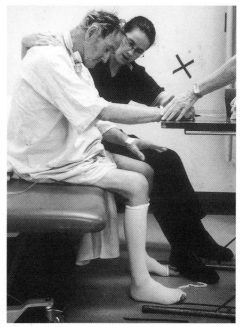

(a)   (b)

cues which must be attended to for successful completion are highlighted. The patient is asked to search for a particular object (concrete goal) rather than being repetitively reminded to turn the head to the left (abstract goal). A close family member who understands the deficit may be able to assist the person to re-orient the head and eyes leftwards. Extraneous stimuli on the right side such as an unattended television or radio should be avoided. Excessive attentional focus may improve quite quickly. Persistent visual inattention complicates rehabilitation.

As soon as possible, the focus changes from a medical and sickness orientation to emphasize exercise and functional training planned around the patient's greatest need, which is to regain effective functioning in daily life. Rehabilitation is specific for each individual's needs, and includes not only a motor training programme, but also programmes designed to overcome specific visual, cognitive, perceptual, swallowing, communication and continence problems. The prevention of complications of immobility and disuse, including reduced endurance, cardiovascular fitness, and the facilitation of psychosocial adjustment to disability and community integration, are central to rehabilitation management of individuals with stroke.

Rehabilitation and the environment in which it occurs is planned to take account of the patient as active learner. The patient's day should provide opportunities to regain self-confidence, take responsibility for unsupervised practice, and regain a sense of time. An overall plan is put in place to motivate the patient and stimulate the individual's learning abilities in both motor and cognitive functions. The therapist's ability to establish contact with the patient through dialogue and positive feedback helps to generate a positive atmosphere and increase the patient's confidence (Talvitie 2000). Furniture, equipment and activities are designed to enable active practice of the necessary tasks outside the protective atmosphere of the rehabilitation unit. Delivery of rehabilitation services is planned to maximize time spent in preparation for the post-discharge phase.

Staff need to be aware that the typical rehabilitation environment is complex, unfamiliar and unpredictable to those who suddenly find themselves in it. Patients have to get to know and interact with a number of different health professionals and other patients. This can be a stressful situation in itself, but after suffering a stroke, a person with a severe disability also has to cope with their own sense of loss and anxiety about the future. For a previously self-sufficient person, adapting both to the disability and to the rehabilitation environment may be difficult and can erode the feeling of competence.

The general role of physiotherapy is to help the person to become physically and mentally active again, with a flexible and strong musculoskeletal system. It is the physiotherapist's role to encourage active participation in the rehabilitation process and to assist the patient to regain the pleasures inherent in being physically and mentally active.

The aims of physiotherapy following stroke are to optimize:

- functional motor performance
- physical fitness, strength and endurance

- interest and motivation
- mental and physical vigour

and to prevent:

- secondary neuromusculoskeletal and cardiovascular disability related to physical inactivity and disuse.

Given our contemporary understanding of brain reorganization and what drives it, plus the emerging empirical evidence of what methods of intervention work and what do not, our recommendations for physiotherapy include the following.

- *Start active task-oriented exercise and training of everyday actions* (sitting balance, reaching and manipulation, sit-to-stand, standing balance and walking) as soon as vital signs are stable, with patient dressed in clothes suitable for exercising.
- *Outline the process of rehabilitation* and discuss the patient's and family's roles in this. Explain the necessity for intensive and repetitive practice.
- *Institute stretching protocols* for at-risk muscles, in particular soleus, shoulder internal rotators and adductors, forearm pronators, wrist and finger flexors, thumb flexors and adductors.
- *Estimate strength of key muscle groups and start repetitive resisted strength training*, for example, lower limb extensors, shoulder flexors, abductors and external rotators, wrist and finger extensors. Use exercise equipment as required.
- *Institute electrical stimulation and EMG feedback* where necessary.
- *Start practice book and check list* of what patient is to practise in order to establish a daily exercise routine.
- *Provide seating* suitable for individual's body dimensions and needs, for example, height-adjustable seat for exercising, suitable chair for sitting, with arm rest (glenohumeral joint in mid-rotation) (see Fig. 5.23).
- *Test and record baseline motor performance* on everyday actions; repeat at intervals, on discharge and follow-up.

The emphasis in rehabilitation research is typically on inpatient care. However, wider issues need to be addressed, especially as long-term disability and social and emotional sequelae of stroke affect *the quality of life after discharge.*

Follow-up services may be poor or non-existent. Many individuals are reported to suffer a loss of rehabilitation gains after they are discharged from rehabilitation (Paolucci et al. 2001). A recent survey in the UK showed a paucity of provision of follow-up services beyond the most basic level of community therapy or support. This was compounded by poor communication between professionals and between patients, carers and professionals, high levels of patient dissatisfaction, and low expectations by professionals of patients' abilities (Tyson and Turner 2000). The significance of this study lies in its methodology which was able to identify not only the shortcomings of services provided but also the reasons for service failure.

Major oversights in post-discharge stroke management are poor access to transport and lack of community exercise facilities for the disabled. There has been little emphasis on the obvious need for individuals with disability to continue with post-rehabilitation exercise and training to not only maintain but also to progress their functional abilities and levels of physical fitness. We know from recent studies of individuals post-discharge that many people, even several years after stroke, are able to make positive gains in strength, fitness, endurance and skill. It has been suggested that the stress of adjusting to the major life change caused by stroke itself may interfere with full potential being achieved during initial inpatient rehabilitation. Patients may have increased motivation to improve function once in their home environment, where the impact of limited functional ability becomes more obvious (Tangeman et al. 1990). Without ongoing or 'top-up' exercise programmes to maintain and improve functional ability, however, rehabilitation gains can be lost once the individual is outside the structure of the rehabilitation setting.

Disability has serious consequences beyond physical function. Difficulty performing essential everyday actions can impose continuing physical inactivity and social isolation on disabled individuals, affecting well-being and quality of life. Psychological sequelae may include loss of self-esteem, fear of walking outside the house, or fear of falling. Social consequences may include role losses, isolation and increased demands on caregivers.

As leisure, sport and social activities are important to quality of life they need to be included as an integral part of planning for discharge and to continue beyond discharge. A community-based stroke group can play an important role; for example, the Stroke Recovery Association of Australia is a social and self-help organization for stroke persons and their families. Weekly group meetings organized by members at different locations offer a rewarding experience for people who have had a stroke, providing emotional support and assisting in the transition back into the community, and in some cases offering a weekly exercise group.

Recent evidence of the effectiveness of task-oriented training and muscle strengthening is promising. It is very likely that an increased understanding of human movement and of the effects of training in a stimulating and challenging environment will begin to give a clearer picture of the potential for brain reorganization and functional recovery after an acute brain lesion.

References

Abercrombie MLJ, Lindon RL, Tyson MC (1964) Associated movements in normal and physically handicapped children. *Dev Med Child Neurol*, **6**, 573–580.

Ada L, O'Dwyer N (2001) Do associated reactions in the upper limb after stroke contribute to contracture formation? *Clin Rehabil*, **15**, 186–194.

Ada L, Westwood P (1992) A kinematic analysis of recovery of the ability to stand up following stroke. *Aust J Physiother*, **38**, 135–142.

Ada L, O'Dwyer NJ, Neilson PD (1993) Improvement in kinematic characteristics and coordination following stroke quantified by linear systems analysis. *Human Mov Sci*, **12**, 137–153.

Ada L, Vattanasilp V, O'Dwyer NJ et al. (1998) Does spasticity contribute to walking dysfunction after stroke? *J Neurol Neurosurg Psychiatry*, **64**, 628–635.

Ada L, Mackey F, Heard R et al. (1999) Stroke rehabilitation: does the therapy area provide a physical challenge? *Aust J Physiother*, **45**, 33–38.

Ada L, Canning C, Dwyer T (2000) Effect of muscle length on strength and dexterity after stroke. *Clin Rehabil*, **14**, 55–61.

Adams JM, Perry J (1994) Gait analysis: clinical application. In *Human Walking* (eds J Rose, JG Gamble), Williams & Wilkins, Philadelphia, 2nd edn, pp 139–164.

Adams R (1990) Attention control training and behaviour management. In *Key Issues in Neurological Physiotherapy* (eds L Ada, C Canning), Butterworth-Heinemann, Oxford, pp 81–97.

Adams RW, Gandevia SC, Skuse NF (1990) The distribution of muscle weakness in upper motoneuron lesions affecting the lower limb. *Brain*, **113**, 1459–1476.

Agahari I, Shepherd RB, Westwood P (1996) A comparative evaluation of lower limb forces in two variations of the step exercise in able bodied subjects. In *Proceedings of 1st Australasian Biomechanics Conference* (eds M Lee, W Gilleard, P Sinclair et al.), University of Sydney, NSW, Australia, pp 94–95.

Ahlsio B, Britton M, Murray V et al. (1984) Disablement and quality of life after stroke. *Stroke*, **15**, 886–890.

Akeson WH, Amiel D, Abel MF et al. (1987) Effects of immobilization on joints. *Clin Orthop Relat Res*, **219**, 28–37.

Andrews AW, Bohannon RW (2000) Distribution of muscle strength impairments following stroke. *Clin Rehabil*, **14**, 79–87.

Andrews AW, Thomas MW, Bohannon RW (1996) Normative values for isometric muscle force measurements obtained with hand-held dynamometers. *Phys Ther*, **76**, 248–259.

Andriacchi TP, Ogle JA, Galante JO (1977) Walking speed as a basis for normal and abnormal gait measures. *J Biomech*, **10**, 262–268.

Andriacchi TP, Andersson GBJ, Fermier RW et al. (1980) A study of lower-limb mechanics during stair-climbing. *J Bone Jt Surg*, **62A**, 749–757.

Anianson A, Gustafsson E (1981) Physical training in elderly men with reference to quadriceps muscle strength and morphology. *Clin Physiol*, **1**, 87–98.

Anianson A, Grimby G, Rundgren A et al. (1980) Physical training in old men. *Age Ageing*, **9**, 186–187.

Annett J (1971) Acquisition of skill. *Br Med Bull*, **27**, 266–271.

Arbib MA, Iberall T, Lyons D (1985) Coordinated control programs for control of the hand. In *Hand Function and the Neocortex* (eds AW Goodwin, I Darian-Smith), Experimental Brain Research Suppl 10, Springer, Berlin, pp 111–129.

Arsenault AB, Winter DA, Martenuik RG et al. (1986) Treadmill versus walkway locomotion in humans: an EMG study. *Ergonomics*, **29**, 665–676.

Arsenault AB, Bilodeau M, Dutil E et al. (1991) Clinical significance of the V-shaped space in the subluxed shoulder of hemiplegia. *Stroke*, **22**, 867–871.

Aruin AS, Latash ML (1996) Anticipatory postural adjustments during self-initiated perturbations of different magnitude triggered by a standard motor action. *Electroencephalogr Clin Neurophysiol*, **101**, 497–503.

Arutyunyan GA, Gurfinkel VS, Mirskii ML (1969) Organization of movements on execution by man of an exact postural task. *Biofizika*, **14**, 1103–1107.

Asanuma H, Keller A (1991) Neuronal mechanisms of motor learning in mammals. *Neuroreport*, **2**, 217–224.

Ashburn A (1995) Behavioural deficits associated with the "pusher" syndrome. *Proceedings of World Congress of Physiotherapists*, Washington, DC, p 819.

Ashworth B (1964) Preliminary trial of carisoprodol in multiple sclerosis. *Practitioner*, **192**, 540–542.

Asmussen E (1953) Positive and negative muscular work. *Acta Physiol Scand*, **28**, 364–382.

Asmussen E (1980) Aging and exercise. In *Environmental Physiology: Aging, Heat and Altitude* (ed J Horvath), Elsevier North-Holland, Amsterdam, pp 419–428.

Asmussen E, Bonde-Petersen F (1974) Storage of elastic energy in skeletal muscles in man. *Acta Physiol Scand*, **91**, 385–392.

Baker LL, Yeh C, Wilson D et al. (1979) Electrical stimulation of wrist and fingers for hemiplegic patients *Phys Ther*, **59**, 495–499.

Balmaseda MT, Koozekanani SH, Fatehi MT et al. (1988) Ground reaction forces, center of pressure, and duration of stance with and without an ankle–foot orthosis. *Arch Phys Med Rehabil*, **69**, 1009–1012.

Barry H, Eathorne S (1994) Exercise and aging: issues for the practitioner. *Med Clin North Am*, **78**, 357–375.

Bassey EJ, Fiatarone MA, O'Neill EF et al. (1997) Leg extensor power and functional performance in very old men and women. *Clin Sci*, **82**, 321–327.

Bateman A, Culpan FJ, Pickering AD et al. (2001) The effect of aerobic training on rehabilitation outcomes after recent severe brain injury: a randomized controlled trial. *Arch Phys Med Rehabil*, **82**, 174–182.

Becher JG, Harlaar J, Lankhorst GJ et al. (1998) Measurement of impaired muscle function of the gastrocnemius, soleus, and tibialis anterior muscles in spastic hemiplegia: a preliminary study. *J Rehabil Res Dev*, **35**, 314–326.

Beckerman H, Becher J, Lankhorst GJ (1996) Walking ability of stroke patients: efficacy of tibial nerve blocking and a polypropylene ankle–foot orthosis. *Arch Phys Med Rehabil*, **77**, 1144–1151.

Beer RF, Given JD, Dewald JPA (1999) Task-dependent weakness at the elbow in patients with hemiparesis. *Arch Phys Med Rehabil*, **80**, 766–772.

Belenkii VY, Gurfinkel VS, Pal'tsev YI (1967) Elements of control of voluntary movements. *Biofizika*, **12**, 135–141.

Bendz P (1993) The functional significance of the fifth metacarpus and hypothenar in two useful grips of the hand. *Am J Phys Med Rehabil*, **72**, 210–213.

Bennett EL (1976) Cerebral effects of differential experience and training. In *Neural Mechanisms of Learning and Memory* (eds MR Rosenzweig, EL Bennett), MIT Press, Cambridge MA, pp 297–287.

Berg K, Wood-Dauphinee S, Williams JI et al. (1989) Measuring balance in the elderly: preliminary development of an instrument. *Physiother Can*, **41**, 304–311.

Berg KO, Maki BE, Williams JI et al. (1992) Clinical and laboratory measures of postural balance in an elderly population. *Arch Phys Med Rehabil*, **73**, 1073–1080.

Berger W, Horstmann G, Dietz V (1984) Tension development and muscle activation in the leg during gait in spastic hemiparesis: independence of muscle hypertonus and exaggerated stretch reflexes. *J Neurol Neurosurg Psychiatry*, **47**, 1029–1033.

Berger RA, Riley PO, Mann RW et al. (1988) Total body dynamics in ascending stairs and rising from a chair following total knee arthroplasty. *Proceedings of the 34th Annual Meeting of the Orthopedic Research Society*, Atlanta, Georgia, p 542.

Bergner M, Bobbitt RA, Carter WB et al. (1981) The sickness impact profile: development and final revision of a health status measure. *Med Care*, **19**, 787–805.

Bernhardt J, Ellis P, Denisenko S (1998) Changes in balance and locomotion measures during rehabilitation following stroke. *Physiother Res Int*, **3**, 109–122.

Bernstein N (1967) *The Coordination and Regulation of Movements*. Pergamon Press, London.

Best TM, McElhaney J, Garrett WE et al. (1994) Characterization of the passive responses of live skeletal muscle using the quasilinear theory of viscoelasticity. *J Biomech*, **27**, 413–419.

Bisiach E, Vellor G (1988) Hemineglect in humans. In *Handbook of Neuropsychology* (eds F Bollar, J Grafman), Elsevier, Amsterdam, pp 195–222.

Blanton S, Wolf S (1999) An application of upper-extremity constraint-induced therapy in a patient with subacute stroke. *Phys Ther*, **79**, 847–853.

Blanpied P, Smidt GL (1993) The difference in stiffness of the active plantarflexors between young and elderly human females. *J Gerontol*, **48**, M58–M63.

Blundell SW, Shepherd RB, Dean CM et al. (2002) Functional strength training in cerebral palsy. A pilot study of a group circuit training class for children aged 4–8 years. *Clin Rehabil* (in press).

Bobath B (1990) *Adult Hemiplegia: Evaluation and Treatment*, 3rd edn, Butterworth-Heinemann, Oxford.

Bobbert MF, van Soest AJK (2000) Two-joint muscles offer the solution, but what was the problem? *Motor Control*, **4**, 48–52.

Bogataj U, Gros N, Malezic M et al. (1989) Restoration of gait during two to three weeks of therapy with multichannel electrical stimulation. *Phys Ther*, **69**, 319–327.

Bohannon RW (1988) Muscle strength changes in hemiparetic stroke patients during inpatient rehabilitation. *J Neurol Rehabil*, **2**, 163–166.

Bohannon RW (1996) Letter: Ipsilateral pushing in stroke. *Arch Phys Med Rehabil*, **77**, 524.

Bohannon RW (1998) Correction of recalcitrant lateropulsion through motor relearning. *Phys Ther Case Reports*, **1**, 157–159.

Bohannon RW (1999) Observations of balance among elderly patients referred to physical therapy in an acute care hospital. *Physiother Theory Pract*, **15**, 185–189.

Bohannon RW, Andrews AW (1990) Correlation of knee extensor muscle torque and spasticity with gait speed in patients with stroke. *Arch Phys Med Rehabil*, **71**, 330–333.

Bohannon RW, Smith MB (1987) Interrater reliability of a modified Ashworth Scale of muscle spasticity. *Phys Ther*, **67**, 206–207.

Bohannon RW, Walsh S (1991) Association of paretic lower extremity muscle strength and standing balance with stair-climbing ability in patients with stroke. *J Stroke Cerebrovasc Dis*, **1**, 129–133.

Bohannon RW, Larkin PA, Smith MB et al. (1986) Shoulder pain in hemiplegia: statistical relationship with five muscles. *Arch Phys Med Rehabil*, **67**, 514–516.

Bohannon RW, Walsh S, Joseph MC (1993) Ordinal and timed balance measurements: reliability and validity in patients with stroke. *Clin Rehabil*, 7, 9–13.

Bohannon RW, Smith J, Hull D et al. (1995) Deficits in lower extremity muscle and gait performance among renal transplant candidates. *Arch Phys Med Rehabil*, **76**, 547–551.

Bortz WM (1982) Disuse and aging. *JAMA*, **248**, 1203–1208.

Bosco C, Tarrka I, Komi PV (1982) Effect of elastic energy and myoelectrical potentiation of triceps surae during stretch-shortening cycle exercises. *Int J Sports Med*, **3**, 137–140.

Bottini G, Sterzi R, Vallar G (1992) Directional hypokinesia in spatial hemineglect: a case study. *J Neurol Neurosurg Psychiatry*, **55**, 562–565.

Bouisset S, Duchenne J-L (1994) Is body balance more perturbed by respiration in seating than in standing posture? *NeuroReport*, **5**, 957–960.

Bourbonnais D, Vanden Noven S (1989) Weakness in patients with hemiparesis. *Am J Occup Ther*, **43**, 313–319.

Bradford J, McFadyen BJ, Winter DA (1988) An integrated biomechanical analysis of normal stair ascent and descent. *J Biomech*, **21**, 733–744.

Branch LG, Meyers AR (1987) Assessing physical function in the elderly. *Clin Geriatr Med*, **3**, 29–51.

Brauer SG, Burns YR, Galley P (2000) A prospective study of laboratory and clinical measures of postural stability to predict community-dwelling fallers. *J Gerontol*, **55A**, M469–M476.

Brinkman JR, Hoskins TA (1979) Physical conditioning and altered self-concept in rehabilitated hemiplegic patients. *Phys Ther*, **59**, 859–865.

Brodal A (1973) Self-observation and neuroanatomical considerations after a stroke. *Brain*, **96**, 675–694.

Broeks JG, Lankhorst GJ, Rumping K et al. (1999) The long-term outcome of arm function after stroke: results of a follow-up study. *Disabil Rehabil*, **21**, 357–364.

Brown DA, Kautz SA (1998) Increased workload enhances force output during pedalling exercise in persons with poststroke hemiplegia. *Stroke*, **29**, 598–606.

Brown P (1994) Pathophysiology of spasticity. *J Neurol Neurosurg Psychiatry*, **57**, 773–777.

Brunnstrom S (1970) *Movement Therapy in Hemiplegia: A Neurophysiological Approach*. Harper and Row, New York.

Brunt D, Liu S, Trimble M et al. (1999) Principles underlying the organization of movement initiation from quiet stance. *Gait Posture*, **10**, 121–128.

Buchner DM, de Lateur BJ (1991) The importance of skeletal muscle strength to physical function in older adults. *Ann Behav Med*, **13**, 91–98.

Buchner DM, Larson EB, Wagner EH et al. (1996) Evidence for a non-linear relationship between leg strength and gait speed. *Age Ageing*, **25**, 386–391.

Burdett RG, Habasevich R, Pisciotta J et al. (1985) Biomechanical comparison of rising from two types of chairs. *Phys Ther*, **65**, 1177–1183.

Burdett RG, Borello-France D, Blatchly C et al. (1988) Gait comparison of subjects with hemiplegia walking unbraced, with ankle–foot orthosis, and with Air-Stirrup Brace. *Phys Ther*, **68**, 1197–1203.

Burke D (1988) Spasticity as an adaptation to pyramidal tract injury. *Adv Neurol*, **47**, 401–423.

Burke D, Gandevia SC (1988) Interfering cutaneous stimulation and the muscle afferent contribution to cortical potentials. *Electroencephalogr Clin Neurophysiol*, **70**, 118–125.

Burke D, Andrews C, Ashby P (1971) Autogenic effect of static muscle stretch in spastic man. *Arch Neurol*, **25**, 367–372.

Burke D, Hagbarth KE, Lofstedt L (1978) Muscle spindle activity in man during shortening and lengthening contractions. *J Physiol*, **277**, 131–142.

Butefisch C, Hummelsheim H, Mauritz K-H (1995) Repetitive training of isolated movements improves the outcome of motor rehabilitation of the centrally paretic hand. *J Neurol Sci*, **130**, 59–68.

Cahill BM, Carr JH, Adams R (1999) Inter-segmental co-ordination in sit-to-stand: an age cross-sectional study. *Physiother Res Int*, **4**, 12–27.

Cailliet R (1991) *Shoulder Pain*. FA Davis, Philadelphia.

Calvanio R, Levine D, Petrone P (1993) Elements of cognitive rehabilitation after right hemisphere stroke. *Behav Neurol*, **11**, 25–57.

Campbell AJ, Robertson MC, Gardner MM et al. (1997) Randomized controlled trial of a general practice programme of home based exercise to prevent falls in elderly women. *BMJ*, **315**, 1065–1069.

Canning CG, Ada L, O'Dwyer N (1999) Slowness to develop force contributes to weakness after stroke. *Arch Phys Med Rehabil*, **80**, 66–70.

Canning CG, Ada L, O'Dwyer NJ (2000) Abnormal muscle activation characteristics associated with loss of dexterity after stroke. *J Neurol Sci*, **176**, 45–56.

Carey JR, Burghardt TP (1993) Movement dysfunction following central nervous system lesions: a problem of neurologic or muscular impairment? *Phys Ther*, **73**, 538–547.

Carey JR, Allison JD, Mundale MO (1983) Electromyographic study of muscular overflow during precision handgrip. *Phys Ther*, **63**, 505–511.

Carey LM (1995) Somatosensory loss after stroke. *Crit Rev Phys Med Rehabil*, **7**, 51–91.

Carey LM, Matyas TA, Oke LE et al. (1993) Sensory loss in stroke patients: effective training of tactile and proprioceptive discrimination. *Arch Phys Med Rehabil*, **74**, 602–611.

Carlsoo S, Dahllof A, Holm J (1974) Kinetic analysis of the gait in patients with hemiparesis and in patients with intermittent claudication. *Scand J Rehabil Med*, **6**, 166–179.

Carolan B, Cafarelli E (1992) Adaptations in coactivation after isometric resistance training. *J Appl Physiol*, **73**, 911–917.

Carr JH, Gentile AM (1994) The effect of arm movement on the biomechanics of standing up. *Human Mov Sci*, **13**, 175–193.

Carr JH, Shepherd RB (1987) *A Motor Relearning Programme for Stroke*, 2nd edn, Butterworth-Heinemann, Oxford.

Carr JH, Shepherd RB (1998) *Neurological Rehabilitation Optimizing Motor Performance*. Butterworth-Heinemann, Oxford.

Carr JH, Shepherd RB (2000) A motor learning model for rehabilitation. In *Movement Science Foundations for Physical Therapy in Rehabilitation* (eds JH Carr, RB Shepherd), PPO-ED Austin, TX, pp 33–110.

Carr JH, Shepherd RB, Nordholm L et al. (1985) Investigation of a new motor assessment scale for stroke patients. *Phys Ther*, **65**, 175–180.

Carr JH, Ow JEG, Shepherd RB (2002) Some biomechanical characteristics of standing up at three different speeds: implications for functional training. *Physiother Theory Prac*, (in press).

Castiello U, Bennett KMB, Paulignan Y (1992) Does the type of prehension influence the kinematics of reaching? *Behav Brain Res*, **50**, 7–15.

Castiello U, Bennett KMB, Stelmach GE (1993) The bilateral reach to grasp movement. *Behav Brain Res*, **56**, 43–57.

Cauraugh J, Light K, Kim S et al. (2000) Chronic motor dysfunction after stroke: recovering wrist and finger extension by electromyography-triggered neuromuscular stimulation. *Stroke*, **31**, 1360–1364.

Chaco J, Wolf E (1971) Subluxation of the glenohumeral joint in hemiplegia. *Am J Phys Med*, **50**, 139–143.

Chae J, Yu D (1999) Neuromuscular stimulation for motor relearning in hemiplegia. *Crit Rev Phys Rehabil Med*, **11**, 279–297.

Chae J, Yu D (2000) A critical review of neuromuscular electrical stimulation for treatment of motor dysfunction in hemiplegia. *Asst Technol*, **12**, 33–49.

Chae J, Bethoux F, Bohinc T et al. (1998) Neuromuscular stimulation for upper extremity motor and functional recovery in acute hemiplegia. *Stroke*, **29**, 975–979.

Chantrain A, Baribeault A, Uebelhart D et al. (1999) Shoulder pain and dysfunction in hemiplegia: effects of functional electrical stimulation. *Arch Phys Med Rehabil*, **80**, 328–331.

Chapman CE, Wiesendanger M (1982) The physiological and anatomical basis of spasticity: a review. *Physiother Can*, **34**, 125–136.

Chari V, Kirby RL (1986) Lower-limb influence on sitting balance while reaching forward. *Arch Phys Med Rehabil*, **67**, 730–733.

Chen C, Chen H, Wong M et al. (2001) Temporal stride and force analysis of cane-assisted gait in people with hemiplegic gait. *Arch Phys Med Rehabil*, **82**, 43–48.

Chen H-C, Schultz AB, Ashton-Miller JA et al. (1996) Stepping over obstacles: dividing attention impairs performance of old more than young adults. *J Gerontol: Med Sci*, **51A**, M116–M122.

Cifu DX, Stewart DG (1996) A comprehensive annotated reference guide to outcome after stroke. *Crit Rev Phys Rehab Med*, **8**, 39–86.

Cirstea MC, Levin MF (2000) Compensatory strategies for reaching in stroke. *Brain*, **123**, 940–953.

Cohen LG, Roth BJ, Wasserman EM et al. (1991) Magnetic stimulation of the human cerebral cortex, an indicator of reorganization in motor pathways in certain pathological conditions. *J Clin Neurophysiol*, **8**, 56–65.

Colebatch JG, Gandevia SC (1989) The distribution of muscular weakness in upper motor neuron lesions affecting the arm. *Brain*, **112**, 749–763.

Colebatch JG, Rothwell JC, Day BL et al. (1990) Cortical outflow to proximal arm muscles in man. *Brain*, **113**, 1843–1856.

Colle FM (1995) The measurement of standing balance after stroke. *Physiother Theory Pract*, **11**, 109–118.

Collin C, Wade D (1990) Assessing motor impairment after stroke: a pilot reliability study. *J Neurol Neurosurg Psychiatry*, **53**, 576–579.

Commissaris DACM, Toussaint HM, Hirschfeld H (2001) Anticipatory postural adjustments in a bimanual, whole-body lifting task seem not only aimed at minimising anterior–posterior centre of mass displacements. *Gait Posture*, **14**, 44–55.

Coote S, Stokes EK (2001) Physiotherapy for upper extremity dysfunction following stroke. *Phys Ther Rev*, **6**, 63–69.

Cordo PJ, Nashner LM (1982) Properties of postural adjustments associated with rapid arm movements. *J Neurophysiol*, **47**, 287–302.

Coslett HB, Bowers D, Fitzpatrick E et al. (1990) Directional hypokinesia and hemispatial inattention in neglect. *Brain*, **113**, 475–486.

Cramer SC, Bastings EP (2000) Mapping clinically relevant plasticity after stroke. *Neuropharmacology*, **39**, 842–851.

Cramer SC, Nelles G, Benson RR et al. (1997) A functional MRI study of subjects recovered from hemiparetic stroke. *Stroke*, **28**, 2518–2527.

Crenna P, Frigo C, Massion J et al. (1987) Forward and backward axial synergies in man. *Exp Brain Res*, **65**, 538–548.

Critchley M (1953) *The Parietal Lobes*. Hafner, New York.

Crompton S, Khemlani M, Batty J et al. (2001) Practical issues in retraining walking in severely disabled patients using treadmill and harness support systems. *Aust J Physiother*, **47**, 211–213.

Crosbie J (1993) Kinematics of walking frame ambulation. *Clin Biomech*, **8**, 31–36.

Crosbie J, Ko V (2000) Changes in the temporal and distance parameters of gait evoked by negotiation of curbs. *Aust J Physiother*, **46**, 103–112.

Crosbie J, Shepherd RB, Squire TJ (1995) Postural and voluntary movement during reaching in sitting: the role of the lower limbs. *J Hum Mov Stud*, **28**, 103–126.

Crosbie J, Vachalathiti R, Smith R (1997a) Patterns of spinal motion during walking. *Gait Posture*, **5**, 6–12.

Crosbie J, Vachalathiti R, Smith R (1997b) Age, gender and speed effects on spinal motion during walking. *Gait Posture*, **5**, 13–20.

Cruz-Martinez A (1984) Electrophysiological study in hemiparetic subjects: electromyography, motor conduction and response to repetitive nerve stimulation. *Electroencephalogr Clin Neurophysiol*, **23**, 139–148.

Culham EG, Noce RR, Bagg SD (1995) Shoulder complex position and glenohumeral subluxation in hemiplegia. *Arch Phys Med Rehabil*, **76**, 857–864.

Dannenbaum RM, Dykes RW (1988) Sensory loss in the hand after sensory stroke: therapeutic rationale. *Arch Phys Med Rehabil*, **69**, 833–839.

Danneskiold-Samsoe B, Kofod V, Munter J et al. (1984) Muscle strength and functional capacity in 78–81-year-old men and women. *Eur J Appl Physiol*, **52**, 310–314.

Darien-Smith I, Galea MP, Darien-Smith C (1996) Manual dexterity: how does the cerebral cortex contribute? *Clin Exp Pharmacol Physiol*, **23**, 948–956.

Davies JM, Mayston MJ, Newham DJ (1996) Electrical and mechanical output of the knee muscles during isometric and isokinetic activity in stroke and healthy subjects. *Disabil Rehabil*, **18**, 83–90.

Davies PM (1985) *Steps to Follow, A Guide to the Treatment of Adult Hemiplegia*. Springer, New York.

Davies PM (1990) *Right in the Middle – Selective Trunk Activity in the Treatment of Adult Hemiplegia*. Springer, Berlin.

Day BL, Steiger MJ, Thompson PD et al. (1998) Effect of vision and stance width on human body motion when standing: implications for afferent control of lateral sway. *J Physiol*, **469**, 479–499.

Dean C, Mackey F (1992) Motor assessment scale scores as a measure of rehabilitation outcome following stroke. *Aust J Physiother*, **38**, 31–35.

Dean CM, Shepherd RB (1997) Task-related training improves performance of seated reaching tasks after stroke: a randomized controlled trial. *Stroke*, **28**, 722–728.

Dean C, Shepherd R, Adams R (1999a) Sitting balance I: trunk–arm and the contribution of the lower limbs during self-paced reaching in sitting. *Gait Posture*, **10**, 135–144.

Dean C, Shepherd RB, Adams RD (1999b) Sitting balance II: reach direction and thigh support affect the contribution of the lower limbs when reaching beyond arm's length in sitting. *Gait Posture*, **10**, 147–153.

Dean CM, Richards CL, Malouin F (2000) Task-related training improves performance of locomotor tasks in chronic stroke. A randomized controlled pilot trial. *Arch Phys Med Rehabil*, **81**, 409–417.

Dean CM, Richards CL, Malouin F (2001) Walking speed over 10 metres overestimates locomotor capacity after stroke. *Clin Rehabil*, **15**, 415–421.

De Deyne PG (2001) Application of passive stretch and its implications for muscle fibres. *Phys Ther*, **81**, 819–827.

Desrosiers J, Bourbonnais D, Bravo G et al. (1996) Performance of 'unaffected' upper extremity of elderly stroke patients. *Stroke*, **27**, 1564–1570.

Dettman MA, Linder MT, Sepic SB (1987) Relationships among walking performance, postural stability, and functional assessments of the hemiplegic patient. *Am J Phys Med*, **66**, 77–90.

De Weerdt W, Spaepen A (1999) Balance. In *Functional Human Movement: Measurement and Analysis* (eds BR Durward, GD Baer, PJ Rowe), Butterworth-Heinemann, Oxford, pp 203–218.

De Weerdt W, Nuyens G, Feys H et al. (2001) Group physiotherapy improves time use by patients with stroke in rehabilitation. *Aust J Physiother*, **47**, 53–61.

Dickstein R, Nissan M, Pillar T et al. (1984) Foot–ground pressure pattern of standing hemiplegic patients. *Phys Ther*, **64**, 19–23.

Dickstein R, Heffes Y, Abulaffio N (1996) Electromyographic and positional changes in the elbows of spastic hemiparetic patients during walking. *Electroencephalogr Clin Neurophysiol*, **101**, 491–496.

Dickstein R, Heffes Y, Laufer Y et al. (1999) Activation of selected trunk muscles during symmetric functional activities in poststroke hemiparetic and hemiplegic patients. *J Neurol Neurosurg Psychiatry*, **66**, 218–221.

Diener HC, Bacher M, Guschlbauer B et al. (1993) The coordination of posture and voluntary movement in patients with hemiparesis. *J Neurol*, **240**, 161–167.

Dieterich M, Brandt T (1992) Wallenberg's syndrome: lateropulsion, cyclorotation and subjective visual vertical in thirty-six patients. *Ann Neurol*, **31**, 399–408.

Dietz V, Berger W (1983) Normal and impaired regulation of muscle stiffness in gait: a new hypothesis about muscle hypertonia. *Exp Neurol*, **79**, 680–687.

Dietz V, Quintern J, Berger W (1981) Electrophysiological studies of gait in spasticity and rigidity. Evidence that altered mechanical properties of muscle contribute to hypertonia. *Brain*, **104**, 431–449.

Dietz V, Quintern J, Berger W (1984) Corrective reactions to stumbling in man: functional significance of spinal and transcortical reflexes. *Neurosci Lett*, **44**, 131–135.

Dietz V, Ketelsen U-P, Berger W et al. (1986) Motor unit involvement in spastic paresis. Relationship between leg muscle activation and histochemistry. *J Neurol Sci*, **75**, 89–103.

di Fabio RP (1997) Adaptation of postural stability following stroke. *Topics Stroke Rehabil*, **3**, 62–75.

di Fabio RP, Badke MB (1990) Extraneous movement associated with hemiplegic postural sway during dynamic goal-directed weight redistribution. *Arch Phys Med Rehabil*, **71**, 365–371.

Dimitrijevic M, Stokic S, Wawro A et al. (1996) Modification of motor control of wrist extension by mesh-glove electrical afferent stimulation in stroke patients. *Arch Phys Med Rehabil*, **77**, 252–258.

Do MC, Bussel B, Breniere Y (1990) Influence of plantar cutaneous afferents on early compensatory reactions to forward fall. *Exp Brain Res*, **79**, 319–324.

Dobkin BH (1999) An overview of treadmill locomotor training with partial body weight support: a neurophysiologically sound approach whose time has come for randomized clinical trials. *Neurorehabil Neural Repair*, **13**, 157–165.

Dromerick AW, Edwards DF, Hahn M (2000) Does the application of constraint-induced movement therapy during acute rehabilitation reduce arm impairment after ischaemic stroke? *Stroke*, **31**, 2984–2988.

Duncan PW (1997) Synthesis of intervention trials to improve motor recovery following stroke. *Topics Stroke Rehabil*, **3**, 1–20.

Duncan PW, Weiner DK, Chandler J et al. (1990) Functional reach: a new clinical measure of balance. *J Gerontol*, **45**, M192–M197.

Duncan PW, Goldstein LB, Horner RD et al. (1994) Similar motor recovery of upper and lower extremities after stroke. *Stroke*, **25**, 1181–1188.

Duncan P, Richards L, Wallace D et al. (1998) A randomized controlled pilot study of a home-based exercise program for individuals with mild and moderate stroke. *Stroke*, **29**, 2055–2060.

Duong B, Low M, Moseley AM et al. (2001) Time course of stress relaxation and recovery in human ankles. *Clin Biomech*, **16**, 601–607.

Dvir Z, Panturin E, Prop I (1996) The effect of graded effort on the severity of associated reactions in hemiplegic patients. *Clin Rehabil*, **10**, 159–165.

Eastlake ME, Arvidson J, Snyder-Mackler L et al. (1991) Interrater reliability of videotaped observational gait-analysis assessments. *Phys Ther*, **71**, 465–472.

Ebrahim S, Barer D, Nouri F (1986) Use of Nottingham health profile with patients after stroke. *J Epidemiol Community Health*, **40**, 166–169.

Edstrom L, Grimby L (1986) Effect of exercise on the motor unit. *Muscle Nerve*, **9**, 104–126.

Elbert T, Pantev C, Wienbruch C et al. (1995) Increased cortical representation of the fingers of the left hand in string players. *Science*, **270**, 305–307.

Eng JJ, Winter CD, Patla AE et al. (1992) Role of the torque stabilizer in postural control during rapid voluntary arm movements. In *Posture and Gait: Control Mechanisms* (eds M Woollacott, F Horak), XIth Int Symposium of Society for Postural and Gait Research. University of Oregon Books, Portland, OR.

Engardt M (1994) Long term effects of auditory feedback training on relearned symmetrical body weight distribution in stroke. A follow-up study. *Scand J Rehabil Med*, **26**, 65–69.

Engardt M, Olsson E (1992) Body weight-bearing while rising and sitting down in patients with stroke. *Scand J Rehabil Med*, **24**, 67–74.

Engardt M, Ribbe T, Olsson E (1993) Vertical ground reaction force feedback to enhance stroke patients' symmetrical body-weight distribution while rising/sitting down. *Scand J Rehabil Med*, **25**, 41–48.

Engardt M, Knutsson E, Jonsson M et al. (1995) Dynamic muscle strength training in stroke patients: effects on knee extension torque, electromyographic activity, and motor function. *Arch Phys Med Rehabil*, **76**, 419–425.

Enright PL, Sherrill DL (1998) Reference equations for the six-minute walk in healthy adults. *Am J Respir Crit Care Med*, **158**, 1384–1387.

Esmonde T, McGinley J, Goldie P et al. (1997) Stroke rehabilitation: patient activity during non-therapy time. *Aust J Physiother*, **43**, 43–51.

Faghri PD, Rodgers MM, Glaser RM et al. (1994) The effects of functional stimulation on shoulder pain in hemiplegic stroke patients. *Arch Phys Med Rehabil*, **75**, 73–79.

Farmer SF, Swash M, Ingram DA et al. (1993) Changes in motor unit synchronization following central nervous lesions in man. *J Physiol*, **463**, 83–105.

Fellows SJ, Kaus C, Thilmann AF (1994) Voluntary movement at the elbow in spastic hemiparesis. *Ann Neurol*, **36**, 397–407.

Feltz DL, Landers DM, Becker BJ (1988) A revised meta-analysis of the mental practice literature on motor skill learning. In *Enhancing Human Performance: Issue, Theories and Techniques* (eds D Druckman, J Swets) National Academy Press, Washington, pp 61–101.

Fiatarone MA, Marks EC, Ryan ND et al. (1990) High-intensity strength training in nonagenarians. *JAMA*, **263**, 3029–3034.

Fiatarone MA, O'Neill EF, Doyle N et al. (1993) The Boston FICSIT study: the effects of resistance training and nutritional supplementation on physical frailty in the oldest old. *J Am Geriatr Soc*, **41**, 333–337.

Fiatarone MR, O'Neill EF, Ryan ND et al. (1994) Exercise training and nutritional supplementation for physical frailty in very elderly people. *N Engl J Med*, **330**, 1769–1775.

Fielding RA, Le Brasseur NK, Cuoco A et al. (2002) High velocity power training increases skeletal muscle peak power in older women. *J Am Geriatr Soc*, **50**, 655–662.

Finch L, Barbeau H, Arsenault B (1991) Influence of body weight support on normal human gait: development of a gait retraining strategy. *Phys Ther*, **71**, 842–856.

Finger S (1978) Environmental attenuation of brain lesion symptoms. In *Recovery from Brain Damage* (ed S Finger), Plenum Press, New York.

Finley FR, Cody KA (1970) Locomotive characteristics of urban pedestrians. *Arch Phys Med Rehabil*, **51**, 423–426.

Fisher SV, Gullickson G Jr (1978) Energy cost of ambulation in health and disability: a literature review. *Arch Phys Med Rehabil*, **59**, 124–133.

Fishman MN, Colby LA, Sachs LA et al. (1997) Comparison of upper-extremity balance tasks and force platform testing in persons with hemiparesis. *Phys Ther*, **77**, 1052–1062.

Fisk JD, Goodale MA (1988) The effects of unilateral brain damage on visually guided reaching: hemispheric differences in the nature of the deficit. *Exp Brain Res*, **72**, 425–435.

Fitts PM, Posner MI (1967) *Human Performance.* Brooks/Cole, Belmont, CA.

Fix A, Daughton D (1988) *Human Activity Profile Professional Manual.* Psychological Assessment Resources Inc, Odessa, FL.

Fleckenstein SJ, Kirby RL, MacLeod DA (1988) Effect of limited knee-flexion range on peak hip moments of force while transferring from sitting to standing. *J Biomech*, **21**, 915–918.

Fletcher GF, Schlant RC (1994) The exercise test. In *The Heart: Arteries and Veins* (eds RC Schlant, RW Alexander), McGraw-Hill, New York, 8th edn, pp 423–440.

Foldvari M, Clark M, Laviolette LC et al. (2000) Association of muscle power with functional status in community-dwelling elderly women. *J Gerontol*, **55A**, M192–M199.

Forssberg H (1982) Spinal locomotion functions and descending control. In *Brain Stem Control of Spinal Mechanisms* (eds B Sjolund,

A Bjorklund), Elsevier Biomedical Press, New York.

Forster A, Young J (1995) Incidence and consequences of falls due to stroke: a systematic inquiry. *BMJ*, **311**, 83–86.

Fowler V, Carr JH (1996) Auditory feedback: effects on vertical force production during standing up following stroke. *Int J Rehabil Res*, **19**, 265–269.

Fowler V, Canning CG, Carr JH et al. (1997) The effect of muscle length on the pendulum test. *Arch Phys Med Rehabil*, **79**, 169–171.

Francisco G, Chae J, Chawla H et al. (1998) Electromyogram-triggered neuromuscular stimulation for improving the arm function of acute stroke survivors: a randomized pilot study. *Arch Phys Med Rehabil*, **79**, 570–575.

Friel KM, Nudo RJ (1998) Restraint of the unimpaired hand is not sufficient to retain spared hand representation after focal cortical injury. *Soc Neurosci Abst*, **24**: 405.

Frontera WR, Meredith CN, O'Reilly KP et al. (1988) Strength conditioning in older men: skeletal muscle hypertrophy and improved function. *J Appl Physiol*, **64**, 1038–1044.

Fuhr P, Cohen LG, Dang N et al. (1992) Physiological analysis of motor reorganization following lower limb amputation. *Electroencephalogr Clin Neurophysiol*, **85**, 53–60.

Furlan M, Marchal G, Vialder F et al. (1996) Spontaneous neurological recovery after stroke and the fate of the ischemic penumbra. *Ann Neurol*, **40**, 216–226.

Gabell A, Nayak VSC (1984) The effect of age on variability in gait. *J Gerontol*, **39**, 662–666.

Gabell A, Simons MA, Mayak USL (1986) Falls in the healthy elderly: predisposing causes. *Ergonomics*, **28**, 965–975.

Gallistel CR (1980) *The Organization of Action: A New Synthesis*. Lawrence Erlbaum, Hillsdale. NJ.

Gardner MM, Robertson MC, Campbell AJ (2000) Exercise in preventing falls and fall related injuries in older people: a review of randomized controlled trials. *Br J Sports Med*, **34**, 7–17.

Gatev P, Thomas S, Kepple T et al. (1999) Feedforward strategy of balance during quiet stance in adults. *J Physiol*, **514**, 915–928.

Gehlsen GA, Whaley MH (1990) Falls in the elderly: part II, balance, strength, and flexibility. *Arch Phys Med Rehabil*, **71**, 739–741.

Gelber DA, Good DC, Laven LJ et al. (1993) Causes of urinary incontinence after stroke. *Stroke*, **24**, 378–382.

Gemperline JJ, Allen S, Walk D et al. (1995) Characteristics of motor unit discharge in subjects with hemiparesis. *Muscle Nerve*, **18**, 1101–1114.

Gentile AM (1987) Skill acquisition: action, movement, and neuromotor processes. In *Movement Science Foundations for Physical Therapy in Rehabilitation* (eds JH Carr, RB Shepherd), Aspen Publishers, Rockville, MD, pp 93–154.

Gentile AM (2000) Skill acquisition: action, movement, and neuromotor processes. In *Movement Science Foundations for Physical Therapy in Rehabilitation* (eds JH Carr, RB Shepherd), PRO-ED Austin, TX, 2nd edn, pp 111–187.

Ghez C (1991) Posture. In *Principles of Neural Science* (eds ER Kandell, JH Schwartz, TM Jessell), Appleton and Lange, Norwalk, CT, 3rd edn, pp 596–608.

Gibson JJ (1977) The theory of affordances. In *Perceiving, Action and Knowing: Towards an Ecological Psychology* (eds R Shaw, J Bransford), Erlbaum, Hillsdale, NJ, pp 67–82.

Gill-Body K, Krebs D (1994) Usefulness of biomechanical measurements approaches in rehabilitation. *Topics Geriatr Rehabil*, **10**, 82–96.

Gioux M, Petit J (1993) Effects of immobilizing the cat peroneus longus muscle on the activity of its own spindles. *J Appl Physiol*, **75**, 2629–2635.

Glanz M, Klawansky S, Stason W et al. (1996) Functional electrostimulation in poststroke rehabilitation: a meta-analysis of the randomized controlled trials. *Arch Phys Med Rehabil*, **77**, 549–553.

Goldie P, Matyas T, Kinsella G (1992) Movement rehabilitation following stroke. Research Report, Department of Health, Housing and Community Services, Victoria, Australia.

Goldie PA, Matyas TA, Evans OM et al. (1996a) Maximum voluntary weight-bearing by the affected and unaffected legs in standing following stroke. *Clin Biomech*, **11**, 333–342.

Goldie PA, Evans O, Matyas T (1996b) Performance in the stability limits test during rehabilitation following stroke. *Gait Posture*, **4**, 315–322.

Goodale MA, Milner AD, Jakobson LS et al. (1990) Kinematic analysis of limb movements in neuropsychological research: subtle deficits and recovery of function. *Can J Psychol*, **44**, 180–195.

Gordon J (2000) Assumptions underlying physical therapy interventions: theoretical and historical perspectives. In *Movement Science Foundations for Physical Therapy in Rehabilitation* (eds JH Carr, RB Shepherd), Aspen Publishers, Rockville, MD, 2nd edn, pp 1–31.

Gottlieb GL, Corcos DM, Jaric S et al. (1988) Practice improves even the simplest movements. *Exp Brain Res*, 73, 436–440.

Gowland C (1982) Recovery of motor function following stroke: profile and predictors. *Physiother Can*, 34, 77–84.

Gowland C, deBruin H, Basmajian JV et al. (1992) Agonist and antagonist activity during voluntary upper-limb movement in patients with stroke. *Phys Ther*, 72, 624–633.

Grabiner MD, Koh TJ, Lundin TM et al. (1993) Kinematics of recovery of a stumble. *J Gerontol*, 3, M97–M102.

Gracies J-M, Wilson L, Gandevia SC et al. (1997) Stretched position of spastic muscles aggravates their co-contraction in hemiplegic patients. *Ann Neurol*, 42, 438–439.

Gracies J-M, Marosszeky JE, Renton R et al. (2000) Short term effects of dynamic lycra splints on upper limb in hemiplegic patients. *Arch Phys Med Rehabil*, **81**, 1547–1555.

Granger CV, Hamilton BB, Sherwin FS (1986) *Guide for the Use of the Uniform Data Set for Medical Rehabilitation*. Project Office, Buffalo General Hospital, New York.

Gregory JE, Morgan DL, Proske U (1988) After-effects in the responses of cat muscle spindles and errors in limb position sense in man. *J Neurophysiol*, 59, 1220–1230.

Gresham G, Duncan P, Stason W et al. (1995) *Post-stroke rehabilitation: clinical practice guidelines, no 16*. US Department of Health and Human Services, Public Health Service, AHCPR 95-0662, Rockville, MD.

Griffin MP, Olney SJ, McBride ID (1995) Role of symmetry in gait performance of stroke subjects with hemiplegia. *Gait Posture*, 3, 132–142.

Grillner S, Shik ML (1973) On the descending control of the lumbosacral spinal cord from 'mesencephalic locomotor region'. *Acta Physiol Scand*, 87, 320–333.

Grimby G (1983) On the energy cost of achieving mobility. *Scand J Rehabil Med Suppl*, 9, 49–54.

Guiliani CA (1990) Adult hemiplegic gait. In *Gait in Rehabilitation* (ed G Smidt), Churchill Livingstone, New York, pp 253–266.

Guyatt GH, Pugsley SO, Sullivan MJ et al. (1984) Effect of encouragement on walking test performance. *Thorax*, 39, 818–822.

Guyatt GH, Sullivan MJ, Thompson PJ et al. (1985) The 6-minute walk: a new measure of exercise capacity in patients with chronic heart failure. *Can Med J*, 132, 919–923.

Hachisuka K, Umezu Y, Ogata B (1997) Disuse muscle atrophy of lower limbs in hemiplegic patients. *Arch Phys Med Rehabil*, 78, 13–18.

Hagbarth K-E, Hagglund JV, Norkin M et al. (1985) Thixotropic behaviour of human finger flexor muscles with accompanying changes in spindle and reflex responses to stretch. *J Physiol*, **368**, 323–342.

Hakkinen K, Komi PV (1981) Effect of different combined concentric and eccentric muscle work regimens on maximal strength development. *J Hum Mov Stud*, 7, 33–44.

Hakkinen K, Komi PV (1983) Electromyographic changes during strength training and detraining. *Med Sci Sports Exercise*, 15, 455–460.

Hakkinen K, Newton RU, Gordon SE et al. (1998) Changes in muscle morphology, electromyographic activity, and force production characteristics during progressive strength training in young and older men. *J Gerontol Biol Sci*, 53A, B415–B423.

Halbertsma JP, van Bolhuis AI, Goeken LN (1996) Sports stretching: effect on passive muscle stiffness of short hamstrings. *Arch Phys Med Rehabil*, 77, 688–692.

Halkjaer-Kristensen J, Ingemann-Hansen T (1985) Wasting of the human quadriceps muscle after knee ligament injuries. 1. Anthropometric consequences. *Scand J Rehabil Med Suppl*, **13**, 5–55.

Hall EJ, Flament D, Fraser C et al. (1990) Non-invasive brain stimulation reveals reorganized cerebral output in amputees. *Neurosci Lett*, **116**, 379–386.

Halligan PW, Marshall JC (1992) Left visuo-spatial neglect: a meaningless entity? *Cortex*, **28**, 525–535.

Hamdorf P, Withers R, Penhall R et al. (1992) Physical training effects on the fitness and habitual activity patterns of elderly women. *Arch Phys Med Rehabil*, 73, 603–608.

Hamm LF, Leon AS (1994) Exercise training for the coronary patient. In *Rehabilitation of the Coronary Patient* (eds NK Wenger, HK Hellerstein), Churchill Livingstone, New York.

Hammond MC, Kraft GH, Fitts SS (1988) Recruitment and termination of electromyographic activity in the hemiparetic forearm. *Arch Phys Med Rehabil*, **69**, 106–110.

Hamrin E, Eklund G, Hillgren A-K et al. (1982) Muscle strength and balance in post-stroke patients. *Uppsala Med Sci*, 87, 11–26.

Harlaar J, Becher JG, Snijders CJ et al. (2000) Passive stiffness characteristics of ankle plantar flexors in hemiplegia. *Clin Biomech*, 15, 261–270.

Harridge SDR, Kryger A, Stensgaard A (1999) Knee extensor strength, activation, and size in very elderly people following strength training. *Muscle Nerve*, 22, 831–839.

Harris ML, Polkey MI (2001) Quadriceps muscle weakness following acute hemiplegic stroke. *Clin Rehabil*, 15, 274–281.

Harvey LA, Herbert RD (2002) Muscle stretching for treatment and prevention of contracture in people with spinal cord injury. *Spinal Cord*, **40**, 1–9.

Hase K, Stein RB (1999) Turning strategies during human walking. *J Neurophysiol*, **81**, 2914–2922.

Hauptmann B, Hummelsheim H (1996) Facilitation of motor evoked potentials in hand extensor muscles of stroke patients: correlation to the level of voluntary contraction. *Electroencephalogr Clin Neurophysiol*, **101**, 387–394.

Hausdorff JM, Rios DA, Edelberg HK (2001) Gait variability and fall risk in community-living older adults: a 1-year prospective study. *Arch Phys Med Rehabil*, **82**, 1050–1056.

Hazlewood ME, Brown JK, Rowe PJ et al. (1994) The use of therapeutic electrical stimulation in the treatment of hemiplegic cerebral palsy. *Dev Med Child Neurol*, **36**, 661–673.

Heilman KM, van den Abell T (1980) The right hemisphere dominance for attention: the mechanism underlying hemispheric asymmetries of inattention (neglect). *Neurology*, **30**, 327–330.

Heilman KM, Bowers D, Valenstein E et al. (1987) Hemispace and hemispatial neglect. In *Neurophysiological and Neuropsychological Aspects of Spatial Neglect* (ed M Jeannerod), Elsevier, Amsterdam, pp 115–150.

Held JM, Gordon J, Gentile AM (1985) Environmental influences on locomotor recovery following cortical lesions in rats. *Behav Neurosci*, **99**, 678–690.

Herbert RD, Balnave RJ (1993) The effect of position of immobilization on resting length, resting stiffness, and weight of the soleus muscle of the rabbit. *J Anat*, **116**, 45–55.

Herbert EP, Landin D (1994) Effects of a learning model and augmented feedback on tennis skill acquisition. *Res Q Exercise Sport*, **65**, 250–257.

Herbert R (1988) The passive mechanical properties of muscle and their adaptations to altered patterns of use. *Aust J Physiother*, **34**, 141–149.

Herbert RD, Sherrington C, Maher C et al. (2001) Evidence-based practice – imperfect but necessary. *Physiother Theory Prac*, **17**, 201–211.

Herman EWM (1992) Spatial neglect: new issues and their implications for occupational therapy practice. *Am J Occup Ther*, **46**, 207–216.

Hermsdorfer J, Mai N (1996) Disturbed grip-force control following cerebral lesions. *J Hand Ther*, **9**, 33–40.

Herzog W, Hasler E, Abrahams SK (1991a) A comparison of knee extensor strength curves obtained theoretically and experimentally. *Med Sci Sport Exercise*, **23**, 108–114.

Herzog W, Koh T, Hasler E et al. (1991b) Specificity and plasticity of mammalian skeleton muscles. *J Appl Biomech*, **16**, 98–109.

Hesse S (1999) Treadmill training with partial body weight support in hemiparetic patients – further research needed. *Neurorehabil Neural Repair*, **13**, 179–181.

Hesse S, Schauer M, Malezic M et al. (1994) Quantitative analysis of rising from a chair in healthy and hemiparetic subjects. *Scand J Rehabil Med*, **26**, 161–166.

Hesse S, Bertelt C, Jahnke MT et al. (1995) Treadmill training with partial body weight support compared with physiotherapy in nonambulatory hemiparetic patients. *Stroke*, **26**, 976–981.

Hesse S, Helm B, Krajnik J et al. (1997) Treadmill training with partial body weight support: influence of body weight release on the gait of hemiparetic patients. *J Neurol Rehabil*, **11**, 15–20.

Hesse S, Schauer M, Petersen M et al. (1998) Sit-to-stand manoeuvre in hemiparetic patients before and after a 4-week rehabilitation programme. *Scand J Rehabil Med*, **30**, 81–86.

Hewson L (1996) *The Stroke Jigsaw: Lorna's Story*. An Integrated Resource Package. University of Newcastle, Newcastle, Australia.

Hill KM, Harburn KL, Kramer JF et al. (1994) Comparison of balance responses to an external perturbation test, with and without an overhead harness safety system. *Gait Posture*, **2**, 27–31.

Hill K, Bernhardt J, McGann A et al. (1996) A new test of dynamic standing balance for stroke patients: reliability and comparison with healthy elderly. *Physiother Can*, **48**, 257–262.

Hill K, Ellis P, Bernhardt J et al. (1997) Balance and mobility outcomes for stroke patients: a comprehensive audit. *Aust J Physiother*, **43**, 173–180.

Hintermeister RA, Bey MJ, Lange GW et al. (1998) Quantification of elastic resistance knee rehabilitation exercises. *J Orthop Sports Phys Ther*, **28**, 40–50.

Hoff B, Arbib MA (1993) Models of trajectory formation and temporal interaction of reach and grasp. *J Motor Behav*, **25**, 175–192.

Hogan N, Winters JM (1990) Principles underlying movement organization: upper limb. In *Multiple Muscle Systems: Biomechanics and Movement Organization* (eds JM Winters, SL-Y Woo), Springer, New York, pp 182–194.

Holden MK, Gill KM, Magliozzi MR (1986) Gait assessment for neurologically impaired patients: standards for outcome assessment. *Phys Ther*, **66**, 1530–1539.

Holt RR, Simpson D, Jenner JR et al. (2000) Ground reaction force after a sideways push as a measure of balance in recovery from stroke. *Clin Rehabil*, **14**, 88–95.

Horak F (1987) Clinical measurement of postural control in adults. *Phys Ther*, **67**, 1881–1885.

Horak F (1997) Invited commentary. *Phys Ther*, **77**, 382–383.

Horak FB, Nashner LM (1986) Central programming of postural movements: adaptation to altered support-surface configuration. *J Neurophysiol*, **55**, 1369–1381.

Horak FB, Esselman ME, Anderson ME et al. (1984) The effects of movement velocity, mass displaced, and task certainty on associated postural adjustments made by normal and hemiplegic individuals. *J Neurol Neurosurg Psychiatry*, **48**, 1020–1028.

Horak FB, Shupert CL, Mirka A (1989) Components of postural dyscontrol in the elderly: a review. *Neurobiol Ageing*, **10**, 727–738.

Horak FB, Henry SM, Shumway-Cook A (1997) Postural perturbations: new insights for treatment of balance disorders. *Phys Ther*, **77**, 517–533.

Hortobagyi T, Tunnel D, Moody J et al. (2001) Low- or high-intensity strength training partially restores impaired quadriceps force accuracy and steadiness in aged adults. *J Gerontol: Biol Sci*, **56A**, B38–B47.

Hu M-H, Woollacott MH (1994) Multisensory training of standing balance in older adults: 1. Postural stability and one-leg stance balance. *J Gerontol: Med Sci*, **49**, M52–M61.

Hufschmidt A, Mauritz K-H (1985) Chronic transformation of muscle in spasticity: a peripheral contribution to increased tone. *J Neurol Neurosurg Psychiatry*, **48**, 676–685.

Hummelsheim H, Mauritz K-H (1993) Neurophysiological mechanisms of spasticity modification by physiotherapy. In *Spasticity: Mechanisms and Management* (eds AF Thilmann, DJ Burke, WZ Rymer), Springer, New York.

Hummelsheim H, Munch B, Butefisch C et al. (1994) Influence of sustained stretch on late muscular response to magnetic brain stimulation in patients with upper motor neuron lesions. *Scand J Rehabil Med*, **26**, 3–9.

Hummelsheim H, Maier-Loth ML, Eickhof C (1997) The functional value of electrical muscle stimulation for the rehabilitation of the hand in stroke patients. *Scand J Rehabil Med*, **29**, 3–10.

Humphreys GW, Riddoch MJ (1992) Interactions between object- and space-vision revealed through neuropsychology. In *Attention and Performance* IX (eds DE Meyer, S Kornblum), Lawrence Erlbaum, Hove.

Hunt SM, McEwen J, McKenna SP (1985) Measuring health status: a new tool for clinicians and epidemiologists. *J Royal Coll Gen Pract*, **35**, 185–188.

Huxham FE, Goldie PA, Patla AE (2001) Theoretical considerations in balance assessment. *Aust J Physiother*, **47**, 89–100

Hyvarinen J, Poranen A, Jokinen Y (1980) Influence of attentive behavior on neuronal responses to vibration in primary somatosensory cortex of the monkey. *J Neurophysiol*, **43**, 870–883.

Iberall T, Bingham G, Arbib MA (1986) Opposition space as a structuring concept for the analysis of skilled hand movements. *Brain Res*, **15**, 158–173.

Ibrahim IK, Berger W, Trippel M et al. (1993) Stretch-induced electromyographic activity and torque in spastic elbow muscles. *Brain*, **116**, 971–989.

Ikai T, Tei K, Yoshida K et al. (1998) Evaluation and treatment of shoulder subluxation in hemiplegia. *Am J Phys Med Rehabil*, **77**, 421–426.

Ikeda ER, Schenkman ML, O'Riley P et al. (1991) Influence of age on dynamics of rising from a chair. *Phys Ther*, **71**, 473–481.

Indredavik B, Slordahl SA, Bakke F et al. (1997) Stroke unit treatment long-term effects. *Stroke*, **28**, 1861–1866.

Ingen Schenau GJ, Bobbert MF, Rozendal RH (1987) The unique action of bi-articular muscles in complex movements. *J Anat*, **155**, 1–5.

Jackson JH (1958) Selected writings. In *John Hughlings Jackson* (ed J Taylor), Basic Books, New York.

Janelle CM, Barba DA, Frehlich SG et al. (1997) Maximizing performance effectiveness through videotape replay and a self-controlled learning environment. *Res Q Exercise Sport*, **68**, 269–279.

Jankowski LW, Sullivan SJ (1990) Aerobic and neuromuscular training: effect on the capacity, efficiency and fatigability of patients with traumatic brain injuries. *Arch Phys Med Rehabil*, **71**, 500–504.

Jeannerod M (1981) Intersegmental coordination during reaching at natural visual objects. In *Attention and Performance* (eds J Long, A Baddeley), vol 9, Erlbaum, Hillsdale, NJ, pp 153–168.

Jeannerod M (1988) *Neural and Behavioural Organization of Goal-directed Movements*. Oxford University Press, Oxford.

Jeannerod M, Michel F, Prablanc C (1984) The control of hand movements in a case of hemianaesthesia following a parietal lesion. *Brain*, **107**, 899–920.

Jenkins WM, Merzenich MM, Ochs MT et al. (1990) Functional reorganization of primary somatosensory cortex in adult owl monkeys after behaviorally controlled tactile stimulation. *J Neurophysiol*, **68**, 82–104.

Jenner JR, Kirker S, Simpson D et al. (1997) Sideways balance after stroke – a serial study of hip abductors and adductors. *Eur J Neurol*, 3, 127.

Johansson BB (2000) Brain plasticity and stroke rehabilitation: the Willis Lecture. *Stroke*, 31, 223–230.

Johansson G, Jarnlo G-B (1991) Balance training in 70-year-old women. *Physiother Theory Pract*, 7, 121–125.

Johansson RS, Westling G (1984) Roles of glabrous skin receptors and sensorimotor memory in automatic control of precision grip when lifting rougher or more slippery objects. *Exp Brain Res*, 56, 550–564.

Johansson RS, Westling G (1988) Programmed and triggered actions to rapid load changes during precision grip. *Exp Brain Res*, 71, 72–86.

Johansson RS, Westling G (1990) Tactile afferent signals in the control of precision grip. In *Attention and Performance* (ed M Jeannerod), Erlbaum, Hillsdale, NJ, pp 677–713.

Johansson RS, Riso R, Hager C et al. (1992a) Somatosensory control of precision grip during unpredictable pulling loads. I. Changes in load force amplitude. *Exp Brain Res*, 89, 181–191.

Johansson RS, Hager C, Riso R et al. (1992b) Somatosensory control of precision grip during unpredictable pulling loads. II. Changes in load force rate. *Exp Brain Res*, 89, 192–203.

Johansson RS, Hager C, Backstrom L (1992c) Somatosensory control of precision grip during unpredictable pulling loads. III. Impairments during digital anesthesia. *Exp Brain Res*, 89, 204–213.

Joyce BM, Kirby RL (1991) Canes, crutches and walkers. *Am Fam Physician*, 43, 535–542.

Judge JO, Underwood M, Gennosa T (1993) Exercise to improve gait velocity in older persons. *Arch Phys Med Rehabil*, 74, 400–406.

Kaminski TR, Bock C, Gentile AM (1995) The coordination between trunk and arm motion during pointing movements. *Exp Brain Res*, 106, 457–466.

Kapanji AI (1992) Clinical evaluation of the thumb's opposition. *J Hand Ther*, 2, 102–106.

Karnath HO, Schenkel P, Fischer B (1991) Trunk orientation as the determining factor of the 'contralateral' deficit in the neglect syndrome and as the physical anchor of the internal representation of body orientation in space. *Brain*, 114, 1997–2014.

Kautz SA, Brown DA (1998) Relationships between timing of muscle excitation and impaired motor performance during cyclical lower extremity movement in post-stroke hemiplegia. *Brain*, 121, 515–526.

Kay TM, Myers AM, Huijbregts MPJ (2001) How far have we come since 1992? A comparative survey of physiotherapists' use of outcome measures. *Physiother Can*, Fall, 268–275.

Keith RA (1980) Activity patterns in a stroke rehabilitation unit. *Soc Sci & Med*, 14A, 575–580.

Keith RA (1995) Conceptual basis of outcome measures. *Am J Phys Med & Rehabil*, 74, 73–80.

Keith RA, Cowell KS (1987) Time use of stroke patients in three rehabilitation hospitals. *Soc Sci & Med*, 24, 529–533.

Kelley DL, Dainis A, Wood GK (1976) Mechanics and muscular dynamics of rising from a seated position. In *Biomechanics V-B* (ed PV Komi), University Park Press, Baltimore, pp 127–134.

Kelly J (2002) Cardiorespiratory fitness and walking ability in acute stroke patients. Master thesis.

Kelso JAS, Buchanan JJ, Murata T (1994) Multifunctionality and switching in the coordination dynamics of reaching and grasping. *Hum Mov Sci*, 13, 63–94.

Kenney WL, Humphrey RH, Bryant CX (eds) (1995) *ACSM's Guidelines for Exercise Testing and Prescription*. Williams & Wilkins, Philadelphia, 5th edn.

Khemlani MM, Carr JH, Crosbie WJ (1998) Muscle synergies and joint linkages in sit-to-stand under two initial foot positions. *Clin Biomech*, 14, 236–246.

Kilbreath SL, Gandevia SC (1994) Limited independent flexion of the thumb and fingers in human subjects. *J Physiol*, 479, 487–497.

King TI (1993) Hand strengthening with a computer for purposeful activity. *Am J Occup Ther*, 47, 635–637.

Kinsella G, Ford B (1980) Acute recovery patterns in stroke patients. Neuropsychological factors. *Med J Aust*, 2, 663–666.

Kirby RL, Price NA, MacLeod DA (1987) The influence of foot position on standing balance. *J Biomech*, 20, 423–427.

Kirker SGB, Simpson S, Jenner JR et al. (2000) Stepping before standing: hip muscle function in stepping and standing balance after stroke. *J Neurol Neurosurg Psychiatry*, 68, 458–464.

Kirsteins AE, Dietz F, Hwang S (1991) Evaluating the safety and potential use of a weight-bearing exercise, Tai-Chi Chuan, for rheumatoid arthritis patients. *Am J Phys Rehabil*, 70, 136–141.

Knutsson E, Richards C (1979) Different types of distributed motor control in gait of hemiparetic patients. *Brain*, 102, 404–430.

Koceja DM, Allway D, Earles DR (1999) Age differences in postural sway during volitional head movement. *Arch Phys Med Rehabil*, 80, 1537–1541.

Kolb B, Gibb R (1991) Environmental enrichment and cortical injury: behavioral and anatomical consequences of frontal cortex lesions. *Cerebral Cortex*, **1**, 189–198.

Komi PV (1973) Relationships between muscle tension, EMG and velocity of contraction under concentric and eccentric work. In *New Developments in Electromyography and Clinical Neurophysiology* (ed JE Desmedt), Karger, Basel, pp 596–606.

Komi PV (1986) The stretch-shortening cycle and human power output. In *Human Muscle Power* (eds NC Jones et al.), Human Kinetics Publishers, Champaign, IL.

Komi PV, Buskirk ER (1972) Effects of eccentric and concentric muscle conditioning on tension and electrical activity of human muscle. *Ergonomics*, **15**, 417–434.

Kopp B, Kunkel A, Flor H et al. (1997) The Arm Motor Ability Test: reliability, validity, and sensitivity to change of an instrument for assessing disabilities in activities of daily living. *Arch Phys Med Rehabil*, **78**, 615–620.

Kopp B, Kunkel A, Muhlnickel W et al. (1999) Plasticity in the motor system related to therapy-induced improvement of movement after stroke. *Clin Neurosci*, **4**, 807–810.

Kornecki S, Kebel A, Siemienski S (2001) Muscular co-operation during joint stabilisation, as reflected by EMG. *Eur J Appl Physiol*, **84**, 453–461.

Kotake T, Dohi N, Kajiwara T et al. (1993) An analysis of sit-to-stand movement. *Arch Phys Med Rehabil*, **74**, 1095–1099.

Kralj A, Jaeger RJ, Munih M (1990) Analysis of standing up and sitting down in humans: definitions and normative data presentation. *J Biomech*, **23**, 1123–1138.

Krebs DE, Wong D, Jevsevar D (1992) Trunk kinematics during locomotor activities. *Phys Ther*, **72**, 505–514.

Krebs DE, Jette AM, Assmann SF (1998) Moderate exercise improves gait stability in disabled elders. *Arch Phys Med Rehabil*, **79**, 1489–1495.

Krichevets AN, Sirokina EB, Yevsevicheva IV et al. (1995) Computer games as a means of movement rehabilitation. *Disabil Rehabil*, **17**, 100–105.

Kuan T, Tsou J, Fong-Chin S (1999) Hemiplegic gait of stroke patients: the effect of using a cane. *Arch Phys Med Rehabil*, **80**, 777–784.

Kukulka CG, Beckman SM, Holte JB et al. (1986) Effects of intermittent tendon pressure on alpha motor neurone excitability. *Phys Ther*, **66**, 1091–1094.

Kumar R, Matter EJ, Mehta AJ et al. (1990) Shoulder pain in hemiplegia. *Am J Phys Med Rehabil*, **69**, 205–208.

Kunkel A, Kopp B, Muller G et al. (1999) Constraint-induced movement therapy for motor recovery in chronic stroke patients. *Arch Phys Med Rehabil*, **80**, 624–628.

Kuo AD, Zajac FE (1993) A biomechanical analysis of muscle strength as a limiting factor in standing posture. *J Biomech*, **26**(suppl 1), 137–150.

Kuster M, Sakurai S, Wood GA (1995) Kinematic and kinetic comparison of downhill and level walking. *Clinical Biomech*, **10**, 79–84.

Kuypers HGJM (1973) The anatomical organization of the descending pathways and their contributions to motor control especially in primates. In *New Developments in Electromyography and Clinical Neurophysiology 3* (ed JE Desmedt), Karger, Basel, pp 38–68.

Kuzoffsky A (1990) *Sensory Function and Recovery after Stroke*. Karolinska Institute, Stockholm.

Kwakkel G, Wagenaar RC, Koelman TW et al. (1997) Effects of intensity of rehabilitation after stroke: a research synthesis. *Stroke*, **28**, 1550–1556.

Kwakkel G, Wagenaar RC, Twisk JWR et al. (1999) Intensity of arm training after primary middle-cerebral-artery stroke: a randomised trial. *Lancet*, **354**, 191–196.

Ladavas E, Del Pesce M, Provinciali L (1989) Unilateral attention deficits and hemispheric asymmetries in the control of visual attention. *Neuropsychologia*, **27**, 353–366.

Ladavas E, Petronio A, Umilta C et al. (1990) The deployment of visual attention in the intact field of hemineglect patients. *Cortex*, **26**, 307–317.

Ladavas E, Menghini G, Umilta C (1994) On the rehabilitation of hemispatial neglect. In *Cognitive Neuropsychology and Cognitive Rehabilitation* (eds MJ Riddoch, GW Humphreys), Erlbaum, London, pp 151–172.

Lance JM (1980) Symposium synopsis. In *Spasticity: Disorder of Motor Control* (eds RG Feldman, RR Young, WP Koella), Year Book, Chicago, pp 485–494.

Landau WM (1980) Spasticity: What is it? What is it not? In *Spasticity: Disorder Motor Control* (eds RG Feldman, RR Young, WP Koella), Year Book, Chicago, pp 17–24.

Landau WM (1988) Parables of palsy, pills, and PT pedagogy: a spastic dialectic. *Neurology*, **38**, 1496–1499.

Landin S, Hagenfeldt L, Saltin B et al. (1977) Muscle metabolism during exercise in hemiparetic patients. *Clin Sci Mol Med*, **53**, 257–269.

Latash LP, Latash ML (1994) A new book by N.A. Bernstein: 'On Dexterity and its Development'. *J Mot Behav*, **26**, 56–62.

Laufer Y, Dickstein R, Resnik S et al. (2000) Weight-bearing shifts of hemiparetic and healthy adults upon stepping on stairs of various heights. *Clin Rehabil*, **14**, 125–129.

Ledin T, Kronhed AC, Moller C et al. (1991) Effects of balance training in elderly evaluated by clinical tests and dynamic posturography. *J Vestibular Res*, **1**, 129–138.

Lee DN, Aronson E (1974) Visual proprioceptive control of standing in human infants. *Percept Psychoanalysis*, **15**, 529–532.

Lee KC, Soderberg GL (1981) Relationship between perception of joint position sense and limb synergies in patients with hemiplegia. *Phys Ther*, **10**, 1433–1437.

Lee RG, van Donkelaar P (1995) Mechanisms underlying functional recovery following stroke. *Can J Neurol Sci*, **22**, 257–263.

Lee RG, Tonolli I, Viallet F et al. (1995) Preparatory postural adjustments in Parkinsonian patients with postural instability. *Can J Neurol Sci*, **22**, 126–135.

Lee WA (1980) Anticipatory control of postural and task muscles during rapid arm flexion. *J Motor Behav*, **12**, 185–196.

Lee WA, Deming L, Sahgal V (1988) Quantitative and clinical measures of static standing balance in hemiparetic and normal subjects. *Phys Ther*, **68**, 970–976.

Lehman JF, Condon SM, Price R et al. (1987) Gait abnormalities in hemiplegia: their correction by ankle–foot orthoses. *Arch Phys Med Rehabil*, **68**, 763–771.

Lemon RN, Bennett KM, Werner W (1991) The cortico-motor substrate for skilled movements of the primate hand. In *Tutorials in Motor Neuroscience* (eds J Requin, GE Stelmark), Kluwer, Dordrecht, pp 477–495.

Leont'ev AN, Zaporozhets AV (1960) *Rehabilitation of Hand Function*. Pergamon Press, London.

Levin MF (1996) Interjoint coordination during pointing movements is disrupted in spastic hemiparesis. *Brain*, **119**, 281–293.

Lexell J (2000) Muscle structure and function in chronic neurological disorders: the potential of exercise to improve activities of daily living. *Exercise Sports Sci Rev*, **28**, 80–84.

Li ZM, Latash ML, Newell KM et al. (1998a) Motor redundancy during maximal voluntary contraction in four-finger tasks. *Exp Brain Res*, **122**, 71–78.

Li ZM, Latash ML, Zatsiorsky VM (1998b) Force sharing among fingers as a model of the redundancy problem. *Exp Brain Res*, **119**, 276–286.

Lieber RL (1988) Comparison between animal and human studies of skeletal muscle adaptation to chronic stimulation. *Clin Orthop Relat Res*, **233**, 19–24.

Lieber RL (1992) *Skeletal Muscle and Function*. Williams & Wilkins, Baltimore, MD.

Liepert J, Tegenthoff M, Malin JP (1995) Changes in cortical motor area size during immobilization. *Electroencephalogr Clin Neurophysiol*, **97**, 382–386.

Liepert J, Miltner WHR, Bauder H et al. (1998) Motor cortex plasticity during constraint-induced movement therapy in stroke patients. *Neurosci Lett*, **250**, 5–8.

Liepert J, Bauder H, Miltner W et al. (2000) Treatment-induced cortical reorganization after stroke in humans. *Stroke*, **31**, 1210–1216.

Liepert J, Uhde I, Graf S et al. (2001) Motor cortex plasticity during forced-use therapy in stroke patients: a preliminary study. *J Neurol*, **248**, 315–321.

Lincoln NB, Gamlen R, Thomason H (1989) Behavioural mapping of patients in a stroke unit. *Int Dis Stud*, **11**, 149–154.

Lincoln NB, Jackson JM, Adams SA (1998) Reliability and revision of the Nottingham Sensory Assessment for stroke patients. *Physiotherapy*, **84**, 358–365.

Lincoln NB, Parry RH, Vass CD (1999) Randomized, controlled trial to evaluate increased intensity of physiotherapy treatment of arm function after stroke. *Stroke*, **30**, 573–579.

Lindboe CF, Platou CS (1984) Effect of immobilization of short duration on the muscle fibre size. *Clin Physiol*, **4**, 183–188.

Lindmark B, Hamrin F (1995) Relation between gait speed, knee muscle torque and motor scores in post-stroke patients. *Scand J Caring Sci*, **9**, 195–202.

Lipshits MI, Mauritz K, Popov KE (1981) Quantitative analysis of anticipatory components of a complex voluntary movement. *Hum Physiol*, **7**, 165–173.

Loewen SC, Anderson BA (1990) Predictors of stroke outcome using objective measurement scales. *Stroke*, **21**, 78–81.

Lord S, Castell S (1994) Physical activity program for older persons. Effect on balance strength, neuromuscular control and reaction time. *Arch Phys Med Rehabil*, **78**, 208–212.

Lord SR, Clark RD, Webster IW (1991) Postural stability and associated physiological factors in a population of aged persons. *J Gerontol*, **46**, M69–M76.

Lundvik GA, Gard G, Salford E et al. (1999) Interaction between patient and physiotherapist: a qualitative study reflecting the physiotherapist's perspective. *Physiother Res Int*, **4**, 89–109.

Lyngberg K, Danneskiold-Samsoe B, Halskov O (1988) The effect of physical training on patients with rheumatoid arthritis: changes in disease activity, muscle strength and aerobic capacity. *Clin Exp Rheumatol*, **6**, 253–260.

McAuley E, Rudolph D (1995) Physical activity, aging, and psychological well-being. *J Aging Phys Activity*, **3**, 67–96.

McComas AJ (1994) Human neuromuscular adaptations that accompany changes in activity. *Med Sci Sports Exercise*, **26**, 1498–1509.

McComas AJ, Miller RG, Gandevia SG (1995) Fatigue brought on malfunction of the central and peripheral nervous systems. In *Fatigue* (eds SG Gandevia et al.), Plenum Press, New York.

McCrum R (1998) *My Year Off: Rediscovering Life after Stroke*. Picador, London.

McGavin CR, Gupta SP, McHardy GJ (1976) Twelve-minute walking test for assessing disability in chronic bronchitis. *BMJ*, **1**, 822–823.

Mackenzie-Knapp M (1999) Electrical stimulation in early stroke rehabilitation of the upper limb within attention. *Aust J Physiother*, **45**, 223–227.

MacKinnon CD, Winter DA (1993) Control of whole body balance in the frontal plane during human walking. *J Biomech*, **26**, 633–644.

McLeod PC, Kettelkamp DB, Srinivasan SR et al. (1975) Measurements of repetitive activities of the knee. *J Biomech*, **8**, 369–373.

McNevin NH, Wulf G, Carlson C (2000) Effects of attentional focus, self-control, and dyad training on motor learning: implications for physical therapy. *Phys Ther*, **80**, 373–385.

Mackey F, Ada L, Heard R et al. (1996) Stroke rehabilitation: are highly structured units more conducive to physical activity than less structured units? *Arch Phys Med Rehabil*, **77**, 1066–1070.

Macko RF, De Souza CA, Tretter LD et al. (1997) Treadmill aerobic exercise training reduces the energy and cardiovascular demands of hemiparetic gait in chronic stroke patients. *Stroke*, **28**, 326–330.

Magill RA (1998) *Motor Learning Concepts and Applications*. McGraw-Hill, New York, 5th edn.

Magill RA (2001) *Motor Learning Concepts and Applications*. McGraw-Hill, New York, 6th edn.

Mahoney FI, Barthel DW (1965) Functional evaluation: the Barthel Index. *Maryland Med J*, **14**, 61–65.

Maki BE, McIlroy WE (1997) The role of limb movements in maintaining upright stance: the "change-in-support" strategy. *Phys Ther*, **77**, 488–507.

Maki BE, McIlroy WE (1998) Control of compensatory stepping reactions: age-related impairment and the potential for remedial intervention. *Physiother Theory Pract*, **15**, 69–90.

Malezic M, Kljajic M, Acimovic-Jamezic et al. (1987) Therapeutic effects of multi-site electric stimulation of gait in motor-disabled patients. *Arch Phys Med Rehabil*, **68**, 553–560.

Malouin F (1995) Observational gait analysis. In *Gait Analysis. Theory and Applications* (eds RL Craik, CA Oatis), St Louis, Mosby, pp 112–124.

Malouin F, Potvin M, Prevost J et al. (1992) Use of an intensive task-oriented gait training program in a series of patients with acute cerebrovascular accidents. *Phys Ther*, **72**, 781–793.

Malouin F, Picard L, Bonneau C et al. (1994) Evaluating motor recovery early after stroke: comparison of the Fugl-Meyer Assessment and the Motor Assessment Scale. *Arch Phys Med Rehabil*, **75**, 1206–1212.

Malouin F, Bonneau C, Pichard L et al. (1997) Non-reflex mediated changes in plantarflexor muscles early after stroke. *Scand J Rehabil Med*, **29**, 147–153.

Mark VW, Kooistra CA, Heilmann KM (1988) Hemispatial neglect affected by non-neglected stimuli. *Neurology*, **38**, 1207–1211.

Martiniuk RB, Leavitt JL, MacKenzie CL et al. (1990) Functional relationships between grasp and transport components in a prehension task. *Human Mov Sci*, **9**, 149–176.

Massion J (1992) Movement, posture, and equilibrium: interaction and coordination. *Prog Neurobiol*, **38**, 35–56.

Mathiowetz V (1990) Effects of three trials on grip and pinch strength measurements. *J Hand Ther*, Oct–Dec, 195–198.

Mathiowetz V, Wade MG (1995) Task constraints and functional motor performance of individuals with and without multiple sclerosis. *Ecolog Psych*, **7**, 99–123.

Mathiowetz V, Weber K, Kashman N et al. (1985) Adult norms for the nine-hole peg test of finger dexterity. *Occup Ther J Res*, **5**, 24–37.

Mauritz K-H (1990) General rehabilitation. *Curr Opin Neurol Neurosurg*, **3**, 714–718.

Mazzeo RS, Cavanagh P, Evans WJ et al. (1998) ACSM Position Stand: exercise and physical activity for older adults. *Med Sci Sports Exercise*, **30**, 992–1008.

Means KM, Rodell DE, O'Sullivan PS (1996) Use of an obstacle course to assess balance and mobility in the elderly. *Am J Phys Med Rehabil*, **75**, 88–95.

Mecagni C, Smith JP, Roberts KE et al. (2000) Balance and ankle range of motion in community-dwelling women aged 64–87 years: a correlational study. *Phys Ther*, **80**, 1004–1011.

Medical Research Council (1976) *Aid to the Examination of the Peripheral Nervous System*. HMSO, London.

Mercer VS, Sahrmann SA (1999) Postural synergies associated with a stepping task. *Phys Ther*, **79**, 1142–1152.

Mercier C, Bourbonnais D, Bilodeau S et al. (1999) Description of a new motor re-education programme for the paretic lower limb aimed at improving the mobility of stroke patients. *Clin Rehabil*, **13**, 199–206.

Mikesky AE, Topp R, Wigglesworth JK et al. (1994) Efficacy of home-based training program for older adults using elastic tubing. *Eur J Appl Physiol*, **69**, 316–320.

Milczarek JJ, Lee Kirby R, Harrison ER et al. (1993) Standard and four-footed canes: their effect on the standing balance of patients with hemiparesis. *Arch Phys Med Rehabil*, **74**, 281–285.

Miller GJT, Light KE (1997) Strength training in spastic hemiparesis: should it be avoided? *NeuroRehabil*, **9**, 17–28.

Millington PJ, Myklebust BM, Shambes GM (1992) Biomechanical analysis of the sit-to-stand motion in elderly persons. *Arch Phys Med Rehabil*, **73**, 609–617.

Miltner W, Bauder H, Sommer M et al. (1999) Effects of constraint-induced movement therapy on patients with chronic motor deficits after stroke: a replication. *Stroke*, **30**, 586–592.

Mizrahi J, Solzi P, Ring H et al. (1989) Postural stability in stroke patients: vectorial expression of asymmetry, sway activity and relative sequence of reactive forces. *Med & Biol Eng & Comput*, **27**, 181–190.

Mngoma NF, Culham EG, Bagg SD (1990) Resistance to passive shoulder external rotation in persons with hemiplegia: evaluation of an assessment system. *Arch Phys Med Rehabil*, **80**, 531–535.

Moritani T (1993) Neuromuscular adaptations during the acquisition of muscle strength, power and motor tasks. *J Biomech*, **26**, 95–107.

Morris DM, Crago JE, DeLuca SC et al. (1997) Constraint-induced movement therapy for motor recovery after stroke. *NeuroRehabil*, **9**, 29–43.

Morrissey MC, Harman ES, Johnson MJ (1995) Resistance training modes: specificity and effectiveness. *Med Sci Sports Exercise*, **27**, 648–660.

Moseley A (1997) The effect of casting combined with stretching on passive ankle dorsiflexion in adults with traumatic head injuries. *Phys Ther*, **77**, 240–247.

Moseley A, Adams R (1991) Measurement of passive ankle dorsiflexion: procedure and reliability. *Aust J Physiother*, **37**, 175–181.

Moseley A, Dean C (2000) Treadmill training with body weight support after stroke. *Aust Synapse*, July, 5–6.

Mountcastle VB, Lynch JC, Georgopoulos A et al. (1975) Posterior parietal association cortex of the monkey: command functions for operations with extrapersonal space. *J Neurophysiol*, **38**, 871–908.

Mudie MH, Matyas TA (1996) Upper extremity retraining following stroke: effects of practice. *J Neurol Rehabil*, **10**, 167–184.

Mudie MH, Matyas TA (2000) Can simultaneous bilateral movement involve the undamaged hemisphere in reconstruction of neural networks damaged by stroke? *Disabil Rehabil*, **22**, 23–37.

Munton JS, Ellis MI, Chamberlain MA et al. (1981) An investigation into the problems of easy chairs used by the arthritic and the elderly. *Rheumatol Rehabil*, **20**, 164–173.

Murphy AJ, Spinks WL (2000) The importance of movement specificity in isokinetic assessment. *J Human Mov Stud*, **38**, 167–183.

Murray MP (1967) Gait as a total pattern of movement. *Am J Phys Med*, **46**, 290–333.

Murray MP, Spurr GB, Sepic SB et al. (1985) Treadmill vs floor walking: kinematics, electromyogram, and heart rate. *J Appl Physiol*, **59**, 87–91.

Myers AM, Fletcher PC, Myers AH et al. (1998) Discriminative and evaluative properties of the Activities-specific Balance Confidence (ABC) Scale. *J Gerontol Med Sci*, **53A**, M287–294.

Nakamura R, Hosokawa T, Tsuji I (1985) Relationship of muscle strength for knee extension to walking capacity in patients with spastic hemiparesis. *Tohoku J Exp Med*, **145**, 335–340.

Nakayama H, Jorgensen HS, Raaschou HO et al. (1994) Recovery of upper extremity function in stroke patients: the Copenhagen Stroke Study. *Arch Phys Med Rehabil*, **75**, 394–398.

Napier JR (1956) The prehensile movement of the human hand. *J Bone Jt Surg*, **38**, 902–913.

Nardone A, Schieppati M (1988) Postural adjustments associated with voluntary contraction of leg muscles in standing man. *Exp Brain Res*, **69**, 469–480.

Nashner LM (1982) Adaptation of human movement to altered environments. *Trends Neurosci*, **5**, 358–361.

Nashner LM (1983) Analysis of movement control in man using the movable platform. In *Motor Control Mechanisms in Health and Disease* (ed JE Desmedt), Raven Press, New York, pp 607–619.

Nashner NL, McCollum G (1985) The organization of human postural movements: a formal basis and experimental synthesis. *Behav Brain Sci*, **8**, 135–172.

Neilson JF, Sinkjaer TA (1996) A comparison of clinical and laboratory measures of spasticity. *Multiple Sclerosis*, **1**, 296–301.

Nelles G, Spiekmann G, Markus J et al. (1999) Reorganization of sensory and motor systems in hemiplegia stroke patients: a positron emission tomography study. *Stroke*, **30**, 1510–1516.

Nelles G, Jentzen W, Jueptner M et al. (2001) Arm training induced plasticity in stroke studied with serial positron emission tomography. *NeuroImage*, **13**, 1146–1154.

Newham DJ, Hsiao S-F (2001) Knee muscle isometric strength, voluntary activation and antagonist co-contraction in the first six months after stroke. *Disabil Rehabil*, **23**, 379–386.

Ng S, Shepherd RB (2000) Weakness in patients with stroke: implications for strength training in neurorehabilitation. *Phys Ther Rev*, **5**, 227–238.

Niam S, Cheung W, Sullivan PE et al. (1999) Balance and physical impairments after stroke. *Arch Phys Med Rehabil*, **80**, 1227–1233.

Nudo RJ, Friel KM (1999) Cortical plasticity after stroke: implications for rehabilitation. *Rev Neurol*, **9**, 713–717.

Nudo RJ, Milliken GW (1996) Reorganization of movement representation in primary motor cortex following focal ischemia infarcts in adult squirrel monkeys. *J Neurophysiol*, **75**, 2144–2149.

Nudo RJ, Wise BM, SiFuentes F et al. (1996) Neural substrates for the effects of rehabilitation on motor recovery after ischemic infarct. *Science*, **272**, 1791–1794.

Nudo RJ, Plautz EJ, Frost SB (2001) Role of adaptive plasticity in recovery of function after damage to motor cortex. *Muscle Nerve*, **8**, 1000–1019.

Nugent J, Schurr K, Adams R (1994) A dose response relationship between amount of weight-bearing exercise and walking outcome following cerebrovascular accident. *Arch Phys Med Rehabil*, **75**, 399–402.

Odeen I (1981) Reduction of muscular hypertonus by long-term muscle stretch. *Scand J Rehabil Med*, **13**, 93–99.

O'Dwyer NJ, Ada L, Neilson PD (1996) Spasticity and muscle contracture following stroke. *Brain*, **119**, 1737–1749.

Ohlsson A-L, Johansson BB (1995) Environment influences functional outcome of cerebral infarction in rats. *Stroke*, **26**, 644–649.

Olney SJ, Monga TN, Costigan PA (1986) Mechanical energy of walking of stroke patients. *Arch Phys Med Rehabil*, **67**, 92–98.

Olney SJ, Richards C (1996) Hemiparetic gait following stroke. Part 1: characteristics. *Gait Posture*, **4**, 136–148.

Otis JC, Root L, Kroll MA (1985) Measurement of plantarflexor spasticity during treatment with tone-reducing casts. *J Pediatr Orthop*, **5**, 682–686.

Oxendine A (1984) *Psychology of Motor Learning*. Prentice-Hall, Englewood Cliffs, NJ, 2nd edn.

Page SJ, Levine P, Sisto S et al. (2001) A randomized efficacy and feasibility study of imagery in acute stroke. *Clin Rehabil*, **15**, 233–240.

Pai Y-C, Patton J (1997) Center of mass velocity position predictions for balance control. *J Biomech*, **30**, 347–354.

Pai Y, Rogers MW (1990) Control of body mass transfer as a function of speed of ascent in sit-to-stand. *Med Sci Sports Exercise*, **22**, 378–384.

Pai Y, Rogers MW (1991) Segmental contributions to total body momentum in sit-to-stand. *Med Sci Sports Exercise*, **23**, 225–230.

Pai Y-C, Rogers MW, Hedman LD et al. (1994) Alterations in weight-transfer capabilities in adults with hemiparesis. *Phys Ther*, **74**, 647–657.

Palmitier RA, An KN, Scott SG et al. (1991) Kinetic chain exercise in knee rehabilitation. *Sports Med*, **11**, 402–413.

Pandyan AD, Johnson GR, Price CIM et al. (1999) A review of the properties and limitations of the Ashworth and modified Ashworth Scales as measures of spasticity. *Clin Rehabil*, **13**, 373–383.

Paolucci S, Grasso MG, Antonucci G et al. (2001) Mobility status after inpatient stroke rehabilitation: 1 year follow-up and prognostic factors. *Arch Phys Med Rehabil*, **82**, 2–8.

Parry RH, Lincoln NB, Vass CD (1999a) Effect of severity of arm impairment on response to additional physiotherapy early after stroke. *Clin Rehabil*, **13**, 187–198.

Parry RH, Lincoln NB, Appleyard MA (1999b) Physiotherapy for the arm and hand after stroke. *Physiotherapy*, **85**, 417–425.

Pascual-Leone A, Torres F (1993) Plasticity of the sensorimotor cortex representation of the reading finger in Braille readers. *Brain*, **116**, 39–52.

Pascual-Leone A, Wassermann EM, Sadato N et al. (1995) The role of reading activity on the modulation of motor cortical outputs to the reading hand in Braille readers. *Ann Neurol*, **38**, 910–915.

Pashley J (1989) Grip strengthening with adapted computer switches. *Am J Occup Ther*, **43**, 121–123.

Patla AE (1993) Age-related changes in visually guided locomotion over different terrains: major issues. In *Sensorimotor Impairments in the Elderly* (eds GE Stelmack, V Homberg), Kluwer, Dordrecht, pp 231–252.

Patla AE (1995) A framework for understanding mobility problems in the elderly. In *Gait Analysis: Theory and Application* (eds RL Craik, CA Oatis), Mosby, St Louis, pp 436–449.

Patla AE (1997) Understanding the roles of vision in the control of human locomotion. *Gait Posture*, **5**, 54–69.

Patla A, Prentice S, Robinson C et al. (1991) Visual control of locomotor strategies for changing direction and for going over obstacles. *J Exp Psychol Hum Percept Perform*, **17**, 603–634.

Patterson RM, Stegink Jansen CW, Hogan HA et al. (2001) Material properties of Thera-Band tubing. *Phys Ther*, **81**, 1437–1445.

Peat M (1986) Functional anatomy of the shoulder complex. *Phys Ther*, **66**, 1855–1865.

Peat M, Dubo HIC, Winter DA et al. (1976) Electromyographic temporal analysis of gait: hemiplegic locomotion. *Arch Phys Med Rehabil*, **57**, 421–425.

Pedersen PM, Wandel A, Jorgenson HS et al. (1996) Ipsilateral pushing in stroke: incidence, relation to neuropsychological symptoms, and impact on rehabilitation. The Copenhagen Stroke Study. *Arch Phys Med Rehabil*, **77**, 25–28.

Pennisi G, Rapisarda G, Bella R et al. (1999) Absence of response to early transcranial magnetic stimulation in ischaemic stroke patients: prognostic value for hand motor recovery. *Stroke*, **30**, 2666–2670.

Perry J (1992) *Gait Analysis. Normal and Pathological Function.* Slack, Thorofare, NJ.

Pierrot-Deseilligny E (1990) Electrophysiological assessment of the spinal mechanisms underlying spasticity. *Electroencephalogr Clin Neurophysiol Suppl*, **41**, 264–273.

Pinniger GJ, Steele JR, Thorstensson A, Cresswell AG (2000) Tension regulation during lengthening and shortening actions of the human soleus muscle. *Eur J Appl Physiol*, **81**, 375–383.

Podsialo D, Richardson S (1991) The timed 'up and go': a test of basic functional mobility for frail elderly persons. *JAGS*, **39**, 142–148.

Pohl M, Mehr-Olz J, Ritschel C et al. (2002) Speed-dependent treadmill training in ambulatory hemiparetic patients. A randomized controlled trial. *Stroke*, **33**, 553–558.

Pollock ML, Foster C, Knapp D et al. (1987) Effect of age and training on aerobic capacity and body composition of master athletes. *J Appl Physiol*, **62**, 725–731.

Pomeroy VM, Dean D, Sykes L et al. (2000) The unreliability of clinical measures of muscle tone: implications for stroke therapy. *Age Ageing*, **29**, 229–233.

Poole JL, Whitney SL (1988) Motor Assessment Scale for stroke patients: concurrent validity and interrater reliability. *Arch Phys Med Rehabil*, **69**, 195–197.

Posner MI, Walker JA, Friedrich FA et al. (1987) How do the parietal lobes direct covert attention? *Neuropsychology*, **25**, 135–145.

Potempa K, Lopez M, Braun LT et al. (1995) Physiological outcomes of aerobic exercise training in hemiparetic stroke patients. *Stroke*, **26**, 101–105.

Potempa K, Braun LT, Tinknell T et al. (1996) Benefits of aerobic exercise after stroke. *Sports Med*, **21**, 337–346.

Powell J, Pandyan AD, Granat M et al. (1999) Electrical stimulation of wrist extensors in poststroke hemiplegia. *Stroke*, **30**, 1384–1389.

Powell LE, Myers AM (1993) The Activities-specific Balance Confidence (ABC) Scale. *J Gerontol Med Sci*, **50A**, M28–34.

Price CIM, Pandyan AD (2001) Electrical stimulation for preventing and treating post-stroke shoulder pain: a systematic Cochrane review. *Clin Rehabil*, **15**, 5–19.

Pritzel M, Huston JP (1991) Unilateral ablation of telencephalon induces appearance of contralateral cortical and subcortical projection to thalamic nuclei. *Behav Brain Res*, **3**, 43–54.

Prudham D, Evans JG (1981) Factors associated with falls in the elderly: a community study. *Age Ageing*, **10**, 141–146.

Putnam CA (1993) Sequential motions of body segments in striking and throwing skills: descriptions and explanations. *J Biomech*, **26**(suppl 1), 125–135.

Rab GT (1994) Muscle. In *Human Walking* (eds J Rose, JG Gamble), Williams & Wilkins, Baltimore, MD, 2nd edn, pp 101–122.

Rasch PT, Morehouse LE (1957) Effect of static and dynamic exercise on muscular strength and hypertrophy. *Appl Physiol*, **11**, 29–34.

Redfern MS, Di Pasquale J (1997) Biomechanics of descending ramps. *Gait Posture*, **6**, 119–125.

Reiter F, Danni M, Lagalla G et al. (1998) Low-dose botulinum toxin with ankle taping for the treatment of spastic equinovarus foot after stroke. *Arch Phys Med Rehabil*, **79**, 532–535.

Richards CL, Malouin F, Wood-Dauphinee S (1993) Task-specific physical therapy for optimization of gait recovery in acute stroke patients. *Arch Phys Med Rehabil*, **74**, 612–620.

Richards CL, Malouin F, Dean C (1999) Gait in stroke: assessment and rehabilitation. *Clin Geriatr Med*, **15**, 833–855.

Riddoch MJ, Humphrey GW (1994) Towards an understanding of neglect. In *Cognitive Neuropsychology and Cognitive Rehabilitation* (eds MJ Riddoch, GW Humphreys), Erlbaum, London, pp 125–149.

Roach KE, Miles TP (1991) Normal hip and knee active range of motion: the relationship to age. *Phys Ther*, **71**, 656–665.

Rodosky MV, Andriacchi TP, Andersson GBJ (1989) The influence of chair height on lower limb mechanics during rising. *J Orthop Res*, **7**, 266–271.

Roebroeck ME, Doorenbosch CAM, Harlaar J et al. (1994) Biomechanics and muscular activity during sit-to-stand transfer. *Clin Biomech*, 9, 235–244.

Rogers MW, Pai Y-C (1990) Dynamic transitions in stance phase accompanying leg flexion movements in man. *Exp Brain Res*, 81, 398–402.

Rogers MW, Pai Y-C (1993) Patterns of muscle activation accompanying transition in stance during rapid leg flexion. *J Electromyogr Kinesiol*, 3, 149–156.

Rogers MW, Hedman LD, Pai Y-C (1993) Kinetic analysis of dynamic transitions in stance support accompanying voluntary leg flexion movements in hemiparetic subjects. *Arch Phys Med Rehabil*, 74, 19–25.

Rogers RL, Meyer JS, Mortel KF (1990) After reaching retirement age physical activity sustains cerebral perfusion and cognition. *JAGS*, 38, 123–128.

Roland PE (1973) Lack of appreciation of compressibility, adynamaesthesia and akinaesthesia. *J Neurol Sci*, 20, 51–56.

Rooney KJ, Herbert RD, Balnave RJ (1994) Fatigue contributes to the strength training stimulus. *Med Sci Sports Exercise*, 26, 1160–1164.

Rosenbaum DA, Vaughan J, Barnes HJ et al. (1992) Time course of movement planning: selection of handgrips for object manipulation. *J Exp Psychol: Learning, Memory, Cognition*, 18, 1058–1073.

Rosenbaum DA, Meulenbroek RGJ, Vaughan J et al. (1999) Coordination of reaching and grasping by capitalizing on obstacle avoidance and other constraints. *Exp Brain Res*, 128, 92–100.

Rosenfalck A, Andreassen S (1980) Impaired regulation of force and firing pattern of single motor units in patients with spasticity. *J Neurol Neurosurg Psychiatry*, 43, 907–916.

Rothstein JM (1997) It is our choice! *Phys Ther*, 77, 800–801.

Rutherford OM (1988) Muscular coordination and strength training: implications for injury rehabilitation. *Sports Med*, 5, 196–202.

Rutherford OM, Jones DA (1986) The role of learning and coordination in strength training. *Eur J Appl Physiol*, 55, 100–105.

Sackett D, Strauss S, Richardson W et al. (2000) *Evidence-based Medicine: How to Teach and Practice EBM*, 2nd edn. Churchill Livingstone, Edinburgh.

Sackley CM, Lincoln NB (1997) Single blind randomized controlled trial of visual feedback after stroke: effects on stance symmetry and function. *Disabil Rehabil*, 19, 536–546.

Sahrmann SA, Norton BJ (1977) The relationship of voluntary movement to spasticity in the upper motor neuron syndrome. *Ann Neurol*, 2, 460–465.

Said CM, Goldie PA, Patla AE et al. (1999) Obstacle crossing in subjects with stroke. *Arch Phys Med Rehabil*, 80, 1054–1059.

Sale DG (1987) Influence of exercise and training on motor unit activation. In *Exercise and Sports Science Reviews 15* (ed KB Pandolf), Macmillan, New York, pp 95–151.

Saling M, Stelmach GE, Mescheriakov S et al. (1996) Prehension with trunk-assisted reaching. *Behav Brain Res*, 80, 153–160.

Sandin KJ, Smith BS (1990) The measure of balance in sitting in stroke rehabilitation prognosis. *Stroke*, 21, 82–86.

Saravanamuthu R, Shepherd RB (1994) The effect of foot placement on the movement pattern of sit-to-stand in the elderly. In *Second World Congress of Biomechanics Abstracts* (eds L Blankevoort, JGM Kooloos), Stichting World Biomechanics, Nijmegen, p 175.

Saunders JB, Inman VT, Eberhart HD (1953) The major determinants in normal and pathological gait. *J Bone Jt Surg*, 35A, 543–558.

Sauvage L, Myklebust B, Crow-Pan J et al. (1992) A clinical trial of strengthening and aerobic exercises to improve gait and balance in elderly male home residents. *Am J Phys Med Rehabil*, 71, 333–342.

Scarborough DM, Krebs DE, Harris BA (1999) Quadriceps muscle strength and dynamic stability in elderly persons. *Gait Posture*, 10, 10–20.

Schenkman M, Berger RA, O'Riley P et al. (1990) Whole-body movements during rising to standing from sitting. *Phys Ther*, 70, 638–651.

Schiene K, Brandt C, Zilles K et al. (1996) Neuronal hyperexcitability and reduction of GABAA receptor expression in the surround of cerebral photothrombosis. *J Cereb Blood Flow Metab*, 16, 906–914.

Schultz AB, Alexander NB, Ashton-Miller JA (1992) Biomechanical analyses of rising from a chair. *J Biomech*, 25, 1383–1391.

Seelen HAM, van Wiggen KL, Halfens JHG et al. (1995) Lower limb postural responses during sit-to-stand transfer in stroke patients during neurorehabilitation. In *Book of Abstracts of the XVth Congress of the International Society of Biomechanics* (eds K Hakkinen, KL Keskinen, PV Komi et al.), University of Jyvaskyla, Jyvaskyla, Finland, pp 826–827.

Seidler RD, Stelmach GE (2000) Trunk-assisted prehension: specification of body segments with imposed temporal constraints. *J Mot Behav*, 32, 379–389.

Sharp SA, Brouwer BJ (1997) Isokinetic strength training of the hemiparetic knee: effects on function and spasticity. *Arch Phys Med Rehabil*, 78, 1231–1236.

Shea CH, Wulf G, Whitacre C (1999) Enhancing training efficiency and effectiveness through the use of dyad training. *J Motor Behav*, **31**, 119–125.

Shelbourne KD, Nitz P (1992) Accelerated rehabilitation after anterior cruciate ligament reconstruction. *J Orthop Sports Phys Ther*, **15**, 256–264.

Shepherd RB (2001) Exercise and training to optimize functional motor performance in stroke: driving neural reorganization? *Neural Plasticity*, **8**, 121–129.

Shepherd RB, Gentile AM (1994) Sit-to-stand: functional relationships between upper body and lower limb segments. *Hum Mov Sci*, **13**, 817–840.

Shepherd RB, Koh HP (1996) Some biomechanical consequences of varying foot placement in sit-to-stand in young women. *Scand J Rehabil Med*, **28**, 79–88.

Sherrington C, Lord SR (1997) Home exercise to improve strength and walking velocity after hip fracture: a randomized controlled trial. *Arch Phys Med Rehabil*, **78**, 208–212.

Sherrington C, Moseley A, Herbert R et al. (2001) Guest editorial. *Physiother Theory Prac*, **17**, 125–126.

Shiavi R (1985) Electromyographic patterns in adult locomotion: A comprehensive review. *J Rehabil Res*, **22**, 85–98.

Shumway-Cook A, Gruber W, Baldwin M et al. (1997) The effect of multidimensional exercises on balance, mobility, and fall risk in community-dwelling older adults. *Phys Ther*, **77**, 46–57.

Shumway-Cook A, Brauer S, Woollacott M (2000) Predicting the probability for falls in community-dwelling older adults using the Timed Up & Go test. *Phys Ther*, **80**, 896–903.

Sidaway B, Yook D, Fairweather M (2001) Visual and verbal guidance in the learning of a novel motor skill. *J Hum Mov Stud*, **40**, 43–63.

Sietsema JM, Nelson DL, Mulder RM et al. (1993) The use of a game to promote arm reach in persons with traumatic brain injury. *Am J Occup Ther*, **47**, 19–24.

Silver KHC, Macko RF, Forrester LW et al. (2000) Effects of aerobic treadmill training on gait velocity, cadence, and gait symmetry in chronic hemiparetic stroke: a preliminary report. *Neurorehabil Neural Repair*, **14**, 65–71.

Simoneau GG, Bereda SM, Sobush DC et al. (2001) Biomechanics of elastic resistance in therapeutic exercise programs. *J Orthop Sports Phys Ther*, **31**, 16–24.

Simpson JM, Salkin S (1993) Are elderly people at risk of falling taught how to get up again? *Age Ageing*, **22**, 294–296.

Sims KJ, Brauer SG (2000) A rapid upward step challenges medio-lateral postural stability. *Gait Posture*, **12**, 217–224.

Singer B, Dunne J, Allison G (2001) Clinical evaluation of hypertonia in the triceps surae muscles. *Phys Ther Rev*, **6**, 71–80.

Singer RN, Lidor R, Cauraugh JH (1993) To be aware or not aware? What to think about while learning and performing a motor skill. *Sport Psychologist*, **7**, 19–30.

Sinkjaer T, Magnussen I (1994) Passive, intrinsic and reflex-mediated stiffness in the ankle extensors of hemiparetic patients. *Brain*, **117**, 355–363.

Skelton DA, Young A, Greig CA et al. (1995) Effects of resistance training on strength, power, and selected functional abilities of women aged 75 and over. *J Am Geriatr Soc*, **43**, 1081–1087.

Skilbeck CE, Wade DT, Hewer RL, Wood VA (1983) Recovery after stroke. *J Neurol Neurosurg Psychiatry*, **46**, 5–8.

Slobounov S, Newell KM (1993) Postural dynamics as a function of skill level and task constraints. *Gait Posture*, **2**, 85–93.

Sluijs EM, Kok GJ, van deer Zee J (1993) Correlates of exercise compliance in physical therapy. *Phys Ther*, **73**, 771–782.

Small S, Solodkin A (1998) The neurobiology of stroke rehabilitation. *Neuroscientist*, **4**, 426–434.

Smeets JBJ, Brenner E (1999) A new view on grasping. *Motor Control*, **3**, 237–271.

Smith GV, Macko RF, Silver KHC et al. (1998) Treadmill aerobic exercise improves quadriceps strength in patients with chronic hemiparesis following stroke: a preliminary report. *J Neurol Rehab*, **12**, 111–118.

Smith GV, Silver KHC, Goldberg AP et al. (1999) Task-oriented exercise improves hamstring strength and spastic reflexes in chronic stroke patients. *Stroke*, **30**, 2112–2118.

Smits JG, Smits-Boone E (2000) *Hand Recovery after Stroke: Exercises and Results Measurements*. Butterworth-Heinemann, Oxford.

Son K, Miller JAA, Schultz AB (1988) The mechanical role of the trunk and lower extremities in a seated weight-moving task in the sagittal plane. *J Biomech Eng*, **110**, 97–103.

Sonde L, Gip C, Fernaeus SE et al. (1998) Stimulation with low frequency (1.7Hz) transcutaneous electrical nerve stimulation (low-TENS) increases motor function of the post-stroke paretic arm. *Scand J Rehabil Med*, **30**, 95–99.

Sonde L, Kalimo H, Fernaeus SE et al. (2000) Low-TENS treatment on post-stroke paretic arm: a three year follow-up. *Clin Rehabil*, **14**, 14–19.

Sorock G, Pomerantz R (1980) A case-control study of falling episodes among hospitalized elderly. *Gerontologist*, **20**, 240.

Spirduso WW, Asplund LA (1995) Physical activity and cognitive function in the elderly. *Quest*, 47, 395–410.

Stapleton T, Ashburn A, Stack E (2001) A pilot study of attention deficits, balance control and falls in the acute stage following stroke. *Clin Rehabil*, 15, 437–444.

Stelmach GE, Worringham C (1985) Sensorimotor deficits related to postural stability: implications for falling in the elderly. *Clin Geriatr Med*, 1, 679–694.

Stephenson R, Edwards S, Freeman J (1998) Associated reactions: their value in clinical practice? *Physiother Res Int*, 3, 69–75.

Stevenson TJ, Garland J (1996) Standing balance during internally produced perturbations in subjects with hemiplegia: validation of the Balance Scale. *Arch Phys Med Rehabil*, 77, 656–662.

Strathy GM, Chao EY, Laughman RK (1983) Changes in knee function associated with treadmill ambulation. *J Biomech*, 16, 517–522.

Stroke Unit Trialists' Collaboration (1997) Collaborative systematic review of the randomized trials of organized in-patient (stroke unit) care. *BMJ*, 314, 1151–1159.

Studenski S, Duncan PW, Chandler J (1991) Postural responses and effector factors in persons with unexplained falls: results and methodologic issues. *J Am Geriatr Soc*, 39, 229–234.

Sun J, Walters M, Svenson N et al. (1996) The influence of surface slope on human gait characteristics: a study of urban pedestrians walking on an inclined surface. *Ergonomics*, 39, 677–692.

Sunderland A, Tinson D, Bradley L et al. (1989) Arm function after stroke. An evaluation of grip strength as a measure of recovery and a prognostic indicator. *J Neurol Neurosurg Psychiatry*, 52, 1267–1272.

Sunderland A, Tinson DJ, Bradley L et al. (1992) Enhanced physical therapy improves recovery of arm function after stroke: a randomised controlled trial. *J Neurol Neurosurg Psychiatry*, 55, 530–535.

Sunderland A, Fletcher D, Bradley L et al. (1994) Enhanced physical therapy for arm function after stroke: a one year follow-up study. *J Neurol Neurosurg Psychiatry*, 57, 856–858.

Sutherland DH, Kaufman KR, Moitoza JR (1994) Kinematics of normal human walking. In *Human Walking* (eds J Rose, JG Gamble), Williams & Wilkins, Baltimore, MD, 2nd edn, pp 23–44.

Svantesson U, Grimby G, Thomee R (1994) Potentiation of concentric plantar flexion torque following eccentric and isometric muscle actions. *Acta Physiol Scand*, 152, 287–293.

Svantesson UM, Sunnerhagen KS, Carlsson US et al. (1999) Development of fatigue during repeated eccentric–concentric muscle contractions of plantar flexors in patients with stroke. *Arch Phys Med Rehabil*, 80, 1247–1252.

Taira M, Mine S, Georgopoulos AP et al. (1990) Parietal cortex neurons of the monkey related to the visual guidance of hand movement. *Exp Brain Res*, 83, 29–36.

Talvitie U (2000) Socio-affective characteristics and properties of extrinsic feedback in physiotherapy. *Physiother Res Int*, 5, 173–188.

Tang A, Rymer WZ (1981) Abnormal force-EMG relations in paretic limbs of hemiparetic human subjects. *J Neurol Neurosurg Psychiatry*, 44, 690–698.

Tangeman PT, Banaitis DA, Williams AK (1990) Rehabilitation of chronic stroke patients: changes in functional performance. *Arch Phys Med Rehabil*, 71, 876–880.

Tardieu G, Shentoub S, Delarue R (1954) A la recherche d'une technique de measure de la spasticite. *Rev Neurol*, 91, 143–144.

Taub E (1980) Somatosensory deafferentation research with monkey: implications for rehabilitation medicine. In *Behavioral Psychology in Rehabilitation Medicine: Clinical Applications* (ed LP Ince), Williams & Wilkins, New York, pp 371–401.

Taub E, Uswatte G (2000) Constraint-induced movement therapy and massed practice. (Letter) *Stroke*, 31, 986–988.

Taub E, Wolf SL (1997) Constraint induced movement techniques to facilitate upper extremity use in stroke patients. *Top Stroke Rehabil*, 3, 38–61.

Taub E, Miller NE, Novak TA et al. (1993) A technique for improving chronic motor deficit after stroke. *Arch Phys Med Rehabil*, 74, 347–354.

Tax AAM, Denier van den Gon JJ, Erkelens CJ (1990) Differences in coordination of elbow flexors in force tasks and in movement. *Exp Brain Res*, 81, 567–572.

Taylor DC, Dalton JD, Seaber AV et al. (1990) Viscoelastic properties of muscle-tendon units. The biomechanical effects of stretching. *Am J Sports Med*, 18, 300–309.

Teixeira-Salmela LF, Olney SJ, Nadeau S et al. (1999) Muscle strengthening and physical conditioning to reduce impairment and disability in chronic stroke survivors. *Arch Phys Med Rehabil*, 80, 1211–1218.

Teixeira-Salmela LF, Nadeau S, McBride I et al. (2001) Effects of muscle strengthening and physical conditioning training on temporal, kinematic and kinetic variables during gait in chronic stroke survivors. *J Rehabil Med*, 33, 53–60.

Telian SA, Shepard NT, Smith-Wheelock M et al. (1990) Habituation therapy for chronic vestibular dysfunction: preliminary results. *J Otolaryngol Head Neck Surg*, **103**, 89–95.

Thepaut-Mathieu C, Van Hoecke J, Maton B (1988) Myoelectric and mechanical changes linked to length specificity during isometric training. *J Appl Physiol*, **64**, 1500–1505.

Thilmann AF, Fellows SJ (1991) The time-course of bilateral changes in the reflex excitability of relaxed triceps surae muscle in human hemiparetic spasticity. *J Neurol*, **238**, 293–298.

Thilmann AF, Fellows SJ, Garms E (1991a) The mechanism of spastic muscle hypertonus. *Brain*, **114**, 233–244.

Thilmann AF, Fellows SJ, Ross HF (1991b) Biomechanical changes at the ankle joint after stroke. *J Neurol Neurosurg Psychiatry*, **54**, 134–139.

Thorstensson A, Oddsson L, Carlson H (1985) Motor control of voluntary trunk movements in standing. *Acta Physiol Scand*, **125**, 309–321.

Tinetti ME, Williams FT, Mayewski R (1986) Fall risk for elderly patients based on number of chronic disabilities. *Am J Med*, **80**, 429–434.

Tinetti ME, Speechley M, Ginter SF (1988) Risk factors for falls among elderly persons living in the community. *N Engl J Med*, **319**, 1701–1707.

Tinetti ME, Liu W, Claus EB (1993) Predictors and prognosis of inability to get up after falls among elderly persons. *JAMA*, **269**, 65–70.

Tinetti ME, Baker DI, McAvay G et al. (1994) A multifactorial intervention to reduce the risk of falling among elderly women living in the community. *N Engl J Med*, **331**, 821–827.

Tinson DJ (1989) How stroke patients spend their days. *Int Disabil Stud*, **11**, 45–49.

Tobis JS, Nayak L, Hoehler F (1981) Visual perception of verticality and horizontality among elderly fallers. *Arch Phys Med Rehabil*, **62**, 619–622.

Topp R, Mikesky A, Wigglesworth J et al. (1993) The effect of a 12-week dynamic resistance strength training program on gait velocity and balance of older adults. *Gerontologist*, **33**, 501–506.

Topp R, Mikesky A, Dayhoff NE et al. (1996) Effects of resistance training on strength, postural control, and gait velocity among older adults. *Clin Nurs Res*, **5**, 407–427.

Treiber FA, Lott J, Duncan J et al. (1998) Effects of Theraband and lightweight dumbbell training on shoulder rotation torque and serve performance in college tennis players. *Am J Sports Med*, **26**, 510–515.

Trombly CA (1992) Deficits of reaching in subjects with left hemiparesis: a pilot study. *Am J Occup Ther*, **46**, 887–897.

Trombly CA (1993) Observations of improvement of reaching in five subjects with left hemiparesis. *J Neurol Neurosurg Psychiatry*, **56**, 40–45.

Tse S, Bailey DM (1991) T'ai Chi and postural control in the well elderly. *Am J Occup Ther*, **46**, 295–300.

Turnbull GI, Chateris J, Wall JC (1996) Deficiencies in standing weight shifts by ambulant hemiplegic subjects. *Arch Phys Med Rehabil*, **77**, 356–362.

Tyson S, Turner G (2000) Discharge and follow-up for people with stroke: what happens and why. *Clin Rehabil*, **14**, 381–392.

van der Lee JH, Wagenaar RC, Lankhorst GJ et al. (1999) Forced use of the upper extremity in chronic stroke patients: results from a single-blind randomized clinical trial. *Stroke*, **30**, 2369–2375.

van der Lee JH, De Groot V, Beckerman H et al. (2001) The intra- and interrater reliability of the action research arm test: a practical test of upper extremity function in patients with stroke. *Arch Phys Med Rehabil*, **82**, 14–19.

Vander Linden DW, Brunt D, McCulloch MU (1994) Variant and invariant characteristics of the sit-to-stand task in healthy elderly adults. *Arch Phys Med Rehabil*, **75**, 653–660.

van der Meche FGA, van Gijn J (1986) Hypotonia: an erroneous clinical concept? *Brain*, **109**, 1169–1178.

van der Ploeg RJO, Fidler V, Oosterhuis HJGH (1991) Hand-held myometry: reference values. *J Neurol Neurosurg Psychiatry*, **54**, 244–247.

Vandervoort AA (1999) Ankle mobility and postural stability. *Physiother Theory Prac*, **15**, 91–103.

Vandervoort AA, Chesworth BM, Jones M et al. (1990) Passive ankle stiffness in young and elderly men. *Can J Aging*, **9**, 204–212.

Vandervoort AA, Chesworth BM, Cunningham DA et al. (1992) Age and sex effects on mobility of the human ankle. *J Gerontol: Med Sci*, **47**, M17–M21.

van der Weel FR, van der Meer AL, Lee DN (1991) Effect of task on movement control in cerebral palsy: implications for assessment and therapy. *Dev Med Child Neurol*, **33**, 419–426.

Van Leeuwen R, Inglis JT (1998) Mental practice and imagery: a potential role in stroke rehabilitation. *Phys Ther Rev*, **3**, 47–52.

van Straten A, de Haan RJ, Limburg M et al. (1997) A stroke-adapted 30-item version of the Sickness Impact Profile to assess quality of life. *Stroke*, **28**, 2155–2161.

van Vliet P (1993) An investigation of the task specificity of reaching: implications for retraining. *Physiother Theory Pract*, **9**, 69–76.

van Vliet P (1999) Reaching, pointing and using two hands together. In *Functional Human Movement: Measurement and Analysis* (eds BR Durward, GD Baer, PJ Rowe), Butterworth-Heinemann, Oxford, pp 159–179.

van Vliet P, Kerwin DG, Sheridan M et al. (1995) The influence of goals on the kinematics of reaching following stroke. *Neurol Rep*, **19**, 11–16.

Vattanasilp W, Ada L (1999) The relationship between clinical and laboratory measures of spasticity. *Aust J Physiother*, **45**, 135–139.

Vattanasilp W, Ada L, Crosbie J (2000) Contribution of thixotropy, spasticity, and contracture to ankle stiffness after stroke. *J Neurol Neurosurg Psychiatry*, **69**, 34–39.

Verfaelli M, Bowers D, Heilman KM (1988) Attentional factors in the occurrence of stimulus–response compatibility effects. *Neuropsychology*, **26**, 435–444.

Verkerk PH, Schouten JP, Oosterhuis HJGH (1990) Measurement of the hand coordination. *Clin Neurol Neurosurg*, **92**, 105–109.

Viallet F, Massion J, Massarino R et al. (1992) Coordination between posture and movement in a bimanual load-lifting task: putative role of a medial frontal region including the supplementary motor area. *Exp Brain Res*, **88**, 674–684.

Visintin M, Barbeau H, Korner-Bitensky N et al. (1998) A new approach to retrain gait in stroke patients through body weight support and treadmill stimulation. *Stroke*, **29**, 1122–1128.

von Schroeder HP, Coutts RD, Lyden PD et al. (1995) Gait parameters following stroke: a practical assessment. *J Rehabil Res Dev*, **32**, 25–31.

Wade DT (1992) *Measurement in Stroke Rehabilitation*. Oxford University Press, Oxford.

Wade DT, Langton-Hewer R, Wood VA et al. (1983) The hemiplegic arm after stroke: measurement and recovery. *J Neurol Neurosurg Psychiatry*, **46**, 521–524.

Wade DT, Wood VA, Langton Hewer R (1985) Recovery after stroke – the first three months. *J Neurol Neurosurg Psychiatry*, **48**, 7–13.

Wade DT, Langton Hewer R, David RM et al. (1986) Aphasia after stroke: natural history and associated deficits. *J Neurol Neurosurg Psychiatry*, **49**, 11–16.

Wade DT, Wood VA, Heller A et al. (1987) Walking after stroke. *Scand J Rehabil Med*, **19**, 25–30.

Wagenaar RC (1990) *Functional Recovery after Stroke*. VU University Press, Amsterdam.

Wagenaar RC, Beek WJ (1992) Hemiplegic gait: a kinematic analysis using walking speed as a basis. *J Biomech*, **25**, 1007–1015.

Wajswelner H, Webb G (1995) Therapeutic exercise. In *Sports Physiotherapy Applied Science and Practice* (eds M Zuluaga, C Briggs,

J Carlisle et al.), Churchill-Livingstone, Melbourne, pp 208–215.

Walker C, Brouwer BJ, Culham EG (2000) Use of visual feedback in retraining balance following acute stroke. *Phys Ther*, **80**, 886–895.

Wall JC (1999) Walking. In *Functional Human Movement: Measurement and Analysis* (eds BR Durward, GD Baer, PJ Rowe), Butterworth-Heinemann, Oxford, pp 93–105.

Wall JC, Nottrody JW, Charteris J (1981) The effects of uphill and downhill walking on pelvic oscillations in the transverse plane. *Ergonomics*, **24**, 807–816.

Walsh EG (1992) Postural thixotropy: a significant factor in the stiffness of paralysed limbs? *Paraplegia*, **30**, 113–115.

Walsh RN, Cummins RA (1975) Mechanisms mediating the production of environmentally induced brain changes. *Psychol Bull*, **82**, 986–1000.

Walshe F (1923) On certain tonic or postural reflexes in hemiplegia, with special reference to the so-called 'associated movements'. *Brain*, **46**, 1–37.

Wanklyn P, Forster A, Young J (1996) Hemiplegic shoulder pain (HSP): natural history and investigation of associated features. *Disabil Rehabil*, **18**, 497–501.

Weiller C, Chollet F, Friston KJ et al. (1992) Functional reorganization of the brain in recovery from striatocapsular infarction in man. *Ann Neurol*, **31**, 463–472.

Weiner DK, Bongiorni DR, Studenski SA et al. (1993) Does functional reach improve with rehabilitation? *Arch Phys Med Rehabil*, **74**, 796–800.

Weiss A, Suzuki T, Bean J et al. (2000) High intensity strength training improves strength and functional performance after stroke. *Am J Phys Med Rehabil*, **79**, 369–376.

Wernick-Robinson M, Krebs DE, Giorgetti MM (1999) Functional reach: does it really measure dynamic balance? *Arch Phys Med Rehabil*, **80**, 262–269.

Westing SH, Seger JY, Thorstensson A et al. (1990) Effects of electrical stimulation on eccentric and concentric torque–velocity relationship during knee extension in man. *Acta Physiol Scand*, **140**, 17–22.

Wheeler J, Woodward C, Ucovich RL et al. (1985) Rising from a chair. Influence of age and chair design. *Phys Ther*, **65**, 22–26.

Whipple RH, Wolfson LI, Amerman PM (1987) The relationship of knee and ankle weakness to falls in nursing home residents: an isokinetic study. *JAGS*, **35**, 13–20.

Whitall J, Waller SM, Silver KHC et al. (2000) Repetitive bilateral arm training with rhythmic auditory cueing improves motor function in chronic hemiparetic stroke. *Stroke*, **31**, 2390–2395.

Whiting HTA (1980) Dimensions of control in motor learning. *Tutorials in Motor Behavior* (eds GE Stelmach, J Requin), North Holland, New York, pp 537–550.

Wiesendanger M, Kazennikov O, Perrig S et al. (1996) Two hands–one action. In *Hand and Brain. Neurophysiology and Psychology of Hand Movements* (eds AM Wing, P Haggard, R Flanagan), Academic Press, Orlando, FL, pp 283–300.

Will B, Kelche C (1992) Environmental approaches to recovery of function from brain damage: a review of animal studies. In *Recovery from Brain Damage: Reflections and Directions* (eds FD Rose, DA Johnson), Plenum Press, New York, pp 79–104.

Williams PE (1990) Use of intermittent stretch in the prevention of serial sarcomere loss in immobilised muscle. *Ann Rheum Dis*, **49**, 316–317.

Williams PE, Catanese T, Lucey EG et al. (1988) The importance of stretch and contractile activity in the prevention of connective tissue accumulation in muscle. *J Anat*, **158**, 109–114.

Wilson B, Cockburn J, Halligan P (1987) Development of a behavioural test of visuospatial neglect. *Arch Phys Med Rehabil*, **68**, 98–102.

Wing AM, Fraser C (1983) The contribution of the thumb to reaching movements. *Quart J Exp Psychol*, **35**, 297–309.

Wing AM, Turton A, Fraser C (1986) Grasp size and accuracy of approach in reaching. *J Motor Behav*, **18**, 245–260.

Wing AM, Lough S, Turton A et al. (1990) Recovery of elbow function in voluntary positioning of the hand following hemiplegia due to stroke. *J Neurol Neurosurg Psychiatry*, **53**, 126–134.

Wing AM, Goodrich S, Virji-Babul N et al. (1993) Balance evaluation in hemiparetic stroke patients using lateral forces applied to the hip. *Arch Phys Med Rehabil*, **74**, 292–299.

Winstein CJ, Gardner ER, McNeal DR et al. (1989) Standing balance training: effect on balance and locomotion in hemiplegic adults. *Arch Phys Med Rehabil*, **70**, 755–762.

Winter DA (1980) Overall principle of lower limb support during stance phase of gait. *J Biomech*, **13**, 923–927.

Winter DA (1983) Biomechanical motor patterns in normal walking. *J Motor Behav*, **15**, 302–330.

Winter DA (1985) Concerning the scientific basis for the diagnosis of pathological gait and for rehabilitation protocols. *Physiother Can*, **37**, 245–252.

Winter DA (1987) *The Biomechanics and Motor Control of Human Gait*, University of Waterloo Press, Waterloo, Ontario.

Winter DA (1991) *Biomechanics and Motor Control of Human Gait: Normal, Elderly and Pathological*. University of Waterloo Press, Waterloo, Ontario.

Winter DA (1995) *A.B.C. of Balance during Standing and Walking*. Waterloo Biomechanics, Waterloo, Ontario.

Winter DA, Patla AE, Frank JS et al. (1990) Biomechanical walking pattern changes in the fit and healthy elderly. *Phys Ther*, **70**, 340–347.

Winter DA, McFadyen BJ, Dickey JP (1991) Adaptability of the CNS in human walking. In *Adaptability of Human Gait* (ed AE Patla), Elsevier Science, Amsterdam, pp 127–143.

Winter DA, Deathe AB, Halliday S et al. (1993) A technique to analyse the kinetics and energetics of cane-assisted gait. *Clin Biomech*, **8**, 37–43.

Winters JM, Kleweno DG (1993) Effect of initial upper-limb alignment on muscle contributions to isometric strength curves. *J Biomech*, **26**, 143–153.

Winward CE, Halligan PW, Wade DT (1999) Somatosensory assessment after central nerve damage: the need for standardized clinical measures. *Phys Ther Rev*, **4**, 21–28.

Wolf SL, Catlin PA, Blanton S et al. (1994) Overcoming limitations in elbow movement in the presence of antagonist hyperactivity. *Phys Ther*, **74**, 826–835.

Wolf SL, Barnhart HX, Ellison et al. (1997) The effect of Tai Chi Quan and computerized balance training in older subjects. *Phys Ther*, **77**, 371–381.

Wolfson L, Whipple R, Judge J et al. (1993) Training balance and strength in the elderly to improve function. *J Am Geriatr Soc*, **41**, 341–343.

Wong AM, Lin Y, Chou S et al. (2001) Coordination exercise and postural stability in elderly people: effect of Tai Chi Chuan. *Arch Phys Med Rehabil*, **82**, 608–612.

Woollacott M, Shumway-Cook A, Nashner LM (1986) Aging and posture control: changes in sensory organization and muscular coordination. *Int J Aging Hum Dev*, **23**, 97–114.

Woollacott M, Inglin B, Manchester D (1988) Response preparation and posture control. *Ann NY Acad Sci*, **525**, 42–53.

Worrell TW, Borchert B, Erner K (1993) Effect of a lateral step-up exercise protocol on quadriceps and lower extremity performance. *J Orthop Sports Phys Ther*, **187**, 646–653.

Wu C, Trombly CA, Lin K et al. (2000) A kinematic study of contextual effects on reaching performance in persons with and without stroke: influences of object availability. *Arch Phys Med Rehabil*, 81, 95–101.

Wulf G, McNevin N, Shea C (1999a) Learning phenomena: future challenges for the dynamical systems approach to understanding the learning of complex motor skills. *Int J Psychol*, 30, 531–557.

Wulf G, Lauterbach B, Toole T (1999b) The learning advantage of an external focus of attention in golf. *Res Quart Exercise Sport*, 70, 120–126.

Wynn-Parry CB, Salter M (1975) Sensory reeducation after median nerve lesions. *Hand*, 8, 250–257.

Yang JF, Winter DA, Wells RP (1990) Postural dynamics in the standing human. *Biol Cybern*, 62, 309–320.

Yekutiel M, Guttman E (1993) A controlled trial of the retraining of the sensory function of the hand in stroke patients. *J Neurol Neurosurg Psychiatry*, 56, 241–244.

Yoshida K, Iwakura H, Inoue F (1983) Motion analysis in the movements of standing up from and sitting down on a chair. *Scand J Rehabil Med*, 15, 133–140.

Yu DT, Chae J, Walker ME et al. (2001) Percutaneous intramuscular neuromuscular electric stimulation for the treatment of shoulder subluxation and pain in patients with chronic hemiplegia: a pilot study. *Arch Phys Med Rehabil*, 82, 20–25.

Yue G, Cole KJ (1992) Strength increases from the motor program: a comparison of training with maximal voluntary and imagined muscle contractions. *J Neurophysiol*, 67, 1114–1123.

Zajac FE (1989) Muscle and tendon: properties, models, scaling, and application to biomechanics and motor control. *Crit Rev Biomed Eng*, 17, 359–411.

Zatsiorsky VM, Li ZM, Latash ML (1998) Coordinated force production in multi-finger tasks: finger interaction and neural network modelling. *Biol Cybern*, 79, 139–150.

Zatsiorsky VM, Li Z, Latash ML (2000) Enslaving effects in multi-finger force production. *Exp Brain Res*, 131, 187–195.

Zattara M, Bouisset S (1988) Chronometric analysis of the posturo-kinetic programming of voluntary movement. *J Motor Behav*, 18, 215–225.

Zorowitz RD (2001) Recovery patterns of shoulder subluxation after stroke: a six-month follow-up study. *Top Stroke Rehabil*, 8, 1–9.

Index

Page references in *italic* refer to figures and those in **bold** refer to tables.

Abstract tasks, 18, 172
Action Research Arm Test (ARA), **205**
Activities of daily life, testing, **205**
Activities Specific Balance Confidence (ABC)
    Scale, 73, 74
Actual Amount of Use Test (AAUT), **205**
Adaptations to motor impairments, 209,
    221–4
  and balance, 48, 49, 61
  classification, 210–11
  standing up, 145
  upper limbs, 173–5
  see also Spatiotemporal adaptations
Aerobic exercise, 88, 119, 254–8
Age-related change
  balance, 45–8
  exercise, 257, 258
  sitting down, 138
  standing up, 138–9
  strength training, 235, 245, 246, 257
  walking, 87–8
Agnosia, spatial, 228–30, 263–4
Aids, walking, 127–8
Amount of Use Scale (AOU), **205**
Ankle
  balance, 35
    exercises, 62, 66, *68*
    falls, 46
    flexibility, 46, 48
    range of motion measurement, 123, 221,
      253
    sitting down, 138, 150
    standing up
      biomechanics, 130, 131, 133–4, 135, 136
      observational analysis, 143, *144*
      training, 146, 147, *152–3*
    walking
      analysis, 89, 90, 92, 93–8
      ankle-foot orthoses, 126–7
      biomechanics, 81, 83, 84, 85–6, 87
      degrees of freedom, 77
      exercises, 113, 115, 116, 245
      falls, 88
      slopes, 86
      stairs, 87
Ankle-foot orthoses (AFOs), 126–7
Anosognosia, 228, 229
Aphasias, 262
Arm
  balance
    age-related change, 45–6
    sitting, 42, *43*, 57–60

    spatiotemporal adaptations, 53
    standing, 38, 39
    walking, 44
  bimanual training, 190–2
  excessive muscle activity, 217, *218*
  persistent posturing, 219
  pulling patient by, 194, 263
  reaching, 159–60
    adaptations, 173–5
    bimanual training, 190
    biomechanics, 161–5
    eliciting muscle activity, 180–6, 204
    motor performance analysis, 171–7
    recovery after stroke, 168–71
    soft tissue stretching, 179–80
    tests, **205**
    training, 57–60, 168–9, 177–9, 180–6,
      204
    and vision, 227
    while sitting, 42, *43*, 57–60
  redundant muscle activity, 219
  shoulder pain, 194, *196*, 197, 263
  sitting balance, 42, *43*, 57–60
  standing balance, 38, 39
  standing up, 130, 139, *144*
  supports for, 197, 198
  walking, 44, 81
Arm Motor Mobility Test (AMAT), **205**
Ashworth Scale, 216, 219, 220–1
Associated movements (synkinesis), 218–19
Astereognosis, 225, 226
Attention
  and balance, 36
  focusing, 16–18, 226
  spatial neglect, 229–30, 263–4
Auditory feedback, 157–8
Autotopagnosia, 228, 229

Balance, 35–7
  age-related change, 45–8
  biomechanical tests, 38, 49, 75
  biomechanics, 38–45, 49–53, 78, 79, 93
  body alignment analysis, 52–3
  central nervous system role, 36
  functional tests, 73–5
  motor performance analysis, 48–54
  need for training, 37
  observational analysis, 50–3
  postural sway, 38, 46–7, 49, 75
  pusher syndrome, 230–1
  responses to loss of, 41, 44–5, 47, 48

Balance (*contd*)
　sensory inputs, 36, 43, 45, 47, 48, 50
　spatiotemporal adaptations, 52–3, *54*
　task contexts, 52–3
　training, 55–6
　　acute phase, 259–60, *261, 263*
　　fall prevention, 47, 55, 119
　　outcome measurement, 73–5
　　sitting, 56–60, 70–1, 259–60, *261, 263*
　　skill maximization, 70–1, *72*
　　soft tissue stretching, 71
　　standing, 60–71, *72*, 259–60, *261*
　　strength, 71–3, **74**, 214, 245
　　supports, *55*, 61, 63, *64, 66*
　　transfer of learning, 45, 55
　visual inputs, 36, 43, 45, 50
　walking
　　biomechanics, 42–4, 78, 79, 93
　　fall avoidance, 77, 119
　　functional tests, 74–5
　　obstacles, 44, 50, 71, 119, *121*
　　training, 66, *67*
Balance reactions, 37
Barthel Index, 26
Berg Balance Scale, 73
Bicycle ergometers, 254, 256, 257
Biofeedback, 181–2, 204, 244
Biomechanical tests
　balance, 38, 49, 75
　sitting down, 157
　standing up, 157
　upper limb function, **205**, 206
　walking, 123
Biomechanics, 3
　balance, 38–45, 49–53, 78, 79, 93
　sitting down, 44–5, 138
　standing up, 44–5, 130–8
　upper limb functions, 161–8, 171–7
　walking, 42–4, 78–87, 89–99
　see also Biomechanical tests
Body alignment, analysis, 52–3
Botulinum toxin, 126, 220, 251–2
Brain reorganization
　functional, 5–8, 169–71, 198
　measurement, 24–7
　rehabilitation environment, 8–24
　sensory training, 227
Brunnstrom stages, upper limb recovery,
　　170–1

Calf muscle length test, 123, *253*
Canes, walking, 127–8
Cardiovascular fitness, 253–8
Chairs, 135–6, *137*, 150
Circuit training, 10, 13, 27, *28–31*
　balance, 72
　strength, 247–8
　walking, **103**
Closed-chain exercises, 237–40, 243
Cognitive impairments, 48, 50, 228–32,
　　263–4
Communication deficits, 262
Community-based support groups, 266
Computerized training
　balance, 67, 70
　upper limb, *183*, 202, *203*

Concentric exercise, 238–9, 240–1
Concrete tasks, 18, 172
Conditioning, physical, 253–8
Constraint-induced movement therapy, 168,
　　169–70, 178, 198, 202, **203**
Cutaneous inputs
　balance, 36, 48
　hand use, 167
　practice, 226
Cycle ergometers, 254, 256, 257

Demonstrating actions, 16, *17*
Dexterity, 159
　critical components, 175–7
　loss of, 214
　tests, **205**
　training, 169, 188–90, 214
Discharge planning, 265–6
Downhill walking, 86
Dynamometry, 213, 249
　joint range, 252
　standing up, 157
　upper limb function, **205**
　walking, 108, 117, *118–19*
Dysphagia, 261
Dystonia, 219, *220*

Eccentric exercise, 238–9, 240–1
Elastic band resistance exercises, 117, *119*,
　　192, 193, 241
Electrical stimulation (ES), 244
　upper limb function, 178, 181–2, 204
　walking, 108, 125–6
Electromyography (EMG)
　excessive muscle activity, 217
　standing up, 136, 138
　upper limb function, 181–2, 204
　walking, 85–6, 91
Environment, for rehabilitation
　　see Rehabilitation environment
Equilibrium reactions, 37
Evidence-based rehabilitation, 24–5
Exercise testing, 257–8
Exercise tolerance, 14, 253

Falls
　and balance, 37
　　age-related change, 46–8
　　exercises, 47, 71
　　functional tests, 74
　　responses to loss of, 41, 44–5, 47, 48
　　strength training, 47, 71, 73
　　walking, 77, 119
　frequency, 48–9
　getting up after, 49, 71, 73
　risk factors, 37, 41, 46, 47, 49, 88, 250
　when standing up, 129, 130
　when walking, 77, 88, 119
Falls Efficacy Scale, 73, 74
Feedback
　augmented, 19
　　sitting down, 157–8
　　standing up, 157–8
　　walking, 108

Feedback (*contd*)
  balance training, 67, 70
  eliciting muscle activity, 108, 181–2, 204,
      244
  rehabilitation environment, 14, 18–20
Fingers
  adaptive movements, 174, *175*
  grasp biomechanics, *162*, 163, 165–7
  motor performance analysis, 172, 174,
      175–6
  sensory perception, 173
  training, 177
    eliciting muscle activity, 181–2, 204
    manipulation, 188, *189*, 190
    strength, 246
    stretching, 179
Fitness tests, 122
Follow-up services, 265–6
Foot
  balance, 36
    age-related change, 46, 47
    single leg support, 65
    sitting, 42, *57*, 58, *59*
    soft tissue stretching, 71
    spatiotemporal adaptations, 53
    standing, 39–41, 60, 62, 63
    walking, 43–4, 48
  sitting balance, 42, *57*, 58, *59*
  sitting down, 150–2
  standing balance, 39–41, 60, 62, 63
  standing up
    biomechanics, 131, 133–4
    eliciting muscle activity, 152–3
    observational analysis, 143, *144*, 145
    soft tissue stretching, 150, *151*
    training, 145–7, 150, 152–3, 154
  walking
    analysis, 89, 92, 93, *95–9*
    ankle-foot orthoses, 126–7
    and balance, 43–4, 48
    biomechanics, 78, 79, 80, 81, 82, 86–7
    exercises, 113, 115
    stairs, 87
Forced use training, 168, 169–70, 178, 198,
      202, **203**
Frames, walking, 126, 127
Fugl-Meyer Scale, 171, 221
Functional brain reorganization, 5–8
  constraint-induced movement therapy, 198
  rehabilitation environment, 8–24
  upper limb, 169–71, 198
Functional electrical stimulation (FES), 204
Functional Independence Measure (FIM), 26
Functional outcomes, 26–7
  aerobic exercise, 257–8
  balance training, 73–5
  sitting down training, **141–2**, 157
  standing up training, **141–2**, 157
  upper limb function, 199–201, **205**, 206
  walking training, **102–3**, 122, 123–5
Functional Reach (FR) Test, 73, 74

Gait *see* Walking
Games
  balance training, 71
  computer, *183*, 202, *203*

Goal setting, 18
Goniometers, 252
Grasp, 159
  adaptive movements, 174, *175*
  biomechanics, 161–8
  motor performance analysis, 172, 174
  sensory perception, 173, 227
  tests for, **205**
  training
    critical components, 175–7
    eliciting muscle activity, 182–3, *184*
    manipulation, 188, *189*, 190
    soft tissue stretching, 179–80
    strength, 192–3, 246
Grip force test, **205**
Group training, 10–13

Hand, 159–60
  adaptive movements, 174, *175*
  bimanual tasks, 160, 163, 177, 178–9,
      190–2
  brain reorganization, 169
  function tests, **205**
  grasp biomechanics, 161–8
  grip force regulation, 173
  motor performance analysis, 172, 174,
      175–7
  recovery after stroke, 168–71
  sensation–motor output relation, 225–6
  sensory function, 160–1, 169, 173, **205**,
      225–6, 227
  shaping, 167
  and standing up, 139, 149
  training, 160, 163, 166–8, 175–7
    bimanual, 190–2
    cutlery use, **192**
    eliciting muscle activity, 180–6
    exercise tasks, 188–90
    strength, 192, 193, 214, 246
  wrist malalignment, *175*, 222
Harness support
  balance training, 55, 61, *64*, 66
  reaching exercises, *12*, 63, *64*
  walking training, 101, 104–6, 124–5
Head
  balance, 35
    body alignment, 53
    sitting, 42, 56–7
    standing, 46–7, 62, *63*
    training, 56–7, 62
    walking, 44
  standing up, 130, 147
Heart rate test, 258
Heel raises, 115–16, *117*
Hemiplegia, denial of, 228, 229
Hip
  balance, 35
    body alignment, 53
    sitting, 42, 53
    soft tissue stretching, 71
    spatiotemporal adaptations, 53, *54*
    standing, 40, 53, 62, *63*, 66, *67–8*
    walking, 44
  sitting balance, 42, 53
  sitting down, 138, 150
  standing balance, 40, 53, 62, *63*, 66, *67–8*

Hip (contd)
  standing up
    age-related change, 139
    biomechanics, 130, 131, 133, 134–5,
      136, 138
    motor performance analysis, 139–40,
      143, 144
    training, 146, 150, 153
  walking
    analysis, 89, 90, 92, 94–8
    biomechanics, 44, 81–2, 83, 84, 85–6, 87
    degrees of freedom, 77
    exercises, 108–11, 113, 115, 245
    slopes, 86
    stairs, 87
Human Activity Profile (HAP), 26, 245
Hyperreflexia, 127, 209, 210, 215–16,
  219–21, 234
Hypertonia, 209–10, 215, 216–17, 220, 221,
  234
Hypotonia, 217

Imagery (mental practice), 23–4
Incontinence, urinary, 261–2
Instructing patients, 16–18, 17
Isokinetic dynamometry
  muscle strength measurement, 157, **205**,
    249
  walking, 108, 117, 118–19
Isokinetic exercise, 237, 240, 243
  walking, 108, 117, 118–19
Isometric exercise, 237
Isotonic exercise, 237–40, 241, 243

Joint malalignment, 175, 222
Joint range measurement, 123, **205**, 221, 252

Kerbs, 86–7, 106
Kinematics
  standing up, 131–3
  walking, 80–2, 86, 90, 91–9
Kinetic chain exercises, 237–40
Kinetics
  standing up, 131–3
  walking, 82–4, 90
Knee
  balance
    sitting, 42, 53
    standing, 60–1, 66, 68
    training supports, 61
    walking, 44
  muscle weakness differentiation, 213
  muscle weakness distribution, 212
  sitting balance, 42, 53
  sitting down, 138, 150
  standing balance, 60–1, 66, 68
  standing up
    age-related change, 139
    biomechanics, 130, 131, 133, 135, 136,
      138
    motor performance analysis, 139–40,
      143, 144
    timed tests, 157
    training, 147, 149, 150

walking
  analysis, 89, 90, 91, 92, 93–8
  balance, 44
  biomechanics, 81, 82, 83, 84, 85–6, 87
  degrees of freedom, 77
  exercises, 113, 115, 245
  falls, 88
  slopes, 86
  stairs, 87

Language deficits, 262
Lateral Step-up Test, 213
Lateropulsion, 230–1
Learning, environment for, 15–24
Leg press exercises, 238
Lifting methods, 262–3, 263
Lower limb
  balance, 35, 37
    age-related change, 45–6, 47
    body alignment, 53
    sitting, 42, 43, 50, 51, 53, 57–60
    sitting down, 44–5
    spatiotemporal adaptations, 53, 54
    standing, 38–41, 49–50, 53, 60–71, 72
    standing up, 44–5
    training, 37, 47, 57–71, 72, 74, 214, 245
    walking, 43–4, 66, 67, 93
  exercises see Lower limb exercises
  muscle weakness differentiation, 213
  muscle weakness distribution, 211–12
  risk factors for falls, 46, 47, 88
  sitting balance, 42, 43, 50, 51, 53, 57–60
  sitting down, 138, 150, 154–6
  standing balance, 38–41, 49–50, 53, 60–71,
    72
  standing up
    age-related change, 139
    balance, 44–5
    biomechanics, 130, 131–4, 135, 136, 138
    functional tests, 157
    motor performance analysis, 139–40,
      143–5
    training, 146, 147–56
  walking
    analysis, 89–99
    balance, 43–4, 66, 67, 93
    biomechanics, 43–4, 78–81, 82–4, 85–7
    degrees of freedom, 77
    falls, 88
    training, 99–121, 123–5, 214, 245–6,
     251
Lower limb exercises
  balance training, 37, 47, 60–2
    outcomes, **74**
    reaching while sitting, 57–60, **74**
    reaching while standing, 62–4, 66–7,
     68–9, **74**
    sideways walking, 66, 67
    single leg support, 65, 66
    skill maximization, 70–1, 72
    soft tissue stretching, 71
    strength, 71–3, **74**, 214
  circuit class, 28–31, 247–8
  pedal machines, 12
  sitting down, 150, 154–6
  standing up, 146, 147–56

Lower limb exercises (*contd*)
  strength training, 237–40, 243, 245–6,
    247–8
    balance, 71–3, **74**, 214
    walking, 111–19, 214, 245–6
  task modification, 22
  walking, 99–106, 123–5
    eliciting muscle activity, 108–11, 125–6
    skill maximization, 119
    soft tissue stretching, 106–8, 251
    strength training, 111–19, 214, 245–6

Manipulation, 159–61
  adaptive movements, 174, *175*
  biomechanics, 161–8
  grip force regulation, 173
  motor performance analysis, 172, 174, 175–7
  recovery after stroke, 168–71
  sensation–motor output relation, 225
  tests of, **205**
  training, 160, 163, 168–71, 175–8
    bimanual tasks, 190–2
    eliciting muscle activity, 180–6
    exercise tasks, 188–90
    strength, 192, 193
Measuring outcomes *see* Outcome
    measurement
Mechanical power, walking, 83–4, 90
Medical Research Council, Motricity Index,
    213, 244
Mental practice, 23–4
Modelling actions, 16, *17*
Moments of force, walking, 82, 83, 90
Motivation, 13–14, 18, 19, 20, 23, 247–8
Motor Activity Log, **205**
Motor Assessment Scale, 73, 204, **205**
Motor impairments, 209
  adaptations to *see* Adaptations to motor
    impairments
  classification, 210–11, *210*
  dexterity, 214
  muscle weakness *see* Muscle weakness
  spasticity, 209–10, 215–21, 224
    aerobic exercise, 254
    ankle-foot orthoses, 127
    strength training, 220, 234
    treadmill training, 123
  walking dysfunction, 77
Motor patterns, adaptive, 223–4
Motor performance
  and sensory function, 225–6
  transfer of learning, 20–1
    aerobic exercise, 253–4
    balance, 45, 55
    strength training, 21, 241–4, 245, 249
Motor performance analysis, 25–6
  balance, 48–54
    sitting down, 140–5
    standing up, 139–45
    upper limb function, 171–7
    walking, 88–99
Motor skills, taxonomy of, 20–1, 52
Motricity Index, 213, 244
Muscle activity
  adaptive changes, 222
  associated movements, 218–19

balance, 35
  age-related change, 45–6, 47
  eliciting, 61
  motor performance analysis, 48, 49, 50
  sitting, 42, *59*
  sitting down, 44–5
  standing, 38–41, 60–1, 68
  standing up, 44–5
  walking, 44
  and body position, 243
  and dexterity, 214
  eliciting, 244
    balance, 61
    mental practice, 23–4
    standing up, 152–4
    upper limb, 178, 180–6, 204
    walking, 108–11, 125–6
  excessive, 217–19
  hand function, 165–7, 168, 171, 180–6,
    204
  persistent limb posturing, 219
  redundant, 217, 218–19
  sitting balance, 42, *59*
  sitting down, 44–5, 138
  standing balance, 38–41, 60–1, 68
  standing up, 44–5, 131–3, 136–8, 152–4
  upper limb function
    biomechanics, 165–7
    motor performance analysis, 171–3
    recovery after stroke, 168, 171
    spasticity, 173
    training, 176, 177, 178, 180–6, 204
  walking, 77, 84–6
    analysis, 91, 93–4
    balance during, 44
    degrees of freedom, 76–7
    eliciting, 108–11, 125–6
    mechanical power, 83–4, 90
    stairs, 87
    support moment of force, 83
Muscle adaptations, 221–4
Muscle co-contraction, 217–18
Muscle contracture, 223, 250–2
  see also Soft tissue stretching
Muscle coordination, dexterity, 214
Muscle fibre changes, 222, 223, 253, 254
Muscle flexibility, 222–3, 249–52
  and aerobic exercise, 254
  see also Soft tissue stretching
Muscle length, 223, 249–52
  passive lengthening *see* Hypertonia
  see also Soft tissue stretching
Muscle spasticity *see* Spasticity
Muscle stiffness, 222–3, 250–2
  and aerobic exercise, 254
  see also Soft tissue stretching
Muscle strength measurement, **205**, 213, 244,
    249
Muscle weakness, 211–13, **215**, 234
  age-related, 45–6, 47
  balance, 45–6, 47, 49, 50, 59, 61, 68
  classification, *210*
  and dexterity, 214
  effects, 235
  eliciting activity *see* Muscle activity, eliciting
  from disuse, 222, 224, 236
  improvement *see* Strength training

Muscle weakness (*contd*)
  measures, **205**, 213, 244, 249
  sitting down, 150
  standing up, 139, 143, 145, 146, 147–50
  upper limb function
    dexterity, 214
    eliciting activity, 180–6
    motor performance analysis, 171–2, 173, *174*
    shoulder pain, 194, 195, 197
    soft tissue stretching, 179, 180
    walking, 77, 88–9, 90, 91, 100

Neglect, spatial, 228–30, 263–4
Nine-hole Peg Test (NHPT), **205**
Nottingham Health Profile, 26, 245

Observational analysis
  balance, 50–3
  sitting down, 140–5
  standing up, 140–5
  upper limb function, 173–5
  walking, 91–9
Obstacle Course Test, 73, 75
Obstacles, 44, 50, 71, 86–7, 119
  practising, 119, *120*, *121*
Open-chain exercises, 237–40, 243
Orthoses, walking, 126–7
Outcome measurement, 24–7
  aerobic exercise, **255**, 257–8
  balance training, 73–5
  sitting down training, **141–2**, 156–7
  standing up training, **141–2**, 156–7
  upper limb function, **199–201**, **205**, 206
  walking training, **102–3**, 121–5

Parallel bars, 127, 128
Passive movement, resistance to (hypertonia),
    209–10, 215, 216–17, 220, 221, 234
Passive stretching, 220, 224, 250, 251, 252
Pelvis
  sitting balance, 42
  standing up, 131, 138, 143
  walking, 44, 81–2, 92, 94, *96*, *98*
Pendulum test, 216, 220–1
Perceptual–cognitive impairments, 48, 50,
    228–32, 263–4
Persistent limb posturing, 219
Physical conditioning, 253–8
Physiological tests, 123, 257–8
Physiotherapists, role of, 264
Pick-up exercises
  balance training, 66–7, 68–9, 70–1, 72
  manipulation practice, 188–9
Post-discharge stroke management, 265–6
Postural reflexes, 37
Postural sway, 38, 46–7, 49, 75
Postural system *see* Balance
Posturing, persistent limb, 219
Power, and strength, 246
Practice, 9–10, 14, 21–4
  repetitive, 23, 243, 246–7, 249
Proprioceptive inputs, 161, 173, **205**, 227
Pusher syndrome, 230–1

Quality of life measures, 26, 245

Ramps, 86, 106, 116, *118*
Reaching, 159–61
  adaptive movements, 173–5
  and balance
    functional test, 73, **74**
    sitting, 41–2, *43*, 50, *51*, 56–60, **74**
    skill maximization, 70–1, *72*
    spatiotemporal adaptations, 53, *54*
    standing, 53, *54*, 62–4, 66–7, 68–9, **74**
  bimanual training, 190
  biomechanics, 161–5
  circuit class, *13*
  critical components, 175–7
  indirectly supervised practice, *12*
  motor performance analysis, 171–7
  recovery after stroke, 168–71
  tests, **205**
  training, 160, 175–7, 178, 180–8, 190
  and vision, 227
Reflex hyperactivity (hyperreflexia), 127, 209,
    210, 215–16, 219–21, 234
Rehabilitation environment, 8–9, 264–5
  acute phase, 259–60
  aims, 264–5
  demonstrating actions, 16, *17*
  exercise tolerance, 14
  feedback, 14, 18–20
  focusing attention, 16–18
  goal setting, 18
  group training, 10–13
  instructing patients, 16–18, *17*
  intervention delivery, 10–15
  making mistakes, 14, 19
  mental practice, 23–4
  motivation, 13–14, 18, 19, 20, 23, 247–8
  patient involvement, 13–14, 20, 264
  physiotherapist's role, 264
  practising, 9–10, 14, 21–4
  recommendations, 265
  repetition, 23
  skill optimization, 15–24
  stroke units, 259
  sub-tasks, 22
  tailored programmes, 14
  task modification, 22
  therapeutic relationship, 20
  transfer of learning, 20–1
  vision, 20
Repetitive practice, 23, 243, 246–7, 249
Resistance exercises, 117, *118–19*, 241
  and spasticity, 173
  upper limb function, 173, 192, 193
Resistance to passive movement (hypertonia),
    209–10, 215, 216–17, 220, 221, 234
Right-sided focus, 263–4

Science-based rehabilitation, 24–5
Seat heights, 135–6, *137*, 146, 150, 154
Self-efficacy, measuring, 26–7
Self-help groups, 265–6
Sensory function
  hand, 160–1, 169, 173, **205**, 225–6, 227
  training, 226–7

Sensory impairments, 224–32
Sensory inputs
    balance, 36, 43, 45, 47, 48, 50
    hand use, 160–1, 167
    testing, 232
    walking, 77
Shoulder
    balance, 53, *54*
    eliciting muscle activity, 184–6, 204
    motor performance analysis, 171, 172, 173,
        174
    pain prevention, 194–7, 204, 263
    range of motion tests, **205**
    reaching, 159, 173, 174
    soft tissue stretching, 179, 180
    standing up, 143, 149
    strength training, 192–3
    subluxation, 195, 197, 204
    walking, 81
Sickness Impact Profile (SIP), 26
Sit to stand *see* Standing up
Sitting balance
    biomechanics, 41–2
    body alignment, 53
    computerized feedback training, 67, 70
    motor performance analysis, 50, *51*, 52–3
    training, 55, 56–60, 70–1, 259–60, *261*,
        263
Sitting down, 129, 130
    age-related change, 138
    balance, 44–5, 73
    biomechanical tests, 157
    biomechanics, 44–5, 138, 140–5
    functional tests, 73, 157
    motor performance analysis, 140–5
    observational analysis, 140–5
    training, 145–6, 150
        feedback, 157–8
        groups, *11*, *12*
        outcomes, **141–2**, 156–7
        skill maximization, 155–6, 249
        soft tissue stretching, 150–2, *151*
        strength, 154–5, 249
Skill acquisition, 15–24
Slide sheets, 262–3, 263
Slings, 197, 198, 202, **203**
Slopes, 86, 106, 116, *118*
Soft tissue stretching, 250
    arm, 179–80
    balance, 71
    hand, 179–80
    passive, 220, 224, 250, 251, 252
    prescription, 252
    sitting down, 150–2, *151*
    standing up, 150–2, *151*
    walking, 88, 106–8, 251
Somatosensory impairments, 48, 50, 225–7
Spasticity, 209–10, 215–21, 224
    aerobic exercise, 254
    ankle-foot orthoses, 127
    strength training, 220, 234
    treadmill training, 123
    upper limb function, 172–3, 217, 218–19
Spatial agnosia, 228–30, 263–4
Spatiotemporal adaptations
    balance, 52–3, *54*
    walking, 100

Spatiotemporal variables
    grasp biomechanics, 163
    walking, 80, 89, 90, 91, 100, 122
Speech disorders, 262
Spine
    balance, *54*
    reaching movements, 173, 174
    standing up, 131, 136, 143, *144*, 150
    walking, 81, 82
Spiral test, **205**
Splints, 61, 202, **203**, 252
Stair walking, *29*, 87
Stand to sit *see* Sitting down
Standing balance
    age-related change, 45–7
    asymmetrical, 61
    biomechanics, 38–41
    body alignment, 53
    compensatory stepping, 41, 47, 48
    computerized feedback training, 67, 70
    motor performance analysis, 48–54
    response to loss of, 41, 47
    spatiotemporal adaptations, 53, *54*
    training, 55, 60–71, 72, 74, 214, 259–60
Standing up, 129
    age-related change, 138–9
    balance, 44–5, 47, 73, **74**
    biomechanical tests, 157
    biomechanics, 44–5, 130–8, 139–45
    chair type, 135–6, *137*, 150
    falls during, 47, 129, 130
    foot placement, 133–4
    functional tests, 73, **74**, 157
    motor performance analysis, 139–45
    muscle activity, 44–5, 131–3, 136–8,
        152–4
    observational analysis, 140–5
    seat height, 135–6, *137*, 146, 150, 154
    speed of movement, 135
    training, 145–50
        circuit class, *28*
        eliciting muscle activity, 152–4
        feedback, 157–8
        focusing attention, *17*
        groups, *11*, *12*
        outcomes, **141–2**, 156–7
        skill maximization, 155–6, 249
        soft tissue stretching, 150–2, *151*
        strength, 154–5, 249
    trunk rotation speed/timing, 134–5
Step test, 122
Stepping
    for balance, 41, 47, 48
    over obstacles, 44, 50, 71, 86–7, 119,
        121
Stepping exercises, 238, 239
    balance, 71, 72, **74**
    group training, *11*
    walking, 112–15, *112*, *114*, *116*
Steps, 86–7
Sticks, walking, 127–8
Strength training, 233–7
    balance, 37, 47, 61, 71–3, **74**, 214, 245
    effects, 235–7, 240, 241–6
    elderly patients, 235, 245, 246, 257
    eliciting muscle activity, 244
    exercise types, 237–41

Strength training (contd)
  prescription, 246–8
  reasons for, 224, 235
  repetitive practice, 243, 246–7, 249
  sitting down, 154–5, 249
  skill maximization, 248–9
  and spasticity, 220, 234
  specificity, 241–4
  standing up, 154–5, 249
  transfer of learning, 21, 241–4, 245, 249
  upper limb, 176, 192–3, 214, 243, 246
  walking, 88, 90, 100, 111–19, 214, 244, 245–6
Stretching exercises see Soft tissue stretching
Stroke management
  acute, 259–60
  post-discharge, 265–6
  recommendations, 265
Stroke units, 259
Sub-tasks, practising, 22
Support groups, 266
Support moment of force (SM), 83
Swallowing difficulties, 261
Synkinesis, 218–19

Tactile inputs, 160–1, 173, **205**, 225, 226
Tai Chi Chuan training, 47
Tardieu Scale, modified, 221
Task modification, 22
Task-oriented training, 18, 172, 231, 243, 249
Task-specific practice, 21, 227
Therapeutic relationship, 20
Thixotropy, 223
Thumb
  adaptive movements, 174
  eliciting muscle activity, 181
  grasp biomechanics, 161–3, 165–7
  manipulation exercises, 188, 190
  motor performance analysis, 172
  sensory perception, 173
  soft tissue stretching, 179–80
Timed 'Up and Go' (TUG) Test, 73, 122
Torque, muscle weakness, 213
Treadmill walking, 90, 101–5, 123–5, 246
  aerobic exercise, 254–6, 257
Trunk
  balance
    body alignment, 53
    sitting, 42, 53, 56–7
    spatiotemporal adaptations, 53
    standing, 40–1, 53, 62
    training, 56–7, 62
    walking, 44
  demonstrating flexion at hips, 17
  muscle weakness distribution, 212–13
  reaching, 163–5
  sitting balance, 42, 53, 56–7
  sitting down, 150
  standing balance, 40–1, 53, 62
  standing up
    biomechanics, 130, 131, 134–5, 136
    observational analysis, 143
    training, 146, 147, 150, 153
  walking, 44, 81, 82, 95

Upper limb, 159–61
  arm supports, 197, 198
  balance
    age-related change, 45–6
    sitting, 42, 43, 57–60
    spatiotemporal adaptations, 53
    standing, 38, 39
    walking, 44
  biomechanical tests, **205**, 206
  biomechanics, 161–8, 171–7
  brain reorganization, 169–71, 198
  excessive muscle activity, 217, 218–19
  learned non-use, 198
  motor performance analysis, 171–7
  muscle weakness differentiation, 213
  muscle weakness distribution, 211, 212
  observational analysis, 173–5
  persistent posturing, 219
  recovery after stroke, 168–71
  redundant muscle activity, 218–19
  sensation–motor output relation, 225, 226
  sitting balance, 42, 43, 57–60
  standing balance, 38, 39
  standing up, 130, 139, 144
  training, 160, 177–80
    bimanual, 160, 163, 177, 178–9, 190–2
    choice of method, 168–9
    circuit class, 13
    computerized, 183, 202, 203
    constraint-induced movement, 168, 169–70, 178, 198, 202, **203**
    cutlery use, 192
    dexterity, 169, 188–90
    electrical stimulation, 178, 181–2, 204
    eliciting muscle activity, 178, 180–6, 204
    feedback, 181–2, 204
    forced use, 168, 169–70, 178, 198, 202, **203**
    manipulation tasks, 188–90
    movement components, 175–7
    outcome measurement, **199–201**, **205**, 206
    reaching practice, 57–60, 186–8
    repetitive practice, 172–3, 177
    shoulder pain, 194–7, 204
    soft tissue stretching, 179–80
    and spasticity, 172–3, 219
    strength, 176, 192–3, 214, 243, 246
  and vision, 227
  walking, 44, 81
Urinary incontinence, 261–2

Verticality misperception, 230–1
Visual attention, 20
Visual impairments, 227–8
Visual inputs
  balance, 36, 43, 45, 50
  hand use, 161, 167, 173, 227
  walking, 77, 227
Visual observation see Observational analysis
Visuospatial agnosia, 228–30, 263–4

Walking, 76–8
  age-related changes, 87–8
  aids, 127–8

Walking (*contd*)
  asymmetrical gait, 100
  balance
    biomechanics, 42–4, 78, 79, 93
    fall avoidance, 77, 119
    functional tests, 74–5
    training, 66, 67
  biomechanical tests, 123
  biomechanics, 42–4, 78–87, 89–99
  causes of dysfunction, 77, 250
  community walking criteria, 76, 77–8
  degrees of freedom, 76–7
  effects of dysfunction, 77–8
  electrical stimulation, 108, 125–6
  falls, 77, 88, 119
  functional tests, 122
  kerbs, 86–7
  kinematics, 80–2, 86, 90, 91–9
  kinetics, 82–4, 90
  moments of force, 82, 83, 90
  motor performance analysis, 88–99
  muscle activity biomechanics, 84–6
  observational analysis, 91–9
  obstacles, 44, 50, 71, 86–7, 119, *121*
  orthoses, 126–7
  sensory inputs, 77, 227
  slopes, 86
  spatiotemporal measures, 122
  spatiotemporal variables, 80, 89, 90, 91,
      100, 243

  speed, 76, 77–8, 80, 121–2, 243, 245
  stairs, 87
  task modification, 22
  task-specific practice, 21
  training, 100–1
    aerobic exercise, 254–6, 257
    for balance, 66, 67
    eliciting muscle activity, 108–11, 125–6
    outcomes, **102–3**, 121–5
    overground, 105–6, 125
    skill maximization, 119
    soft tissue stretching, 88, 106–8, 251
    strength, 88, 90, 100, 111–19, 214, 244,
        245–6
    treadmill, 90, 101–5, 123–5, 246
    walking backward, 110–11
    walking forward, 105–6
    walking sideways, 109–10
Weightbearing exercises, 111–17, 238–40,
    243
Wheelchairs, one-arm drive, 128
Work capacity, 253
Wrist
  adaptive movements, 174, *175*
  components of actions, 175–6
  malalignment, *175*, 222
  training, 177
    manipulation, *189*, 190
    muscle activity, 181–2, 204
    strength, 193, 246